Unending Work
and Care

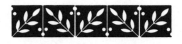

Juliet M. Corbin

Anselm Strauss

Unending Work and Care

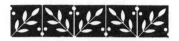

Managing Chronic Illness at Home

Jossey-Bass Publishers

San Francisco • London • 1988

UNENDING WORK AND CARE
Managing Chronic Illness at Home
   by Juliet M. Corbin and Anselm Strauss

Copyright © 1988 by: Jossey-Bass Inc., Publishers
                      350 Sansome Street
                      San Francisco, California 94104

                      &

                      Jossey-Bass Limited
                      28 Banner Street
                      London EC1Y 8QE

Library of Congress Cataloging-in-Publication Data

Corbin, Juliet M., date.
   Unending work and care.

   (A Joint publication in the Jossey-Bass health
series and the Jossey-Bass social and behavioral
science series)
   Bibliography: p.
   Includes index.
   1. Chronic diseases—Social aspects.   2. Chronic
diseases—Psychological aspects.   3. Chronically ill—
Home care—Psychological aspects.   4. Chronically ill—
Family relationships.   I. Strauss, Anselm L.   II. Title.
III. Title: Managing chronic illness at home.   IV. Series:
Jossey-Bass health series.   V. Series: Jossey-Bass social
and behavioral science series.   [DNLM: 1. Chronic Dis-
ease—nursing.   2. Chronic Disease—psychology.   3. Home
Care Services—nurses' instruction.   WY 115 C791u]
RC108.C67   1988   649.8   87-46343
ISBN 1-55542-082-6

Manufactured in the United States of America

The paper in this book meets the guidelines for
permanence and durability of the Committee on
Production Guidelines for Book Longevity of the
Council on Library Resources.

JACKET DESIGN BY WILLI BAUM

FIRST EDITION

Code 8806

A joint publication in
The Jossey-Bass Health Series
and
The Jossey-Bass
Social and Behavioral Science Series

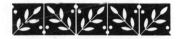

Contents

ix

Preface

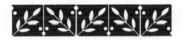

    Unending Work and Care illustrates how victims of chronic illness and their spouses struggle with the simultaneous challenges of managing serious illness and conducting their personal lives. What makes this book different from other books concerned with the care of the chronically ill is that it examines how chronic illness is managed at home, how the management of home care and the illness itself affect the lives of married couples, and how the domestic adjustments made to accommodate chronic illness, in turn, affect the management of the illness. Our major focus, then, is on effectively managing chronic illness at home and the relationship of the psychological experiences of couples to the success of that undertaking.

    In our research for this volume, we undertook to study the experiences of many couples at home and at work, we accomplished this through intensive interviews. Our aim was to establish a body of grounded information about the problems such couples are up against in their personal lives. The research also addressed a pressing policy question: How can the chronically ill be helped to manage their illnesses more effectively? Policy planning and decisions about managing chronic illness are sometimes unrealistic and, therefore, ineffective, because they are developed by people whose experiences and perspectives are far removed from those of the chronically ill and their families. The principal field of battle lies in the homes of the chronically ill, so the more we know about what happens there, the better our policies can be.

The genesis of the research for this book goes back to the late 1960s, when Anselm Strauss began to interview and observe chronically ill people, both in hospitals and in their homes. Several years later, he coauthored a book entitled *Chronic Illness and the Quality of Life* (1984), which contains an outline of a social/ psychological framework for working with chronic illness. This framework was used in studies of pain management techniques devised for the chronically ill by hospital staffs and, later, of medical technology's affects on the care of hospitalized patients. We have drawn from that past research in developing the study reported in this new volume.

Research on chronically ill people who manage their own illnesses has increased in recent years. Consequently, there is now a considerable body of social and behavioral science literature that reports on the results of these studies. However, little of this research has focused on the actual work of managing illness at home, and even less has examined the roles played by the partners of the chronically ill. In the course of our research, however, we have realized that the key players in the drama of accommodating chronic illness at home are the ill people and their spouses, rather than the assisting medical staff. And, we have found that the psychological experiences of marital partners—considered separately and together—are crucial to the degree of success they have in managing illness. Hence, this biographical—or social/psychological—data will receive extensive attention in this volume.

Who Should Read This Book?

This book is designed to serve three different groups of readers. First, practitioners in the health care field will be interested in this book—especially those who deal with the chronically ill outside of acute-care hospitals, including nurses, social workers, psychologists, physicians, and home-care agency personnel. A second group of readers are professionals who are involved in establishing health-care policy. This group includes government administrators, legislators, and policy researchers. The third group of readers who will find this book useful are social scientists concerned with health matters—especially medical sociologists and medical anthropologists—as well as sociologists who specialize in the area of work and professions. Readers of this volume will find not only new substantive information pertaining to their respective interests but also the further development of a theory arising from an ongoing research program, of which this book represents the most recent publication (Glaser and Strauss, 1965, 1968; Strauss and Glaser, 1970; Fagerhaugh and Strauss, 1977; Strauss and others, 1984; Strauss, Fagerhaugh, Suczek, and Wiener, 1985; Fagerhaugh, Strauss, Suczek, and Wiener, 1987).

Overview of the Contents

This book begins with an introductory chapter, in which the prevalence of chronic illness and some of its salient properties are discussed. In this chapter, we also outline the structure of the entire book and discuss in some detail the nature of the case presentations and commentaries that appear in the latter half of the volume. Chapter Two addresses the diagnostic phase of chronic illness. This phase is sometimes prolonged, is often stressful for the sufferer and his or her family, and can involve a subtle interplay of lay and professional views of illness.

The five remaining chapters in Part One are each devoted to fairly abstract analytic formulations. Chapter Three presents the concept of "trajectory," which pertains both to the course of the illness and to the working relationships of the people who attempt to control and shape that course. Trajectories involve adapting home-care and professional responsibilities in accordance with what we term *trajectory phases*—namely, acute, comeback, stable, unstable, deteriorating, and dying stages of illness. Chapters Four and Five pertain to the social/psychological concerns and experiences that arise from and accompany the management of chronic illness. In Chapter Four, we detail major issues—such as how both immediate and long-range personal and familial plans are altered by chronic illness and how these changes engender stress—and present a framework of concepts for understanding these phenomena. Chapter Five focuses on some basic biographical processes, such as how the chronically ill and their intimates come to terms with physical and social limitations and how these limitations may result in a partial reshaping of their life-styles and identities. In Chapter Six, we discuss the intricate relationship that exists among three types of work: home care, the tasks of everyday life, and social/ psychological accommodation of chronic illness. Chapter Seven examines how this work gets done, to the extent that it does get done, especially through the alignment of responsibilities between marital partners and their realignment in the face of chronic illness. The theoretical framework developed in Chapters Three through Seven is illustrated frequently with case examples and quotations from our interviews of couples.

In Part Two, this theoretical framework is utilized as we discuss the various types of trajectory phase in considerable detail. Each chapter covers a different phase of chronic illness. In Chapter Eight, we discuss the comeback phase. Rather than regard this phase as a period of simple physical recovery, we demonstrate that subtle psychological and social aspects are crucial to getting well again. These include grappling with and solving questions such as: How close will I come to returning to who I was before? What exactly will my capabilities be? How fast will my recovery be? How quickly will I assess my situation?

Chapter Nine is devoted to a period that we call the stable trajectory phase. This phase is easily mistaken as an easy time for the ill person, during which her or his illness, regimens, work, and social arrangements are all stabilized. Nevertheless, when the illness is serious, the symptoms intrusive, or the regimens difficult, stability cannot be assumed by the victim or the spouse. It has to be struggled with to be maintained.

Chapter Ten discusses the unstable trajectory phase, including what is entailed in terms of work, social arrangements, and identity impact when chronic illness or its symptoms cannot be easily stabilized. In Chapter Eleven, we discuss the phases of deterioration and dying. We pay particular attention to the complexities of some victims' deterioration, both in terms of managing home care and the social/psychological impact of accommodating deterioration itself. Chapter Twelve focuses on the spouses of the chronically ill and what they must live through. In the final chapter, Chapter Thirteen, we summarize the contents of the volume, elaborate on the meaning of the term *trajectory,* and discuss the relationship of our research to the body of social and behavioral science literature on the chronically ill.

Acknowledgments

We wish to acknowledge the following friends and colleagues for sharing stimulating and helpful conversations or work sessions with us during the course of our research for this volume: Gay Becker and Sharon Kaufman, Department of Social and Behavioral Sciences, University of California, San Francisco; Shizuko Fagerhaugh, Department of Social and Behavioral Sciences, University of California, San Francisco; Barbara Suczek, Department of Sociology, San Francisco State University; and Carolyn Wiener, Department of Family Nursing, University of California, San Francisco. All of the aforementioned colleagues were members of an earlier research team of which Anselm Strauss was also a member. We would also like to express our appreciation to Elihu Gerson and Leigh Star, Tremont Research Institute; Leonard Schatzman, Department of Social and Behavioral Sciences, University of California, San Francisco; Fritz Schuetze, Department of Social Work, University of Kassel, West Germany; Peter Conrad, Department of Sociology, Brandeis University; and Lloyd Gross and Laurens White, two San Francisco physicians who referred chronically ill patients to us at the outset of our study. We also wish to thank the Visiting Nurses and Hospice of San Francisco and the Veteran's Administration Medical Center in Palo Alto, California, for their cooperation.

San Francisco   Juliet M. Corbin
March 1988   Anselm Strauss

The Authors

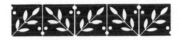

Juliet M. Corbin is a lecturer in the Department of Nursing, San Jose State University, and a research associate in the Department of Social and Behavioral Sciences, University of California, San Francisco. She received her B.S.N. degree (1963) from Arizona State University, her M.S.N. degree (1972) from San Jose State University, and her D.N.S. (1981) from the University of California, San Francisco.

Corbin has taught courses on research and on chronic illness, and she has served as a consultant in these same areas. Her research has focused on chronic illness and the sociology of work. Currently she is studying the integrative role of head nurses and nurse managers who work on a psychiatric ward at a Veteran's Administration hospital. She has had considerable experience as a nurse, working both in hospitals and, more recently, in the homes of the chronically ill. She has also been a postdoctoral research fellow in the Department of Social and Behavioral Sciences, University of San Francisco.

Corbin has authored or coauthored several research articles and chapters in edited collections. She is presently writing another book (with A. Strauss) on chronic illness and health policy.

Anselm Strauss is professor emeritus of sociology, University of California, San Francisco. He received his B.S. degree in biology (1939) from the University of Virginia, and his M.A. and Ph.D. degrees in sociology (1942 and 1945) from the University of Chicago.

Strauss's main research activities have been in medical sociology of work/professions. His research program in medical sociology goes back over two decades and includes studies on dying in hospitals, the management of pain in hospitals, the impact of medical technology on the care of hospitalized patients, and the problems of living with chronic illness. In 1981 he received the Distinguished Medical Sociologist of the Year award from the Medical Sociology section of the American Sociological Association. He received the Cooley Award (1980) and Mead Award (1985) from the Society for the Study of Symbolic Interaction, and was named the 30th Annual Research Scholar of the Year of the University of California, San Francisco (1987). Strauss is a fellow of the American Association for the Advancement of Science (1980). His publications include *Psychiatric Ideologies and Institutions* (1964, with others), *Awareness of Dying* (1965, with B. Glaser), *The Discovery of Grounded Theory* (1967, with B. Glaser), *Time for Dying* (1968, with B. Glaser), *The Politics of Pain Management* (1977, with S. Fagerhaugh), *Chronic Illness and the Quality of Life* (2nd. ed.) (1984, with others), *The Social Organization of Medical Work* (1984, with others), *Qualitative Analysis* (1987), and *Hazards in Hospital Care* (1987, with others).

He has been a visiting professor at the University of Cambridge (England), the University of Paris, the University of Manchester, the University of Constance, the University of Adelaide, and the University of Hagen.

Unending Work
and Care

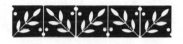

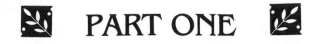

PART ONE

Understanding
the Course and Impact
of Chronic Illness

Part One of *Unending Work and Care* consists of seven chapters that build cumulatively to present an overall theoretical framework for interpreting the data gathered around the central issue of how chronic illness gets managed at home. This framework consists of a set of related concepts. It is important to understand that all of these concepts—with one exception, which is carefully adapted to our materials—have been developed through the authors' careful, sensitive, and lengthy interaction with the information derived from their interviews and observations. In common parlance, the theoretical formulations are grounded in the data. Readers can gain additional confidence in the applicability (or validity) of these formulations through two modes of checking. One is through scrutiny of the supporting data, that is, the words and phrasing of the interviewees themselves, which appear in these chapters. The second mode is through a comparison of whatever personal experiences are similar to, akin to, or in some degree different from but still related to the experiences of our interviewees.

A set of grounded, related concepts is requisite for understanding in more than a descriptive or intuitive sense what is involved in our interviewees' experiences and actions. The researchers' problem is to be both theoretically and interactionally sensitive, to walk a fine line between keeping interpretative distance from the people they are studying and at the same time seeing things as they do insofar as that is possible.

1

The central concept, the one around which all the others revolve, is that of trajectory. To begin with, it embodies a sociological
perspective on events that are ordinarily and primarily interpreted in
medical terms or a combination of medical and psychological terms.
Our concept embraces both the temporal physiological phenomena
of a course of disease and the equally important and temporal
sociological phenomena of the unfolding of sequential work and
work relationships that are related to attempts at controlling, or at
least shaping, the course of the disease. Related subconcepts
discussed in these pages include trajectory phases, projections of the
disease course and work course, and schemes for handling the
immediate as well as the projected future. Accompanying the
unfolding of the trajectory are a host of biographical consequences,
which in turn cycle back to affect to some degree the trajectory work
and the illness itself. These include the changed relationships of
body, self, and sense of biographical time. In some measure the body
is now failed or failing and thus is affecting one's social performances and perhaps even one's appearance. A set of biographical
processes corresponds to this disturbance in one's relations with
body and self. We refer to these as contextualizing the illness,
coming to terms, reconstituting identity, and recasting biography,
respectively. Each of those processes involves a great deal of a
particular type of work, one that we call biographical work.

The work that is most central to the concerns of this book,
however, is the work of managing the illness itself. In hospitals,
patients are the recipients of the staff's work—and that managerial
medical and nursing work is almost the only type of work that goes
on; indeed, hospital wards are organized in those terms. At home,
however, the managerial work takes place in a much more varied
context. That context prominently includes the work of everyday
life (housekeeping, rearing children, and so forth) and the biographical work referred to above. For this reason we shall discuss
the complexly patterned relationships among these three lines of
work.

Finally, in Part One of this book we address the difficult
theoretical and phenomenological issue of just how the work gets
carried out—what its mechanics are. In responding to this issue we
draw on the well-known sociological concept of alignment,

adapting it to our purposes but elaborating on it in some detail. We discuss alignment as a process, with disalignments occurring over time and thus necessitating the creation of realignments. These realignments, as well as keeping alignments stable, are achieved not only through overt interactions but through self-interactions: before, during, and after the overt interactions themselves. To understand the directions of all these interactions, as well as their occurrences, requires us to relate them in theoretical terms to impinging conditions, whether these are immediately interactional or related to family structure or even to the larger macrostructure.

Chapters One through Seven, then, provide more than a backdrop for the illustrative case materials of Part Two: they are a necessary instrument for illuminating and relating those materials.

1

The Effect
of Chronic Illness
on People's Lives

The Problem and Its Scope

Why study chronic illness? Because according to national statistics it is now the prevalent form of illness, the major health problem facing our nation and, in fact, all industrialized countries today. Indeed, as almost everyone knows, health care costs now constitute a large and even alarming percentage of national expenditures. Currently, there is a concentrated effort to reduce these costs through various legislative, financial, legal, and organizational mechanisms.

Meanwhile, there are no accurate measures of the social costs and human suffering associated with chronic illnesses. Yet for purposes of effective and humane long-term health planning and policy decisions, this kind of information—quantified or not—is also crucial (Cluff, 1981).

The Human Cost of Accommodation

It is to the issue of the social and psychological consequences of chronic illness that this book is addressed. Using our research results, we shall explore what chronic illness means in terms of human costs to the ill and their spouses. What are the costs accrued by the continuous accommodations that couples are forced to make

5

in response to the inevitable demands placed upon them by the illnesses and their management? By *accommodation* we mean the day-to-day struggle of spouses to keep some sense of balance and give meaning to their respective lives as they attempt to manage a severe illness. This struggle involves a constant juggling of time, space, energy, money, jobs, activities, and identities.

For example, there is the paradox of coping with the horrors of mutilating surgery and at the same time feeling grateful to be alive. Or the paradox of balancing the effects of radiation therapy on malignant cells with a concern about the healthy cells that it might also be killing. Or living with the paranoia that arises in response to the vagueness of one's doctor's answers when questioned about the future—who is putting me on, about what, when, and what are they really saying?—yet having to trust the doctor because he or she has needed skills. Or making choices among activities because one no longer has the energy or ability to do all that could be done before the illness. Or having "slip backs" in rehabilitation progress because complications with the illness develop, and then questioning the value of beginning the therapy all over again.

The well spouse, while indirectly weighing such concerns, also has personal concerns: balancing the value of live-in help against the invasion of privacy that comes with that help; responding to the mate's need for assistance and care yet feeling somewhat resentful that as the caretaking spouse, one can never become tired or ill because there is no one else to take over; willingly using one's life savings for the medical care of the ill person, while at the same time wondering what lies ahead for one's own future once all that money is gone; wanting to break away from the stress and strain of a relationship torn apart by illness, yet feeling the weight of a legal and moral commitment.

When both partners are ill, the human costs become even greater. In fact, the need for resources then may be multiplied; a partner barely able to take care of him- or herself may not be available to care for the other or for household matters. More expensive services closer to home may have to be used. When there is a choice among options, usually the least stressful path is chosen because neither partner can manage otherwise. Accommodations must be made over and over again because of the frequently—and sometimes continually—changing nature of illness, as well as the illness-related changes in the couple's lives. Furthermore, the accommodations reach into almost every aspect of their lives. As one woman so eloquently put it, "It impacts sex; it impacts money, friendship networks, work; it impacts the quality of your quiet time together, how relaxed you are, everything! I can't think of a single thing it does not affect."

The Failed Body

Exploring the reasons for constant accommodation will bring us to a very deep issue: the failed body—and having a chronic illness or disability may well be equated with having a failed body. Illness aside, whatever one chooses to do, physically or mentally, usually assumes that one has a functioning body capable of carrying out the desired activity. It also assumes a body that is physiologically functioning as nature intended. Usually one walks, works, plays, engages in the activities of daily living, touches and is touched, all without undue consideration of the role the body plays in carrying out those actions or the image that the body presents to oneself and others. One delights in the sensations of the touch of another, the warmth of the sun, the chill of the wind, and the feeling of fatigue after heavy but enjoyable physical or mental activity. Yet in the course of the daily hustle and bustle of life these things are hardly noticed. Usually, not until the body is overexerted in some way—as with unaccustomed exercise or activity, or when it hurts as with a headache, or when it does not function quite right as when one is tired or a blemish develops on the face—usually not until then does a person stop long enough to take notice.

Naturally, with aging one becomes aware that the body doesn't quite perform or look as it used to. However, the changes are so slow that one hardly notices them. For the most part, strenuous activities are gradually let go of or replaced by substitutes. Gray hair and wrinkles are accepted as more or less inevitable. One may not like the changes, but life goes on.

During periods of acute illness or temporary injury, activities may be limited, and the strain of illness may show on one's face.

Annoying though this may be, the temporary nature of the situation makes such periods bearable for most people. In fact, some may enjoy the unexpected respite from daily activities.

However, when body failure is due to chronic illness or permanent injury, then performance may be curtailed and the way one looks may be permanently altered. The degree to which either or both of these situations occur depends upon the severity of the illness or injury, the symptoms it presents, the possibility and degree of comeback, the variations in symptoms, and the type of activity one wishes to engage in. It is these manifestations of disease, injury, or symptoms—in the form of decreased performance, altered external or internal appearance, limited activity, and potential death—to which the ill and their spouses must accommodate. Indeed, the metaphors people use when speaking of failed bodies are often related to the bodily manifestations of illness or injury: "I feel like a prisoner in my own body," "my broken body," and so forth. One of the main themes of this book is the fateful and variegated impact of failed bodies on the lives of the ill and their partners.

The Work of Managing

Managing an illness or disability and accommodating to the associated bodily manifestations require a considerable amount of work by all involved. To this work we turn next. To understand its subtleties and varied implications, we have found very useful a theoretical perspective developed by some sociologists of occupations and work (e.g., Hughes, 1971; Becker, Geer, Hughes, and Strauss, 1964; Dalton, 1954; Freidson, 1976). For the most part, their concept of work has focused on the characteristics of work associated with occupations or professions, that is, what kinds of work go with what kinds of occupations, and what difference the work makes in what goes on among representatives of the same or different occupations. In short, the theoretical concern is primarily with the outcomes for occupations and workers. However, there is little focus on the work process itself. More recent publications in this research tradition, however, have been looking more closely at how work is actually carried out (Becker, 1982; Gerson, 1983;

Glaser, 1978; Glaser and Strauss, 1965, 1968; Strauss, Fagerhaugh, Suczek, and Wiener, 1985; Fagerhaugh, Strauss, Suczek, and Wiener, 1987; Star, 1983, 1985; Fujimura, 1987; Bendifallah and Scacchi, 1987).

In this book we shall pay much attention to work, viewing it as a complex process. Hence, we shall examine the different kinds of work involved in managing illness over time, the tasks related to each kind of work, how the tasks are done or not done, by whom, under what conditions, and with what consequences. Work is here defined as a set of tasks performed by an individual or a couple, alone or in conjunction with others, to carry out a plan of action designed to manage one or more aspects of the illness and the lives of ill people and their partners.

Why a focus on work? First, it allows one to distinguish the many different types of work required to manage illness within the context of couples' lives and then to break each type down into its various task components. This in turn allows one to readily see what actions are involved, who does them, and how the tasks vary in amount, type, degree of difficulty, and amount of time it takes to complete them—all in relation to the phase of the illness, its severity, and the complexity of the lives of those doing the work. The focus on work also directs attention to how the tasks might change according to any contingencies that arise in the course of the illness or the partners' lives and then affect their management of the illness. Second, illness management when performed in a place outside the home (as in a hospital) or at home by trained personnel is considered work in the traditional sense of tasks performed for pay by members of given professions or occupations. Management by the ill and family surely is also work. Third, the ill and their families use the language of work when speaking of illness management and its associated aspects. Since our focus on work is derived from the data, it surely should have some degree of pertinence to this area of study.

Moving now to the work itself, just what types of work are involved in managing an illness? There are many, each made up of its associated tasks. For example, Strauss, Fagerhaugh, Suczek, and Wiener (1985) in a study of hospital care discuss the following types of work: diagnostic work, work with machinery and other technologies, comfort work, clinical safety work, sentimental (or psycho-logical) work. These types include the tasks of controlling symp-toms; monitoring, preventing, and managing crises; carrying out regimens; and managing limitations of activity. Then there are types of work related to the illness or care of the ill but not directed at managing the illness itself. These types include (1) stretching the limitations of activity—the rehabilitation process, or performing the activities of daily living—especially when done by someone other than the ill person, and (2) preventing or living with social isolation.

But illness work when done in the home does *not* take place apart from the couple's lives, lives requiring other types of work if they are to go on with more or less success despite the illness. For example, there are biographical types of work—the work involved in defining and maintaining an identity. Contextualizing the illness into one's biography (making it part of ongoing life); coming to terms with the illness itself, the limitations it imposes, and the possibility of death; and restructuring new conceptions of the self in light of the illness and bodily changes it brings are three types of biographical work. (For a more detailed discussion, see Chapters Four and Five.)

Other types of work are related to individuals' everyday lives but have a less direct impact on their identities. These types include occupational work, tasks related to obtaining and maintaining a paid position; marital work, tasks involved in maintaining a marriage, including the sentimental and affectional; domestic work, tasks involved in running and keeping up a home; and child-care work, tasks involved in raising a child (see Chapter Six). Implicated in both illness and biographical work is still another very important type of work: the handling of social situations by the ill person and partner. Also immensely important is information work, which involves the quest for, the receiving of, and the passing of information. Without this, many of the other types of work could not be done.

Taken together, all these types of work can add up to a considerable work load for both spouses. They must be done if life is to go on, but they must be coordinated so that time, energy, and other resources are allotted for each. This requires the performance of still another, higher-level order of work termed "articulation work" (Strauss, Fagerhaugh, Suczek, and Wiener, 1985; Strauss, in press; Fujimura, 1987; Bendifallah and Scacchi, 1987; Gerson and Star, 1986). Articulation work is the organization and coordination of the varied types of work that are necessary to operationalize any plan of action be it the management of illness or the building of a house. It includes identifying the types of work and associated tasks to be done, giving priority to tasks in terms of their importance, making arrangements for who will do them and when, calculating the need for resources and obtaining and maintaining them and assuming and delegating responsibility for tasks (see Chapters Six and Seven).

Finally, the work must be done by someone. When managing illness in the home, the work is divided among the ill, their spouses, health professionals, paid assistants, children, other kin, friends, and others. Generally speaking, who does what work, and when, varies according to the type of work to be done, the skill and knowledge level needed for its performance, and the physical and mental ability of people available to carry it out, as well as by daily variations of mood, fatigue level, convenience, and boredom.

Understanding work and biography in relation to illness/disability and failed bodies is, then, central to understanding the management of illness and the associated life experienced by the ill and their spouses.

The History of the Research

Our research grew out of the need perceived by both authors for a study of chronic illness management carried out in the home. One of the authors had recently completed a study of chronic illness and pregnancy and was struck by the desire of the respondents to talk about the illness itself as well as its relationship to the pregnancy. During lengthy discussions, the women in the study often talked not only about their ups and downs (both physical and emotional) with the illness but also about how it affected their lives and their marital relationships.

The other author's involvement in the study being reported on here came about as a natural outgrowth of some years of research on chronic illness in general and on medical work in hospitals (Strauss and others, 1984; Strauss, Fagerhaugh, Suczek, and Wiener, 1985; Fagerhaugh, Strauss, Suczek, and Wiener, 1987). He had noted that while patients were hospitalized for the acute periods associated with their chronic illnesses, most of the daily management of chronic illness actually took place in the home and was performed there by the ill person, often in association with his or her spouse. Then, too, this author's own experiences over the last years in managing a chronic illness also made him realize the importance and need for such a study.

The study began with a focus primarily on the well partners of ill people. Partners were chosen because we noted, after reviewing the literature on chronic diseases and disabilities, that they often experience grave consequences from illnesses just as do their ill mates. Yet in terms of assistance offered by society or indeed really available for dealing with their own health, with caretaking, and with other problems, there still remains an enormous gap between the degree of need experienced by couples and the actual provision of relevant services (Lubkin, 1986; Estes, 1986). However, it became very clear after the first interviews that to understand the impact of illness on one partner of a dyadic relationship, it is also necessary to grasp its meaning for the other partner. Thus, the project immediately grew to encompass a study of both partners.

Data were collected from in-depth interviews with sixty couples, at least one and sometimes both of whom had a chronic illness or disability. About fifty couples were people whose names were obtained through the San Francisco Visiting Nurse Association and the Palo Alto Veterans Administration Medical Center, Palo Alto, California. The remaining interviewees were students, friends, or those referred by private physicians. The interviewees included almost the whole spectrum of socioeconomic strata (from working class to upper-middle class) except the extremely impoverished and the extremely wealthy. The major illness conditions represented included diabetes, cancer, spinal cord injury, stroke, and cardiovascular disease. Other types of conditions sampled were muscular dystrophy, arthritis, Alzheimer's disease, kidney disease, severe migraine headaches, chronic obstructive lung disease, lupus erythematosus, schizophrenia, and chronic pain due to injury.

An unstructured interview format was used in order to allow the respondents to bring out those aspects of illness management that were important or problematic to them. As the researchers became more sensitive to nuance and more analytically astute, so did their interview probes and questions. In six cases, it was impossible to interview the ill partner because of too great a physical or mental impairment. Only one ill mate refused to participate. Each partner was interviewed separately for two to three and sometimes more hours. Most interviews took place in the respondents' homes, thus enabling the interviewer to observe the context in which the illness management took place and the couple's interaction in their natural habitat. Some interviewing was done in the hospital setting, especially that of paraplegics and quadriplegics.

In addition, we analyzed a number of published autobiographies and biographies (by spouses), which proved especially useful for cuing us to more subtle variants of biographical processes in our interviews, as well as stimulating our thoughts about those processes. We have included occasional quotations and one case analysis from these materials.

Every social scientist who studies chronic illness faces a sampling problem concerning the range or types of illnesses to be sampled. This is perhaps rendered less difficult if the researcher confines his or her study to a single illness (which most have done) (e.g., Commaroff and McGuire, 1981; F. Davis, 1963; M. Davis, 1973; Gerhardt and Briesekorn-Zinke, 1986; Gussow and Tracy, 1965; Locker, 1983; Schneider and Conrad, 1983; Speedling, 1982; Waddell, 1982). However, sampling methods used in comparative research encompassing several chronic illnesses have been recently questioned on two grounds by Peter Conrad (1987). First, chronic illness is not a sociological concept but rather a quasi-medical one. In addition, given the great variety of symptoms and associated experiences of the ill, does it make any sense "to lump [them] together and call [them] chronic illness?" Conrad believes this masks too many important differences among the illnesses and "the problem is that it creates such an amorphous category that shades and distinctions among illnesses are lost." Conrad's tentative

solution is to suggest a taxonomy of types of chronic illness such
as "lived with illness" and "mortal illness."

Our solution was different. We reasoned that to maximize
both similarities and differences of spousal experience and couples
working together, we should study a spread of illnesses among
dimensions of symptoms, including pain, discomfort, visibility,
importance for identity, indicative of decline or dying to the ill,
uncertainty of the illness course, and uncertainty of symptomatic
appearance and disappearance. We reasoned also that the interviews
should include some spread of socioeconomic strata, age, and
ethnicity and include at least some healthy spouses who were
husbands and some couples where both partners had illnesses.
(There are also three homosexual partnerships that we know of
among our interviewees; their relationships and work reflect the
same general patterns as those of marital partners.)

This mode of sampling has been termed "selective sampling" (Schatzman and Strauss, 1973, p. 297), and it is used
frequently in qualitative research. Our procedure was to begin with
selective sampling and then, as analysis proceeded and quite early
in the data collection, to move to "theoretical sampling." This
involves choice of phenomena to study as directed by one's
emerging theoretical formulations. The technique is discussed fully
in our previous publications (Glaser and Strauss, 1967; Glaser, 1978;
Strauss, Fagerhaugh, Suczek, and Wiener, 1985; Strauss, 1987) so we
will not repeat its logic and details here except to touch on one
issue. Theoretical sampling is directed by evolving theoretical
formulations and feeds back into their further evolution; it also
builds on and incorporates comparative analysis of (both) similarities and differences among the phenomena being studied. This
makes for a broad and rich range of descriptive material (included
in an ensuing monograph) and also for effective theoretical
interpretations of that material.

The data were analyzed by means of the grounded theory
method (Glaser and Strauss, 1967; Glaser, 1978; Strauss, 1987). In
this mode of qualitative analysis, incoming data are constantly
compared for similarities and differences against previous data, in
the form of incidents and actions that are analytically represented
as categories. The previously collected data are coded further so that

eventually all categories are linked one to the other through relationships of conditions, interactions, strategies, and consequences; then they are arranged in hierarchical fashion until the rudiments of a grounded theory are formed. The theory is then refined and delimited until it forms an orderly, integrated, dense, and parsimonious representation of the substantive area under study.

Case Studies and the Structure of Unending Work and Care

Unending Work and Care has a somewhat unusual structure. It should be helpful if we briefly discuss that structure and its rationale. As mentioned in the preface, there is first of all an introductory chapter on chronic illness, next a lead-in chapter on the diagnostic question, and then five chapters (Three through Seven) in which we develop a cumulative theoretical framework. These seven chapters comprise Part One of the book. In Part Two we apply this theoretical framework to case materials and develop it further.

Why this format? When the central issues addressed in our study were nearing resolution, we reasoned as follows. As sociologists (one of us is also a nurse), we have listened intently to our interviewee-informants and interpreted their words and actions in as precise, informed, and systematic analytic terms as we could. Our main contribution to the understanding of these materials is twofold: to capture the experiential sense of the ill and their spouses and at the same time to make interpretive or analytic sense that illuminates their experiences. This is the familiar stance of some (certainly not all) sociologists. But the specific issue that confronts analysts when they are finally ready to organize their materials for others' eyes is how in presentation and style to relate the "natives'" experiences and the analyses. Alas, these are often poles apart.

On this issue there is a basic, though often unrecognized, disagreement among qualitative researchers. Some prefer to keep their analyses to a minimum and to present relatively large amounts of direct quotations from interviews or field notes. This style of presentation tends to be associated with a relatively sparse conceptualization of the data and a belief in the benefits of direct inspection of data. After all, this allows better judgment of the interpreter's credibility and is additionally useful when the interviewees are eloquent or the events are striking or can be described in detail.

Our position is not entirely opposed to this, even when quotation of raw qualitative data approaches, at its most extreme, a kind of superior journalism; but surely that mode of presentation is not the only conceivable or useful one. Our aims in this book are analytic. This means that even the cases in it are not merely presented as oral histories. We shall be a presence on virtually every page, but our interpretations are grounded in the words (mostly) and actions of the people studied. This style of presentation and grounded analysis runs the probable risk of disturbing either those who are more accustomed to reading large chunks of raw data with interpretive commentary fore, aft, and perhaps a bit in between or those who simply do not recognize that the relationship of analysis and data is a very difficult one to balance. Yet unless one eschews scientific aims, the relationship must be confronted, and perhaps the more explicitly the better.

The most explicit form is the interweaving of data and theory—in any fashion judged best suited to the joint aims of giving "understanding" and formulating theory. Why theory? The answer seems self-evident until one considers that some social scientists have eschewed scientific aims in favor of quasi-esthetic ideals of research and may also value either the "research findings" or a deep psychological-social understanding of the people and groups they are studying more than theory itself. Science? Yes, perhaps, but not much—if at all—directed toward constructing a complex, cumulative body of theory. This, too, is an arguable matter. Our position is that theory is cumulative but findings in social science are mostly not; they tend to change when social conditions change, whether within a few years or decades. Genuinely grounded theory is not discarded; it gets modified or refashioned and so can both direct research efforts and profit by them.

Because we have put a great deal of effort into further developing several theoretical formulations that had previously evolved from our research and that of our research associates (Glaser and Strauss, 1965, 1968; Fagerhaugh and Strauss, 1977; Strauss,

Fagerhaugh, Suczek, and Wiener, 1985), we decided to place these theoretical formulations front and center in this book. Nevertheless, these analytic materials must be in constant contact with substantive data and sprinkled with enough quotations from the interviews to remind you—and us—that our analyses are firmly grounded in the respondents' realities. The analytic chapters in Part One, devoted to developing a series of theoretical formulations (theory), are built around more numerous concepts than are ordinarily found in sociological works. (Although more is not necessarily better!) And though each chapter takes up from a different perspective the issue of work in relation to illness, nevertheless each draws on preceding chapters and increasingly integrates the total theoretical formulation.

These chapters should, we reasoned, also inform Part Two. This part should probably satisfy readers who are accustomed to reacting to qualitative research presentations in terms of the researchers' capturing of the respondents' views, either in their own words or at least in the researchers' descriptions. A key issue, then, was in what form we should present our data and how we should bring the analyses into contact with these data. We opted for the use of case histories. As used by social scientists (by some journalists, too), case histories convey in relatively compact form each actor's experiences and views of events, people, institutions, and himself or herself. We have quite literally built the chapters in Part Two around case histories. (Case histories also appear in Chapters Six and Seven.) Some cases are short; others are quite long. The various styles of presenting them flow organically from how the two researchers (or sometimes the one who was actually writing the chapter or case) sensed that the combined analytic-substantive materials should be shaped in order to convey effectively both the data and theory. A close inspection of the cases should show anyone curious enough to make this inspection that the interweaving of those two aspects is rather varied. Sometimes we have used the conventional presentation of single interviews ordered by chronological sequence. We have used excerpts from interviews as husband and wife talked separately to the same substantive issues or different issues. We have summarized some interviews with only occasional quotations. In two case presentations we have used essentially an

itemized chronological listing of items. We have summarized an
entire autobiography by Agnes de Mille (1981) describing her
recovery from a stroke, and included in the running account, along
with a theoretical commentary, a number of short quotations. We
have also used sequences of letters. And so on.

As for the theoretical side of these cases, an inspection of
them will show a variety of presentational forms. Conventionally,
some cases are preceded by a theoretical statement designed to guide
readers to see what we have seen in the materials in addition to what
they may also see. Then, after the case presentation, we have usually
provided a short summary of it. Sometimes a chapter introduction
(as in Chapter Eight) is quite extensive, giving new theoretical
material that is nonetheless conscientiously related to previous
theoretical formulations. This introductory section is meant to
enrich the reading of the two or three or more cases that follow, with
the cases designed to bring out varied conditions, interactions,
strategies, and consequences. This, however, requires that each case
should still have its own specific introduction or that some other
format be used. For instance, in presenting de Mille's story, our
focus is on describing and interpreting evolving phases of her
illness and associated experiences; thus there is both a lengthy
introduction, which pertains to phases, and a weaving in of
concepts from the theoretical introduction and concepts discussed
in earlier chapters. When we wished to show the conditions,
consequences, etc., that pertain to the phenomena of alignment,
disalignment, and realignment of spouses' actions in relation to
work performance, then we used another format. Excerpts from the
interviews are each followed by analytic commentary—sometimes
longer, sometimes shorter than the excerpts—with the whole
leading cumulatively to a better empathetic grasp of what the
couple was up against and, at the same time, an increasingly better
understanding of how alignment and work performance are related.

Finally, to enhance the linkage between description and
theory that virtually every page of this monograph exemplifies, we
chose the cases by means of theoretical sampling, which was
described earlier in this chapter.

It is somewhat more difficult to preselect a theoretically
satisfying range of interviews on the basis of evolving theory than,

perhaps, with a combination of field observations and interviews. We have compensated for that in this study by determining how potentially to maximize theoretical variation through the choice of different kinds of illnesses, hoping there would be sufficient variation among them and within them to give a wide range of theoretical samples. In addition, we have made explicit and implicit comparisons among cases within each chapter (as in Chapter Eight on comeback) as well as across chapters. Readers will judge for themselves whether this strategy proved successful. Here it is only necessary to recognize the strategy as one among several meant to paint a vivid, yet believable, descriptive picture while also allowing extensive analytic commentary. In aiming for the latter, we have sought to emphasize equally the similarities and differences in related phenomena under study.

In all of this discussion, we have been referring to case histories—meaning cases with a temporal aspect or story line. This is in contrast to another kind of case presentation, the case study. The aim of the two types of case are different (Strauss and Glaser, 1970). Generally speaking, the purpose of using a case history is to exemplify a set of interpretations or, in the hands of some social scientists, simply to give an evolving picture of people, careers, etc., with perhaps only implicit interpretations of the case history. In contrast, a case study focuses on analytic abstractions for the purpose of description or verification or generation of theory. In case studies, as opposed to case histories, the narrative line is subordinated to abstract purpose. Most sociological and anthropological monographs are case studies or contain case studies. Yet often case histories are woven into these case studies. If the researchers are to achieve maximum integration of theoretical formulations in their case studies, they must choose among their case histories, using them in accordance with the theoretical points they wish to make.

In *Unending Work and Care* we have not only selected the case histories on theoretical grounds but have taken pains to develop and apply to case histories theory that is (1) quite extensive in amount, (2) at a relatively high level of generality, (3) drawn both from our previous research and from the specific data of the current study, and (4) formulated with much conceptual density. We have done this while developing the theory with a fairly high degree of systematization and cumulative thrust throughout the book. In short, the basic choice concerning the book's structure arose from such considerations, as did the presentational style. The same is true for each chapter and each individual case or cluster of cases. The chief accomplishment of this particular architecture, we trust, is that it underscores two main responsibilities of sociologists. The first is to further the understanding of nonsociologists (practitioners, policymakers, reformers in the substantive area under study; also the people studied if they happen or wish to read the work; even interested segments of the lay public; and of course other social scientists). The sociologist's second responsibility is to colleagues; here we would emphasize less the findings (though they are surely relevant to the discipline) than the theoretical formulations, the guiding theoretical perspectives—both specific and general—and the potential contribution that new concepts can make to further sociological theorizing and research.

Summary

This chapter introduces the reader to the content and structure of the book. It describes the constant accommodations that those with chronic illness must make in their lives and the social and psychological costs accrued by those adjustments. It points out how body failure, through performance failure, lies at the core of those adjustments and that the work of managing chronic illness is more than just a matter of "illness management." It also encompasses a great deal of what we have termed biographical work. All of the work, illness and biographical, takes place within a context of everyday living.

The research upon which this book is based started out as a study of well partners only and then evolved into an examination of the experiences of couples. We explain some of the other methodological decisions that we made, such as why we have presented many case histories and what we mean by theoretical sampling.

Most importantly, this chapter emphasizes that the purpose of *Unending Work and Care* is not only to describe experience but to develop a theory about chronic illness management and notes how we have sought to strike a balance between the two. Thus, the first part of the book focuses primarily on our theory, while the second part places the experiences of our couples within the context of that theory.

2

The Onset and Diagnosis
of Chronic Illness:
A New Life Course Begins

Most people regard chronic illness when it occurs to themselves as an unanticipated event. Like natural disasters, chronic illness is something that happens to other people. Yet such illness is very much a reality in the lives of many Americans; furthermore, it is not confined to the elderly but can occur at any age.

How does chronic illness make its presence known? How does someone know that he or she is about to encounter a situation that will ultimately change the course of his or her life forever? The answer is one doesn't. For most people, that awareness comes only with the onset of symptoms, symptoms that sometimes strike without warning.

When I was fifty-two years old, I was occasionally very tired at the end of the afternoon. EKGs and an EKG stress test turned up no heart disease. Meanwhile, I was having some heartburn. My internist finally suspected an esophygeal hernia, and a diagnostic test confirmed that hunch. Since there is nothing to be done about that, I resigned myself to living with the ailment, whose manifestations seemed to come and go. When I was fifty-six, the symptoms worsened until my wife asked me pointedly: 'Do you think you might be having a heart attack?' I stubbornly and foolishly continued to believe in the heartburn diagnosis. From my description of the greatly intensifying symptoms, the physician suspected a heart condition, took an EKG, and diagnosed me as in the throes of a myocardial infarction.

The Diagnostic Quest

Chronic illness seldom develops overnight. Its beginnings are often insidious, with cellular changes going unnoticed for many years. Eventually, these changes are manifested, usually in the form of symptoms. When symptoms appear some people seek medical attention immediately. Others wait until the symptoms become undeniable, so visible or alarming that they can no longer be ignored. Slight symptoms are discounted. Not until the person has a heart attack or is hospitalized are those overlooked symptoms recalled and given meaning:

> You never noticed any symptoms before? I would say no. Well, I did in a way. I was helping this carpenter, carrying some boards upstairs. When we got up there I noticed a little shortness of breath. Then I had to go upstairs to pick up another bundle of two-by-fours. I couldn't breathe. I didn't know what hit me. I said: "Well, I don't know if I want to work anymore after today." This is before I went to the hospital with a collapsed lung.

Some people never really pick up on any significant symptoms. Rather, their illnesses are discovered during routine physical checkups or when they seek treatment for acute or other chronic conditions:

> We were going to buy a house, and he went and had a physical for the loan. The doctor said, "Wonderful healthy guy." The next day he [the doctor] called and said, "Your husband must see a doctor right away. His urine is syrupy." That is how the diabetes came about.

Sometimes the spouse, other kin, or close friends notice and bring to attention symptoms or changes in behavior, and then go on to suggest that medical evaluation be sought.

We shall term the search for the meaning of symptoms or other manifestations of disease a diagnostic quest. The quest has three phases: (1) the prediagnostic, (2) the announcement, and (3) the postdiagnostic, or filling-in. Its duration may be long or short. It involves many types of work. A person may pass through all the phases or skip the first if the onset of illness is sudden and acute, as with a heart attack. The diagnostic quest may be repeated at any time during the illness course when there is a need to gather further diagnostic information. For example, when there is a notable change in the nature and/or number of symptoms.

Prediagnosis

The main actions taken during the prediagnostic phase are aimed at uncovering the source of symptoms and/or other physiological changes. Variations in the duration of this phase are due to the nature of the symptoms, the skill and knowledge of the interpreting physician, when and how symptoms are reported, technological factors, and organizational factors.

For instance, symptoms may or may not be alarming. They may or may not be noticed. They may be denied for a while or acted upon immediately. They may be discounted or not discounted. They may be slight or intense. Some symptoms are elusive, while others mimic a variety of diseases. Some temporarily disappear or improve with treatment or on their own only to reappear at a later date in a more intensified form. Others may be noticeable only at certain times, only after certain activities, or only to some people. Other symptoms or disease manifestations are clearly indicative of disease, thus making diagnosis easy. Still others can be attributed to a variety of factors—from physical overexertion to mental stress—making diagnosis more difficult.

Physicians possess different degrees of knowledge and skill in reading and interpreting disease signs. Some physicians are better diagnosticians than others. Sometimes they have insufficient data upon which to base a diagnosis. At other times they misinterpret symptoms, gather insufficient data, or attribute them to other causes. Hence there is nondiagnosis, diagnostic error, or delayed diagnosis. These wrong paths can lead to lost time and, as we all know, to disaster and eventually even to malpractice suits.

Occasionally, a person who is experiencing symptoms will try to uncover their source by conducting library research or talking to other people who have similar symptoms, either before, instead of, or in addition to undergoing a traditional medical evaluation. This process may enhance, hinder, or delay the physician's diagnosis. Then, too, while the use of available technology may improve and hasten the diagnostic process, sometimes it hinders or retards it. The latter may occur when the technology is not sophisticated enough to determine the cause of the symptoms or when the test results are inconclusive or when there are technological errors (false positives or negatives) that mislead or confuse diagnosis. "On the mammograms it shows that one breast is almost twice as large as the other, and they said, 'No cancer.' So . . . nobody called me up and said, 'Maybe there is something going on. We need to go inside and take a look.' They just said, 'Your mammograms are clear.' "

If procedures or tests are improperly conducted, they give false information. If the ill are uncooperative or develop complications during testing, interpretations may be difficult to make or test repetitions may be necessary, thus confusing or prolonging the diagnostic process. Sometimes many tests are needed, and they must take place sequentially for diagnostic reasons or the patient's comfort, this too will prolong the diagnostic search.

The organizational structure within which the testing or examining takes place also affects its duration. If appointments are difficult to make or get, then more time is consumed. Time will also be extended if scheduling must be postponed because of backup, confusion, or time conflicts, or when record keeping is faulty or records are lost.

The work done during the uncovering phase of the diagnostic search is of several different types. Its aim, of course, is to arrive at a correct and timely diagnosis. It includes a kind of detective work aimed at discovering the underlying disease process. This may be broken down into many different types of tasks, such as making arrangements and preparing for the actual physical examination or tests and for their reading and interpretation. The diagnostic work may also include measures to manage symptoms. Other types of work can include comfort work—sentimental types of work such as tasks directed at lowering anxiety and fright, and symptomatic and biographical reviews—and error work—that is, correcting, assessing, and monitoring for errors (Fagerhaugh, Strauss, Suczek, and Wiener, 1987). Parts of this total work may take place in a hospital, clinic, doctor's office, or even in the home.

The work is normally divided among the physician and other health professionals, technicians and laboratory assistants, and the ill and their spouses or other kin. Each is responsible for the performance of certain tasks and for informing the others of the manner, time frame, and accuracy in which they are done. For example, the physician's work includes performing patient examinations, ordering appropriate tests, and interpreting their results. Laboratory assistants and technicians must maintain their equipment in working order, take precautions to maximize patient safety and minimize technical errors, and maintain a schedule. Patients are responsible for reporting symptoms accurately, carrying out necessary preparations, arranging work and other schedules so that they themselves are available, cooperating during the testing, and maintaining their composure while others carry out their own work. Spouses also have work to do. If the ill person cannot drive or needs the sympathetic presence of a significant other, the spouse may be called upon to perform these tasks. Therefore, he or she may also have to schedule time away from work or arrange for child care. Sometimes spouses are called upon to help interpret instructions or to assist with preparations. They too must cooperate during the testing by not interfering and by doing composure work on themselves and on their ill partners when tests are painful, dangerous, or humiliating.

Information work is also vital to the diagnostic process. For example, information is passed along in the form of communication about symptoms by the patient. Information is gathered by the physician and others through examinations, interviews, and testing as part of the gathering of clinical evidence. Professionals and patients exchange information when making arrangements for tests, explaining when, where, and how those tests are to be conducted, discussing what preparation is needed, and communicating during the actual test procedure. If, during the diagnostic quest, the proper questions are not asked or the information exchanged is incomplete or misleading, then errors and delays may result. Sometimes during the diagnostic search a health professional may, intentionally or unintentionally, drop some hints about a potential diagnosis. This may cause a patient or spouse to ask questions in an attempt to confirm suspicions. At other times, all information is withheld from the patient until the test are completed and all the evidence is in. Occasionally, of course, the type of disease is evident from the onset, and the diagnostic search is done simply to confirm it.

To discover the source of symptoms and bring that search to its natural conclusion with a diagnosis requires a great deal of coordination by a great many people at each level of involvement. Each person, including the patient and his or her spouse, must make decisions; juggle tasks, time, and costs; make arrangements; and coordinate activities with the others, within their primary work settings, whether at home, in the hospital, or in the clinic.

Diagnostic Limbo

People's reactions and feelings during the diagnostic period may vary from unconcern to real fear (Schneider and Conrad, 1983). For those who believe they have potentially serious symptoms, this period can become what might be termed a diagnostic limbo because their lives and the lives of their significant others seem suspended in time as they await the news that will confirm or disprove fears and control symptoms.

Biographically related work may be temporarily interrupted while the patient undergoes possibly numerous, dangerous, humiliating, painful, or uncomfortable but necessary tests and examinations. The waiting time during which diagnostic data are being analyzed and confirmed may be filled with thoughts of death, images of disability and impaired function, discomfort resulting from symptoms and side effects of tests, even panic: "Is it cancer? Is it malignant? If it isn't why does it hurt? Those kinds of things go through your mind." The body once taken for granted has now become the center of focus. Even before suspicions are confirmed, some people begin to wonder if their body has failed them.

The degree to which people feel they are in diagnostic limbo varies, depending upon the degree of bothersomeness and intrusiveness of symptoms, their suspicions regarding the type and severity of the disease, the stage of life they are in, the degree to which biographically related work is interrupted, and their interpretations of how the potential disease may disrupt life in the future.

Some people never feel like they are in limbo for their symptoms are not bothersome, or the possible disease does not seem terribly threatening, or the symptoms are defined as merely a side effect of aging. While indicative of physiological changes in some cases, the symptoms are judged by the physician as not important enough yet to do anything about. Under these conditions, both physician and patient may decide to wait and see what develops.

However, many of those who feel they are in a diagnostic limbo or distrust their diagnosis will express fear and anxiety. Some engage in "diagnosis shopping": they seek a variety of medical opinions, rejecting those that don't confirm what they want to believe. Some people bargain: "Please, God, don't let it be serious or what I think it is." Others deny the potential seriousness of the symptoms or make light of them. Still others delay in making appointments or fail to keep their appointments. Some read everything they can find and/or question others about their symptoms or the suspected disease. Many fill time by engaging in occupational, social, or other activities that will keep their minds too busy to dwell on frightening images of disease and on their potentially threatening future.

The Announcement

When clinical evidence is sufficient for the physician to arrive at a diagnosis, tentative though it may be, an announcement follows. Its timing and style take many forms, depending upon the degree of certainty of the diagnosis, the nature of the illness and its prognosis, the physician's interactional style, the ill person's degree of suspicion, and what the physician anticipates the patient's reaction will be to the news.

The announced diagnosis may be made tentatively or with certainty. The physician may present the diagnosis immediately after gathering the evidence or delay the announcement. Sometimes all known information is given to both partners and sometimes only part of it is given. Sometimes only one partner is given the announcement, while the other is kept temporarily or permanently in at least partial ignorance of the diagnosis. The information given may be clearly understood or partly misunderstood, its full implications coming perhaps at a later date. Sometimes the announcement is made bluntly, with little compassion or understanding of its impact. However, it also can be made with gentleness and compassion.

Upon hearing the diagnosis, reactions range from shock and disbelief—"not my body," "not me" (Rosenberg, 1980, p. 49)—to relief that a diagnosis has finally been arrived at. Time may seem to stand still while the ill person or the couple attempt to process the information they have been given. The past, the future, and even the present may seem to merge into the overwhelming moment of the announcement. Of course, while some grasp the diagnosis and its implications immediately, others need time to absorb all of this:

> The doctor impressed upon us that this is a permanent injury. But even then there was that denial. I think the real turning point—the time we had to face it—is when he went into rehabilitation. Because we were seeing people with spinal cord injuries that had been injured for ten years and coming back for their annual checkup. That made us realize that people do live this way for a very long time.

When no diagnosis or a highly provisional one is given because evidence is inconclusive or erroneous, then the no-diagnosis announcement may also be shocking and traumatizing. The limbo state and perhaps the diagnostic search continue until a diagnosis is actually offered and accepted (Kotarba, 1979, 1983). The state and search may even continue indefinitely since the ill have no certainty about cause, prognosis, or even the preferable treatment for their symptoms. "Give me a diagnosis even if there is no treatment, otherwise I will think that I am crazy or imagining all of this."

Postdiagnosis

In most cases there is sufficient evidence upon which to base a diagnosis. However, there is not always enough evidence to arrive at the proper treatment. An ill person may feel that he or she has insufficient information upon which to make decisions among treatment options. Or the onset of the illness may have been sudden (as with stroke), leaving little doubt about its cause but considerable doubt about the extent of its resulting damage. Or the diagnosis may have been tentative because the evidence was not totally conclusive, leaving room for doubt. Under these conditions, the diagnostic quest continues, with the aim of filling in the information gaps.

This "filling in" attempts to answer the question how much, how far, and what does "it" mean? The work may or may not involve more tests or even surgery. It may involve more reading, talking to others, and sifting and sorting information, by physicians, ill people, and spouses alike. This period of filling-in may be long or short, depending upon the amount and type of information needed, its availability, the speed with which it is acquired, the individual's physical ability to tolerate the testing, whether or not physical or biographical complications hinder the process, and how long each involved party is willing to persist in the search.

The diagnostic limbo may continue into this postdiagnostic phase because often there are still many unanswered questions and uncertain elements. Armed with a diagnosis but uncertain about the extent of physiological involvement or what form of treatment should be undertaken, some people relate their situation to what they have heard or read about others who have the same or similar diagnoses. Images of the illness and its potential course may lessen and give rise to images ranging from unrealistic optimism to questions about an uncertain future. The situation also can precipitate images of bodily failure and possible death.

This abrupt passage from totally healthy to seriously ill aroused a dizziness, a kind of shaking of the world. . . . I could no longer rely on the sensations of my body. . . . Once the status of my eye tumor was confirmed, the potential generality of the tumor in my body had to be tested. The next six days the geographical processing through the hospital area reflected the checking of my body "map." The qualification of "negative" as the check of one part of the body was balanced with the anxiety about the next test—a marathon of tumor check and tumor denial. . . . I came to see my position between birth and death more clearly. I felt threatened, paralyzed by anxiety. . . . But deep in me I could not believe that my life was really in danger.

Summary

The diagnostic period can be traumatic, especially if it is prolonged or ends with the confirmation of a physically or mentally crippling or life-threatening illness. Uncertain about the length or quality of life in the future, the newly diagnosed and their spouses embark upon a new life course that requires, if the illness is serious, that they learn—through experience or otherwise—not only what the diagnosis will mean in terms of their lives but what they might do to maintain some control over the ultimate path it will take.

Theory. The diagnostic period that almost always accompanies chronic illness is conceptualized as the diagnostic quest. The three phases of this quest are the prediagnostic, the announcement, and the postdiagnostic, or filling-in. Each phase may be long or short and requires many types of diagnostic-related work, including work by victim and spouse. Diagnostic limbo is the biographical uncertainty and resulting setting aside of the present and future biography that so often accompany this period.

Applications. This chapter reminds practitioners not only to be alert to the physical strain that is so often a part of the diagnostic period but also to consider the biographical impact when planning interventions. In the light of physical discomfort, biographical uncertainty, and often crushing identity blows that accompany this period, perhaps the most important types of work to be done by health professionals, aside from the diagnostic work itself, are identity work and comfort work—both physical and emotional. The specifics and focus of these types of work naturally vary with the diagnostic subphase and individual reactions.

3

Illness Trajectories

The unfolding of a chronic illness may be thought of as a voyage of discovery. Like a ship, it travels upon a course. And although one may set out with an image of the probable path an illness will take and a plan for controlling that path, the actual passage may bear little resemblance to those first conceptions. The ups and downs and twists and turns a chronic illness takes as it moves along over time and the types of work required to keep it on the projected course can only become known through the intimate contact of living with and managing the illness on a daily basis. Much like a sailor who learns the ways of the sea and the adaptability of his vessel, so an ill person comes to learn about the illness and the body's response to it. Then just when he or she thinks the course of the illness is under control, contingencies related to both illness and life in general arise somehow to alter that course, affect its management, and impact upon the lives of those doing the work of managing. This change often necessitates the projection of a new image of the illness course, a revision in the plan for controlling it, a restructuring of the division of the work needed to carry out that plan, and perhaps a reorganization of the lives of those most affected by it.

The *work* needed to manage an illness leads to a sociological perspective on these matters. While encompassing the *course of illness,* this perspective is very different from the medical one represented by that term. The distinction between a course of illness and what we shall call an *illness trajectory* will be central to our analysis (Glaser and Strauss, 1968; Fagerhaugh and Strauss, 1978; Strauss, Fagerhaugh, Suczek, and Wiener, 1985). "*Course of illness* is . . . both a commonsense and professional term. In contrast, *trajectory* refers not only to the physiological unfolding of a . . . disease but to the *total organization of work* done over that course, plus the *impact* on those involved with that work and its organization" (and then the consequences of that impact for the work itself) (Strauss, Fagerhaugh, Suczek, and Wiener, 1985). Thus the illness course is only one aspect or part of a trajectory, albeit a central feature of it.

The term *trajectory* focuses us on the active role that people play in shaping the course of an illness. This course is shaped not only by the nature of an illness and a person's unique response to it but also through actions taken by health personnel as well as the ill, their wives or husbands, and any others involved in its management. Ultimately, however, it is the couple who carry out the day-to-day work involved in illness management, who work out the problems accompanying that work, and who in the end are most affected by the consequences of the illness and illness work.

In sum, the term *trajectory* captures implicated aspects of the temporal phases, the work, the interplay of workers, and the nonmedical features of management along with relevant medical ones. In that last regard, it captures aspects of the experiences of everyone involved in the management drama, experiences that are anxious, puzzled, and painful, as well as those that are brighter. In some sense, illness is more or less (though sometimes very much less) fateful. The trajectory concept adds the aspect of fatefulness, of "undergoing and experiencing" (Dewey, 1934), to what sociologists ordinarily call action schemes and medical people call treatment and plans or programs.

The Nature of Illness Trajectories

The Physician's Trajectory Projection and Scheme. An illness trajectory may be said to begin with the onset of symptoms, with the actions taken to manage them, and with the search for a diagnosis to play a part in shaping the eventual course of the illness. However, not until there is some certainty about a diagnosis and some filling-in of the individual's physiological response to the disease can decisions be made about the course that the disease might take and the best mode of management.

The physician uses information gained through the diagnostic process coupled with his or her knowledge of the disease to project an image of the probable course that the illness will take in the specific individual. This projected image we shall term a *trajectory projection*. How accurate that projection is depends upon how clear the diagnosis is, how much information is available about how far the illness has progressed, how much is known about the amount of bodily damage, and the physician's skill in interpreting that information.

Having arrived at a trajectory projection, the physician decides upon a plan of action, or a *trajectory scheme*. The purpose of this scheme is to manage the symptoms and control the course of the illness itself. What particular scheme will be selected and how well it will work depend a great deal upon the nature of the chronic illness, the clarity of the diagnosis, the technology available to treat the illness, the ill person's physiologic response to that treatment, and how well the plan is (or can be) carried out in the home.

For instance, in arriving at a treatment plan, the physician considers the type of illness and its specific properties. That includes whether the illness generally progresses slowly or quickly; whether it is more debilitating or less debilitating; whether it is life-threatening even with management or not life-threatening with good control and management; whether it presents many symptoms or few symptoms; whether the symptoms are highly visible, less visible, or invisible; whether the illness is incapacitating or not; and whether it occurs in infancy, middle age, or old age.

Also impacting upon decisions made about management schemes are the more encompassing structural conditions affecting illness management. (The discussion of these conditions is adapted from Gerson and Strauss, 1975, pp. 12-18.) For instance, chronic illnesses are long-term, meaning that they require organizations suitable for providing the type of care needed over time. Most hospitals are set up to provide short-term and acute care. Few facilities, except perhaps nursing homes, provide the long-term and specialized care needed to manage chronic illness. Thus, whether the patient is cared for at home or elsewhere depends mainly upon what options are available for the type of care needed.

The prognoses of chronic illnesses are often uncertain,

making difficult the development of long-term treatment and other plans. Sometimes only during the evolving course of a disease does sufficient information become available to provide a reasonable estimation of what is going on and what can be done about it. Then, too, the unpredictable nature of some illness-related crises often makes preventative treatment a game of chance rather than skill. In addition, since chronic illnesses are often episodic, with acute flare-ups followed by quiescence or periods of remission, even the most thoroughly worked out treatment plans become ineffective and outdated as an illness progresses through its various phases.

Chronic diseases also require proportionately large efforts at palliation. Therefore, physicians must pay considerable attention to developing the types of treatment plans that will ensure patients and their families quality as well as quantity of life. Also, chronic illnesses are often multiple diseases: not uncommonly a person has two or more illnesses simultaneously. This complicates formulation of the treatment scheme because the physician must take into consideration the number of regimens a person is on, their possible interactive effects, and the ability of the ill person to carry them out.

In addition, chronic diseases are disproportionately intrusive upon the lives of patients and their families. Though the primary consideration of the physician is control of the illness and symptoms, he or she must consider that if regimens are to be long-term, then they must be adaptable to the lives of patients and their families and be as nonintrusive as possible. Many chronic illnesses also require a wide variety of ancillary services. In assessing the options available for treatment, the physician must consider the availability and costs of these services. The best treatment plan won't work if the ill person doesn't have a means of transportation, must travel long distances, or simply cannot afford to pay for all the needed services.

Moreover, chronic diseases imply potential conflicts of authority among patients, medical personnel, and funding agencies. Some options for treatment may be closed because nursing services that would make home care possible or more convenient are not available. Or funding sources won't provide money for the families of those caring for ill people in the home on a continuous and long-term basis in order to obtain temporary respite services.

Also affecting consideration of the management scheme is conflict between patient and physician over certain aspects of the trajectory scheme, especially if they are in direct opposition to valued aspects of the patient's life. Chronic illnesses are also expensive. When considering options the physician must balance the costs of tests, drugs, hospitalization, and long-term treatments, such as dialysis, against their long-term value. Repeated tests, expensive drugs, and costly treatments can tax a family's and society's financial resources.

Space-age technology has spilled over into medicine. New forms or combinations of chemotherapy, antibiotics, and cardiac drugs save lives and improve treatments. Nonetheless, illnesses remain chronic because so often there is no cure, only control and palliation. Thus, in devising schemes for trajectory management, the physician has at his or her disposal only those options that are technically feasible. For some diseases and at some stages of illness, those options are limited.

Moreover, people respond differently to treatments. What works for one person may not work for another. Some people can tolerate a wider range and number of side effects than other people can. Some are willing to undergo extensive rehabilitation programs. Others will settle for greater disability rather than suffer intense pain in pursuit of only possible improvement. So in considering options for treatment, the physician also has to tailor the treatment to the individual.

The most effective treatment plans fail if ill people fail to carry them out as they are prescribed. Therefore, before advocating a particular plan, the physician may consider the factors that might affect the ill person's willingness to comply with it. These factors include the number of regimens, their complexity and cost, degree of assistance needed, biographical considerations that might conflict with the regimens, and whether or not the ill person believes the regimens actually work (Corbin and Strauss, 1985; Conrad, 1987).

Having arrived at a trajectory scheme, physicians use different styles and timing in presenting their specific treatment plans, depending on the physician and the patient. A physician may present a treatment plan along with the diagnosis or delay the plan until the shock of the diagnosis is deemed over. A physician may present the plan all at once or in parts, with a clear explanation of why it is needed or without any explanation. A choice of options may or may not be given. All of these decisions are affected not only by the physician's medical judgment and assessments of the patient's personality but by the physician's own personal beliefs and social ideologies. Finally, trajectory schemes, like trajectory projections, are not static. They must constantly be revised in accordance with perceived changes in the phases of an illness.

The Couple's Trajectory Projection. Before embarking on a voyage, whether by choice or not, most people have some vision of where they are going. Thus, before embarking upon the management of chronic illness, the ill and their spouses project some vision of the possible course that the illness may take.

Trajectory projections (the couple's as well as the physician's) have many properties. The type and nature of these properties are directly related to the degree and type of information and to the interpretations and understanding possessed by each person. How these properties come to combine for each individual will form the basis upon which his or her vision of the future course of the illness is projected and his or her trajectory projection is made. Because of this, each spouse's trajectory projection may differ from the other's and also from the physician's.

One of the properties of a trajectory projection is that the nature of imagery can vary for the respective parties. For instance, the imagery may include a temporal span ranging anywhere from the present to the distant future. The imagery may also be ambiguous or unambiguous and accurate or inaccurate. It may be seen as reversible or irreversible, and it may include projections of improvement or decline, including the amount, rate, and degree of either. The imagery may also embrace the expectedness of change— getting better or worse; moreover, that change and any accompanying complications may be seen as preventable or not preventable. In addition, as the illness progresses, the well spouse may view the illness and the work involved in its management as having either a slight or an enormous impact on the couple's respective and mutual identities and other aspects of their biographies.

Another property of trajectory projections is that they can be shaped. This shaping is a deliberate attempt to influence another person's projected images of the illness course. Shaping occurs through manipulation of the amount and timing of information given and to whom it is given. Shaping may be done by the physician or by either partner, with or without the physician's assistance. Usually shaping occurs because of a desire to protect the other person from undue fear and anxiety or to keep the other person from giving up the hope necessary to continue illness management. Withholding information may be temporary or permanent. When temporary, it may be given all at once or parceled out in small cues until the other is gradually brought to full awareness. How much information is given, by whom, and when are matters usually determined by one person's judgment as to the other's physical and emotional tolerance for that information. Withholding, distorting, or giving selective information to the dying is only one instance of keeping them "out of awareness" (Glaser and Strauss, 1964).

The actual mechanics of trajectory shaping can vary. For example, the physician can shape the ill person's and/or spouse's trajectory projection in the following ways. When making the announcement, the physician may make his or her own trajectory projection either implicit or explicit, reveal it entirely or only partially, and give it to both partners simultaneously or to each separately. The physician may also give the same or different information to each partner. Moreover, one spouse can shape the other's projection by entering into alliances with the physician regarding what and when to tell the other. Similarly, the couple may share information acquired from sources other than the physician completely, partially, or not at all. Then, too, sometimes an ill person becomes suspicious and attempts to elicit informational clues.

Yet another property affecting the formation of trajectory projections is the perceptions of various participants in the drama of the availability of internal and external resources for managing the illness. Various people have different internal and external resources that come into play, enabling them to work at illness management and, if necessary, to fight or hang on doggedly. The greater the resources, the less likely a person is to give up. While physicians know a great deal about the nature of particular illnesses, by contrast they usually know very little at first about an individual patient's capacity to draw upon internal and external resources. These resources include motivation to live, physical and emotional strength to fight back, family and friends, financial security, and knowledge of how to obtain the most up-to-date and competent care.

Still another property of trajectory projections is that the imagery of the future is not held constant in terms of either the illness course or its impact. An upward or downward change in the illness, the development of serious complications, or a change in either partner's biography may bring about new visions of the future or a retrieval of ones that had been set aside. Thus, the trajectory projection may be redefined as foreshortened, lengthened, or leveling off. These redefinitions may come about as sudden prophecies of the future in response to a new insight into old information or newly acquired information. They may develop slowly as the illness evolves, as for example with a patient's extraordinarily good physiological responses to a given drug, surprising even to the physician who prescribed them. Or: "After about a year, he said, 'Well, you need another mastectomy. You have lumps in your right breast so you should get one.' At that point I could see myself being whittled to pieces. I thought the first time was going to take care of the problem, but obviously it didn't."

Sometimes trajectory projections are frozen, at least temporarily, in time: ill people or their spouses cling to their images of the future course of an illness—usually favorable—despite possible evidence to the contrary. A trajectory's projection may be frozen through denial of the future or an unwillingness to accept its reality. While freezing, it may hinder treatment. It may also enhance or at least make the treatment more bearable: "You have to have hopes and dreams to continue the fight." And of course, frozen projections can enhance or impede pursuit of desired nonmedical activities and goals.

The fading in and out of focus of the trajectory projection is yet another of its properties. This property tends to come to the forefront during acute episodes or temporary setbacks of the illness to become the "overriding trajectory projection," and with it, bring to mind the fears and anxieties about one's life normally associated with that projection. When the illness is quiescent or in a relatively stable phase, the projection tends to fade into the shadows. Although it is not the center of immediate attention, it is still there, affecting, perhaps in a less direct way, how each partner feels, thinks, and acts in the present and plans for the future. For example, a man wants to retire early and travel with his diabetic wife before she develops complications that will preclude their doing this.

The Couple's Trajectory Scheme. The ill person alone or with his or her spouse may accept, reject, or negotiate the physician's trajectory scheme in whole or in part, permanently or temporarily. For the most part, this is because the physician's scheme is strictly medical. The physician presents what he or she believes is the plan most likely to control the illness and manage the symptoms. Although the physician may consider the possible biographical impact of the treatment plan when weighing treatment options, he or she usually gives these considerations lower priority primarily because most physicians do not know their patients well enough to make such judgments. The present illness may have brought about a physician's first encounter with a particular patient.

Many people, however, give major consideration to biographical implications when making decisions about whether or not to accept one or another treatment plan or option. That is, many evaluate the plan or options not only in terms of their perceived potential effects on the illness course and the presenting symptoms but also in terms of their perceived potential impact upon ill people's lives and often their spouses' lives.

While some people readily accept the treatment plan and don't question it until they begin to live with some of the consequences, other people project what that scheme will mean in terms of their lives and make decisions based on those implications. In the end, even if they go with the physician's proposed plan, they want to know what the options are, what will happen "if," what choices they have, and how much time they have within which to explore options and make their decisions. When multiple biographical implications are considered, then deciding upon the trajectory scheme can become a lengthy and complex process. The decisions that the ill and their spouses finally arrive at can be just as crucial as those made by physicians. In short, the couples form their own versions of the trajectory scheme. The scheme that they form often encompasses strategies to manage the illness symptoms and control its course and also to manage their lives in light of the illness and the functional disability it brings.

However, a couple may agree or differ over the scheme. This is so because each partner views the proposed scheme in light of his or her perceptions of its impact on each individual and on the couple. If the couple's respective trajectory projections differ or their visions of the potential impact of the illness and the physician's management scheme upon each one's own life and their mutual lives differ, then in all probability their perceptions of the most appropriate trajectory scheme for controlling *both* the illness and their lives will also differ.

One major property of trajectory schemes is that they are not fixed for the duration of the illness. Rather, the schemes of both physicians and couples change in response to illness phasing and accommodate any illness and biographical contingencies that arise over time. Furthermore, couples may add to, modify, or change the schemes proposed by their physicians to bring them into better accord with their own cultural and religious beliefs. Or they may change the schemes to bring them more into line with their own trajectory projections, which may differ considerably from those of their physicians. For example, acupuncture, herbal medicines, natural foods, mineral baths, and other forms of alternative treatments may be used in combination with, as supplements to, or instead of a doctor's treatment plan. Shopping around for more palatable or reasonable-sounding treatments is another form of choice that may lead to supplementing or abandoning the first physician's plan. For example, Chinese patients living in the United States frequently supplement their physician's plans with herbal medicine or Chinese foods traditionally perceived to have special curative properties (Louie, 1975).

Trajectory Shapes and Phases

The shape that an illness trajectory eventually takes is not contingent upon physiological fate alone. Each trajectory takes form and is shaped by the interplay among the illness itself, the individual's particular response to it, and any illness or biographical contingencies that arise to affect it, as well as by the physician's and couple's trajectory projections and action schemes for managing both the illness and their lives. These factors taken together create the dynamics that affect illness management and its eventual impact on the course of the illness and the lives of those closely affected by the illness and its management.

Although a future image of an illness course and its impact can be and is projected, because of the fate and contingency possibilities the ultimate shape of a trajectory cannot be known until the end of a person's life. Nevertheless, theoretically we can look back on the evolution of anyone's trajectory, noting its shape up to the present moment. For example, the illness course of someone with, say, sinusitis may be a relatively straight line, with occasional dips marking allergy seasons or colds. The trajectory shape would thereby reflect an even course in terms of the "work" involved in managing the illness and the illness's and work's impact on the person's life. Such a stable trajectory with occasional acute phases might look something like this:

Figure 1. Sinusitis Trajectory.

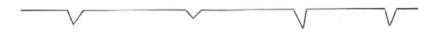

The trajectory shape of someone with cardiac disease might be different, showing first an acute phase, then a minute upward trend as the individual begins to recover, and finally plunging rapidly downward to end in death, the illness work and impact corresponding naturally to the ups and downs of the course. This type of multiphased trajectory might resemble the one portrayed in Figure 2.

The trajectory shape of a stroke victim might begin with an acute episode, be followed by slow recovery, and then stabilize, though at a lower level of functioning than before the stroke. Such a trajectory might look like Figure 3.

Figure 2. Cardiac Disease Trajectory.

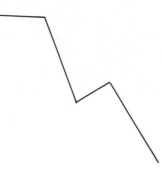

Figure 3. Stroke Trajectory.

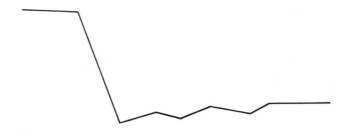

The trajectory shape of someone with cancer in which there are active periods, followed by remissions and short stable phases and then by further physical deterioration, ultimately ending in death, might be graphed this way:

Figure 4. Cancer Trajectory.

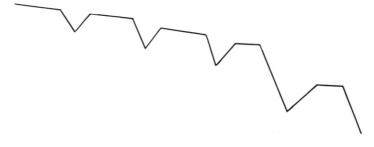

Trajectory shapes have two important properties: *variability* and *phasing*. First of all, they are not only variable in form but also in duration as well as in the work to be done and its impact. Variability is determined by a combination of (1) the nature of the illness and the person's physiological and emotional response to it and (2) management schemes instituted by health professionals and the ill.

Second, any trajectory can analytically be broken down into phases, which give it its shape. The phases are acute, comeback, stable, unstable, and downward. Basically, phases correspond to the physical and physiological status of the illness. Phasing is analytically and practically important because it denotes the type of management work to be done and what the potential physical and emotional impact might be.

However, when one examines phasing closely, one can see that it is more complicated than it appears at first glance. This is because a person may be improving physically but not emotionally adapting to the illness and the changes made by it in his or her life; or a person may believe the illness is stable and because of this be on an emotional high, while the illness is actually steadily moving downward physiologically. Furthermore, one might say that a person had a "partial comeback," the term *partial* indicating that the person is making only moderate physical recovery or indicating that while the person is making considerable physical recovery, he or she has failed to make a corresponding emotional adjustment.

Phases may also be analytically broken down into subphases, which can be described in several ways. For example, one might describe a comeback in terms of an early, middle, or late comeback; or in terms of the physical and emotional stages that the ill person passes through during a comeback; or in terms of variations in the course of a comeback: Is it a steady forward climb, or are there periods of little or no progress, or short dips and drops interspersed within the overall upward climb? Usually an ill person passes through several such subphases.

Phases, their combinations, and their subphases are easier to describe analytically than overall shapes because of the formers' variability. Since we are examining illness management in the home, we shall examine the comeback, stable, unstable, and downward phases—most directly in Chapters Eight, Nine, Ten, and Eleven. Management of a trajectory as it passes through several phases can also be seen in the long cases presented in Chapters Six and Twelve. Acute trajectory phases will be only briefly discussed since management of these usually takes place in the hospital. We turn now to a brief discussion of specific phases.

An acute phase is one in which the afflicted individual is physically or mentally affected by an illness to a degree that necessitates immediate medical attention and hospitalization to prevent further deterioration and/or death. The work is directed at bringing about physiological or mental stabilization and promoting recovery. Biographical types of work may be held in abeyance until the acute episode has passed, though a person may wonder at this time how life will change because of the illness.

Comeback denotes the physical *and* emotional recovery that take place following an acute illness phase. The course is overall an upward one; management is directed at getting physically well and also at regaining all or part of any functional ability that may have been lost as a result of the illness, and at coming to terms with the illness and any residual disability. Examples of illnesses or disabling conditions that may require a period of comeback are myocardial infarction, stroke, and spinal cord injury. Comeback is characterized by questions such as Will I come back? How far will I come? How long will it take before I peak? When will I know? How much work is necessary to get there? In a comeback trajectory the present is seen as overbearing, and the future is put on hold while one awaits answers to the foregoing questions.

A stable phase is one in which there is very little change in the course of the illness either upward or downward. An illness may be in remission, quiet, or simply slowly changing over the years, showing few if any outward manifestations. Management is aimed at maintaining that stability, and except for the occurrence of minor complications, it is usually routine. Chronic sinusitis, back conditions, spinal cord injuries, well-controlled diabetes, a remission phase of multiple sclerosis or arthritis are examples of illnesses and debilitating conditions that can be in a stable period. Questions asked during a stable phase of a trajectory include How long will the phase last? How do I keep it this way? How will I know if a change begins? In a stable trajectory, one hopes the present is unending and views the future as open.

In an unstable phase an illness or chronic condition, though not acute and sometimes briefly stabilized, is persistently out of control. Because normal management tactics are not effective, management is aimed at discovering the source of the instability and/or alternative tactics that will bring and keep the conditions under some degree of control. Because of the erratic nature of the illness, normal living may be seriously hampered. Sometimes people are hospitalized during this phase, but often they remain at home. Questions here might be Will they ever find out why this is happening or how to control it? What does this mean in terms of my life? How much longer can I go on living this way?

A downward trajectory phase indicates that the course of an illness is slowly or rapidly descending. This can be the result of a progressive disability, as with diseases such as Parkinson's, or is present when someone is defined as "dying." Increased incapacitation and/or death is seen as overarching, with the present viewed as only temporary and the exact state of the future still unknown. The questions most often asked in this phase are How fast? How far? When will it end? How will it end? How will I know? What can I do to slow it down, to prepare for the inevitable? Management is aimed at controlling the rate and extent of descent.

One more note about trajectories before we move on to Chapter Four. A person may have more than one illness trajectory, with the second trajectory either related or not related to the first. The management and impacts of each trajectory will be different, and the management scheme envisioned for one may enhance or detract from the ultimate course and management of the other.

Summary

Theory. In this third preliminary chapter, we continued to outline some basic theoretical conceptions for better understanding illness management in the home. The lay and health professional concepts of illness can be reconceptualized sociologically as a trajectory. The term *trajectory* denotes not only the potential physiological development of an illness but also the *work* involved in its management, the *impact* of illness, and the changes in the lives of the ill and their families that in turn affect their management of the illness itself. A vision of the potential path that an illness and its associated work might follow is termed a trajectory projection, whereas an envisioned plan to manage all of that is called a trajectory scheme. Afflicted people and their families, as well as health professionals, have such projections and schemes. Because trajectories can take different paths, they assume various shapes. What gives a given trajectory its shape are the phases that it passes through. These phases include acute, comeback, stable, unstable, and downward. Each may have subphases, and each may combine or alternate with one or more other major phases.

Applications. Management of an illness on the part of practitioners should involve much more than consideration of how to manage symptoms and control the course of an illness. It should also take into account the *work* to be done by trajectory *phase* and the impact of that work, as well as the illness itself, on the lives of the ill and their spouses. Successful trajectory management rests upon a meshing of the trajectory projections and schemes of health professionals with those of the ill and their partners. Only through open and honest information work on the part of all the participants can this meshing occur.

4

Experiencing Body Failure and a Disrupted Self-Image

The following quotation touches on the main themes of this chapter: body, biography, conceptions of self, and time.

> I am fundamentally denied. Present living is felt not to be enough because I cannot use my special gifts. Being multiple sclerotic I am kept from the lecture room, as from everything else. I no longer experience myself as competent. I feel outside life, as if it were passing me by, because I have no vital engagement in it. . . . Reflecting on the past and future aggravates the emptiness and futility of the present. Because I am unable to make significant contact with my environment, there is contraction of self. . . . My distinctive powers are negated and I am unfree [Birrer, 1979, p. 22].

When a severe chronic illness comes crashing into someone's life, it cannot help but separate the person of the present from the person of the past and affect or even shatter any images of self held for the future. Unless the illness is mild or its effect on activity is relatively negligible, who I was in the past and hoped to be in the future are rendered discontinuous with who I am in the present. New conceptions of who and what I am—past, present, and future—must arise out of what remains. Is there any question, then, that to achieve a relatively full and subtle understanding of the reciprocal impact of chronic illness and illness management and of biographical phenomena will require a complex set of concepts and the drawing of connections among them?

49

When chronic illness appears, the resulting perceptions of body failure refer to (1) the body's inability to perform an activity, (2) the body's appearance, and (3) the body's physiological functioning at the cellular level. The first perception hits directly at action: "I can no longer do many of those meaningful activities, such as teach, that I used to do." The second and third perceptions pertain less directly to action. Rather, they reflect a "because" view: "Because of the way I perceive that I look now or anticipate I will look in the future," or "Because of how I feel about what is happening inside of me," "I no longer feel I want to do, can do, or will be able to do."

A failed body often leads the ill person to wonder what he or she did or what someone or something else did to cause the situation. But the real meaning of body failure, as well as the self-reflection that follows, is more profound. The perception touches the inner core of a person's being. As such, that perception creates a situation to which the afflicted person and his or her family must accommodate if they are to move beyond the present and open up the future once again.

Accommodation refers not merely to the day-to-day struggle of managing the illness and its symptoms in and around any mental or physical limitations that occur but also refers to actions aimed at achieving a sense of control and balance over life, as well as giving life continuity and meaning despite the illness and the changes it brings. Accommodation, if successful, must therefore also take place in terms of the ill person's biography.

We use the term *biography* to refer to a *life course:* life stretching over a number of years and life evolving around a continual stream of experiences that result in a unique—if socially constituted—identity.

It is crucial to take biographies of the ill into consideration when examining the management of illness by them and their spouses. First, a life course can often be interrupted and possibly changed profoundly by a chronic illness. Second, an illness constitutes only one part of the total self. Hence illness management must be examined in the context of that more encompassing life. In short, biography (the life course and all that it implies) is affected by the management and in turn affects the management.

Though some chronically ill people make illness the main focus of their lives, others are able eventually to integrate the illness to varying degrees into the fabric of their being. Although the illness may periodically move into the foreground (as during illness crises or when it interferes with much wanted activity), for the most part it remains part of the texture of a biography—something to be managed and taken into consideration but certainly not the only aspect of life. Ill people are also wives, husbands, engineers, parents, and friends. The ill are far more than just ill, even if being ill affects their performing many tasks, poses serious biographical risks, and brings serious biographical consequences (Bury, 1982; Charmaz, 1980, 1983, 1984, 1985; Schuetze, 1981; Reimann, 1987). Naturally, the more frequent and severe the symptoms, the more difficult it is to push an illness into the background and the greater are its biographical consequences.

One observation we made early in our research is that neither the husbands nor the wives ever spoke only of the illness. They made it part of their life stories and placed it in a biographical context—what had been going on before, what life was like in the past, what hopes and dreams were interrupted or changed. In addition, the spouses talked about their children, current interests, and mundane problems, just as healthy people do.

Thus biographical processes are central to taking action for retaining or regaining some degree of control over a life rendered discontinuous by chronic illness. These processes enable the ill to incorporate into their lives the illness and the changes it has brought. Through these processes their lives are given shape and meaning in response to the phasing of the illness and any contingencies it brings. In order to understand when, where, how, and with what consequences this takes place, it is necessary to examine at some length several critical issues in relation to biography. However, we need first to consider major dimensions of biography itself.

Three Major Dimensions of Biography

Being multiple sclerotic I find that my body is
something more than an overcoat, the purely material

encasement of what I really am. In this state I cannot
avoid the reality that I am my body. I am not consoled
by the remark that my illness has only to do with my
physical shell; I know, as you cannot, that my whole
existence is stricken by calamity [Birrer, 1979, p. 19].

When illness brings about a failed body, the foundations of
one's existence are shaken to some degree. Unless care is taken to
support and repair that foundation, it can eventually bring down
with it the whole self-structure it supports.

Biography, as used in this book, has three constituent
elements: (1) *biographical time,* (2) *conceptions of self,* and (3) *body.*
Conceptions of self refers to personal identity, a self-classification
in terms of who I am at this point in my life's course. These
conceptions are formed through the integration of various aspects
of self into a more inclusive whole (Mead, 1934). For each aspect of
myself, I must perform various bundles of tasks in relation to
biographical management. As a teacher, I teach classes, grade
papers, counsel students. All of the tasks related to various aspects
of myself take place over biographical time, for they are part of my
past, present, and future. When the self feels integrated, it is because
all of these aspects have been (at least for this period of life)
successfully articulated. In turn, continued performance of self-
related tasks requires an appropriately functioning body.

We have coined the term *biographical body conceptions* (or
BBC) to represent those three interrelated concepts: conceptions of
self (identity), arising directly or indirectly through body, as they
evolve over the course of biographical time. These three concepts
together form what we have chosen to term the *BBC chain* because
the combination of the three *working together* gives structure and
continuity to who a person is at any point along the biographical
time line. The effects of illness on the BBC chain are central in the
lives of the chronically ill.

Biographical Time. One can hardly speak of biography
without a discussion of time in relation to it (Fischer, 1983). One
lives in the present, comes from the past, and moves toward the
future. Past experiences influence the interpretation of who one is
at present, while the past and an unfolding present together form

the basis for who one shall be in the future (Mead, 1934). Then, too, all the tasks related to various aspects of the self, though measured in clock time (be it minutes, hours, weeks, or years), must be articulated into the stream of biographical time.

Time perceptions are given expression by the adjectives or metaphors used to describe an event experientially in terms of time. Time perceptions, of course, imply a consciousness of time experienced at any point along the biography. For example, in diagnostic limbo, time slows to a painful or even terrifying crawl. Time conceptions, on the other hand, are expressed in terms of temporal perceptions and clock time but also in terms of a longer biographical arc. For example, one might say, "When I was young, time seemed to pass so slowly; now it passes so quickly" or "I want to accomplish so much with my life, but I know I will never be able to finish all that I've planned in one lifetime."

Conceptions of Self. Conceptions of self are complex and intricately linked with biographical time. Aspects of the self not only change over life courses but differ with regard to the different situations and social relationships in which people find them-selves—that is, at any given moment in time (Strauss, 1959). For example, I am a different mother to my adolescent than I was to the same child when he was a baby. And I will be a different mother to that same child when he is an adult. Furthermore, I am a different mother to each of my children and take a different perspective on each depending on the social *and* biographical situation in which I find myself.

People become unique individuals precisely because their life courses and associated experiences are different. Those experiences become touchstones for the interpretation of events and situations. Yet while one interprets those events and situations—regardless of whether they involve interactions with inanimate objects or with other people—one constantly adjusts conceptions of self and, therefore, one's actions. (See Chapter Seven for an elaboration of this point.)

Body. As briefly noted earlier, the body is the medium through which conceptions of self are formed. First of all, it is through the body that people take in and give off knowledge about the world, objects, self, and others (Merleau-Ponty, 1962). For the most part, this is an unconscious process (Whitehead, 1923). It takes place through both contact (by means of sensations such as sight, sound, smell, touch, taste) with the environment and perceptions that arise from that contact. Second, communication occurs through the body. Communication entails cooperative activity with others and is the basis of shared significant symbols (Mead, 1934), giving meaning to what one feels, sees, hears, smells, and touches. Third, the body itself, as one of these significant symbols, can become an object—distinct in all its parts yet integrated into a whole (Mead, 1934; Joas, 1983; Gadow, 1982). As an object to oneself, the body can be viewed as others see it and reflected upon in its parts and as a whole in terms of its appearance and ability to perform. Fourth, to others, one's body can—and usually does—become a social object, sexual, admired, stigmatized (Goffman, 1963; Kaufman and Becker, 1986; Schmitt, 1984; Schneider and Conrad, 1983; Davis, 1972)—and some of these resulting responses become interpreted by oneself, and consequently so do one's views of one's body and self. Fifth, a body is required to perform tasks associated with the various aspects of the self. This body must be physically and mentally capable of carrying out those tasks.

Thus, while one engages in activities and tasks, conceptions of self are being formed and reformed. That is, one performs or doesn't perform, performs successfully or unsuccessfully, receives rewards, praise, or criticism for performance; and while doing so, one is constantly evaluating, though not always consciously, one's performance, which always involves some aspect of the body. On the basis of these evaluations, a total conception of the self is formed, a conception that is constantly changing and evolving over one's lifetime (Becker and Strauss, 1956; Strauss, 1969; Erikson, 1959).

However, by conceptions of self we mean not merely self-esteem (how one feels about oneself) but rather the views held of oneself in relationship to the whole of identity—who one is. These views evolve in accordance with an ability to perform the tasks associated with various aspects of the self. Such views are often expressed in metaphorical terms by the ill to describe impacts that illnesses have had upon their lives. For example, consider the lines quoted from Birrer (1979): "Because I am unable to make significant contact with my environment, there is contraction of self. . . . My distinctive powers are negated and I am unfree." Here we find two expressions involving her conceptions of self—"contraction of self" and "I am unfree"—meaning that she has lost many aspects of herself because of illness, and so her very self has become constricted. Because of her body's failure, she is unfree, no longer having the power of sufficient control over her body to regain those aspects of the self so as to be the person she was before her illness or had then hoped to be.

As we have been noting, the centrality of the body lies in its capacity for action—its ability to act upon the environment as well as to be acted upon—and in the images formed of the self in relationship to the performance of action. That action and those images occur as a person attempts to carry out all of the various tasks associated with the different aspects of the self over time. We call that action pertaining to tasks *performance*—again, crucial in the lives of the healthy as well as the ill.

Performance

Performance as Action. As suggested by Mead, action is a process that occurs in stages involving both physical and mental responses. As long as action is unimpeded, it occurs in an almost reflexive manner (Dewey, 1921; Mead, 1934). That is, a stimulation is received and the individual responds quickly, almost without thought. However, when action becomes problematic, the mental processes of reflective thought are brought into play. For instance, when a driver applies his brakes but finds they aren't working, he has to think quickly of what he can do to avoid a potential collision. Similarly, a person recently disabled has to "concentrate" on each step taken, until the activity eventually may become relatively automatic.

Action, in short, involves both a body and a mind. However, these are not separate and distinct entities as is commonly assumed in lay thinking. Rather, both are required for completion of the act—with mental processes and physical processes each coming into focus during various stages of the act. For performances, we need a body—but not just *any* body. Performance requires a body in which both the mental and physical processes are working in harmony toward the completion of an act. A startling demonstration of this in terms of illness was revealed in the plight of a victim of a neurological phenomenon that rendered her completely insensitive to stimulation from her body. Yet she learned to "will" her body to do many normal things successfully. To do this, she needed for many months to look at a relevant body part and *will* it to do the movement.

The Many Aspects of Performance. Performances may be routine or problematic, depending upon the nature of the work to be done and the context in which it occurs. Playing scales on the piano is a routine and simple task for the concert pianist. However, playing a new and difficult piece may be problematic at first. Playing a fast piece may be problematic even for a skilled pianist if he or she has recently suffered from a heart attack (as one of our interviewees explained).

A performance may also be simple or complex. It may require one person, or two people, or more. It may require more emphasis on the physical processes or on the mental processes; or it may require equal emphasis, as when one plays a difficult piano piece. Its duration may be variable. A performance may begin with a mental rehearsal about what one is to do in advance of the physical part of the act, or it may not. And completion of the physical portion of an act may be followed by a mental review of one's performance, or it may not. A performance may be conducted with one or more parties to the performance not aware of certain aspects of the performance—usually the mental processes that condition the physiological or visible aspects. Or a performance may be conducted with none of its aspects hidden. And it may be carried out because of a commitment to a person, place, or thing, or it may be done out of sheer desire.

In addition, the term *performance* denotes both the capacity for action and appearance. *Appearance* is used here in a double sense: first, the appearance of action—what I or others think of what I did; and second, appearance in terms of physical features—the way I look to myself and others. Each of these aspects of appearance (action and person) involves the body (Stone, 1962; Goffman, 1963). Action and appearance relate to performance as conditions that define a person's perception of the purpose as well as to anticipated consequences of his or her performance.

Performance, then, may be usefully broken down into the following dimensions: (1) for oneself, (2) for others, (3) before others, (4) with others, (5) through others, (6) appearance of the performance, and (7) appearance of the performer. However, any performance may include a combination of dimensions. We shall see many examples presently. In regard to these dimensions and their combinations, one might therefore ask: What are the conditions that bring out that dimension or combination of dimensions; what interactional tactics are involved; and what are the consequences for each person involved?

It stands to reason that successful performances, whether they be for oneself or another, whether they involve appearances or not, can act as identity boosters that enhance conceptions of the self. On the other hand, failed performances can erode or shatter conceptions of the self. Of course, one reason for failed performances is body failure due to chronic illness. We turn now to the ill and their body-biographical difficulties.

Body Failure and Failed Performances

When there is body failure due to chronic illness, the resulting limitations in activity or changes in appearance can vary greatly. Each limitation in activity or change in appearance corresponds to the body part or function affected. The degree and kind of body failure depends in turn upon the type and severity of the illness or injury, the symptoms it presents, the methods of treatment (such as mutilating surgery), the possibility of comeback, the variations of symptoms within a day or week, the type of activity one wishes to engage in, and more globally the type of activity necessitated by one's life-style (Strauss and others, 1984; Schneider and Conrad, 1983; Speedling, 1982).

A failed body may lead to failed performances because of limitations in capacity for activity or changes in appearance and also because of altered sensations, such as the phantom pain experienced by amputees, or because of no sensation in certain parts of the body, as in paralysis. Failed performances may also be accounted for by distortions or interruptions in the communication process, whereby a person absorbs and processes information and is unable to make thoughts and feelings known, as in aphasia. Then, too, performances may fail because of altered perceptions of objects; for instance, things may appear fuzzy around the edges, and this can affect action toward them. Altered perceptions of space can also cause performance failure; for example, one man with Parkinson's disease now finds that he is sometimes unsure where he is placing a glass on the counter.

Sometimes a person is not sure about the cause of a failed performance. Is it due to body failure or to the anticipation of body failure? (As the man with Parkinson's said, "Is it my illness or is it my mind playing tricks on me?") For those with chronic mental illness, the cause of failed performance usually is deemed functional unless they are also clearly physically ill.

As a consequence of body failure, accommodation in the form of altered, modified, or omitted performances must occur in accordance with body limitations. Just as an illness condition can vary over time, so can the type and degree of corresponding body failure. Sometimes, as with arthritis (Wiener, 1975a; Locker, 1983), the degree of body failure can vary quite drastically in one day, making performance accommodation an ongoing process.

In a failed performance, then, there may be perceived failure in one's performance *for self, for others, before others, through others,* or *with others,* as well as in the *appearance* of the performance or the performer. The breakdown may occur in either the mental or physical parts of the process. It may occur in regard to the appearance of a performance or the level of performance features themselves. Holding to the perspective of G. H. Mead (1932, 1934), we can say that one can fail in one's performance for, with, and before others even if they are not present. This is because one holds within oneself the attitudes of others toward oneself and can bring these attitudes into consciousness through reflexive action and in doing so pass a negative judgment upon the self. The degree and type of body failure create the trajectory-related context for failed performances, while biographical experience comes into play by acting as a condition for the performance and at the same time giving meaning to it.

Failed self-performances are reinforced by failed performances for, before, and with others and by the others' responses. This means that limitations in activity and negative appearance features have to be coped with strategically in regard to other people's responses. To minimize performance failure, ill people use a variety of tactics and props, for example, taking angina pills surreptitiously before engaging in an activity with someone else, especially if it must be a mutual performance, or pausing on a walk to look at an interesting object or scene to ease the pain of angina. The ill also use a variety of tactics to conceal or minimize negative appearance features or to highlight positive appearance features that might detract other people's attention from the negative features. (One interviewee showed the researcher how she uses attractive jewelry and scarves to conceal her tracheotomy.) Just as symptoms or limitations may be handled during a performance to minimize performance failure, preventive action may be taken before a performance for the same reason. An instance of this is the timing of medications to decrease pain or other visible symptoms so that their peak action coincides with a performance.

Sometimes self-performance tactics are used to handle others' responses to negative appearance features or appearance performances. In his book *Stigma*, Goffman (1963) relates how when people would say to a woman, "I see you lost a leg," she would reply acidly with a comment such as, "Yes, I checked it in with an insurance company." Davis (1972) describes in his article "Deviance Disavowal" how the visibly handicapped will handle negative appearance features or appearance performances during the course of interaction by skillfully shifting the focus of interaction away from the negative aspects to more positive aspects of the self. For example, they can engage in such interesting conversation that the listener's attention is drawn away from their blindness or prominent skin blemish.

Though an ill person may perceive a performance as a failure, others may not. For example, a sufferer of Parkinson's disease said that while he must constantly rely on the assistance of others, there is no way he can repay them for what they do, though they don't help him with the expectation of getting something in return. Still another example comes from *One Step at a Time* by

Lenor Madruga (1979), who recounts the horror she felt at having to descend from an airplane in a stair chair in front of the friends waiting for her. Returning home after a drastic operation performed at a distant medical center, she wished to appear before them as the lively, self-sufficient, and self-confident fashion model who had left for treatment some weeks before. She wanted to come off the airplane under her own power, for their sake as well as for her own, but she could not. Though her friends did not perceive her assisted descent as a failed performance, she did—and on three dimensions: performance for self, for others, and before others.

Paradoxically, occasionally performance failure based on body failure is completely misunderstood or not believed by a "normal," healthy person. Thus, a young girl was accused by her public school teachers of laziness because she could not learn her lessons, the teachers never believing that greatly defective reading vision was the real explanation.

It is important to understand that spouses may take part in an ill mate's performances in various ways. They may put on performances of their own, covering their fatigue or their own illness when providing care to the other, or hiding their disappointment at the other's performance.

As for the ill person, failing to perform competently or at all often elicits a sense of panic, despair, frustration, impatience with slow progress, and a railing at fate. Such feelings of failure can hit directly at identity, shattering the BBC chain to some degree, permanently or temporarily.

The Disturbed BBC Chain. The impact of body failure and consequent performance failure can be measured by the impact it has on each dimension of the BBC (self-conceptions, biographical time, body conceptions). Since each dimension exists in a tightly bound relationship with the others, the consequences of body failure with regard to one aspect are further felt with the other two. It is the combined impact on all three that profoundly affects biographical continuity and meaning. (See, for example, the plight of the radically destabilized woman in Chapter Ten or the woman dying of throat cancer in Chapter Eleven.) The conditions determining the degree to which each BBC dimension is affected arise from both trajectory and biographical sources. With every major change in the trajectory that brings about a change in the degree of body failure, whether for better or worse, there may be an accompanying change in the BBC dimensions. One's cumulative experience gives further meaning to those failed performances.

Trajectory-related conditions include (1) the type of trajectory phase, (2) the subphase within a type, (3) the severity of illness and the associated number and type of symptoms, and (4) the degree to which the symptoms can be controlled. Biography-related conditions include (1) the life stage, (2) the salient aspect(s) of self loss, (3) the ability to learn new ways of living within the limitations imposed by body failure, and (4) the ability to come to terms with losses. Both sets of conditions—trajectory and biographical—whether alone or together, act upon each dimension of the BBC to affect the BBC chain.

Impact on Biographical Time. When severe chronic illness occurs, it breaks into the stream of biographical time, interrupting and possibly forever changing past performances from those of the present and future. Accordingly, time conceptions are likely to be altered for dealing with and taking into consideration these changes. (Who I am now and will be is not who I was and thought I would be.) New biographical projections that correspond with the trajectory projections must be arrived at.

Simultaneously, clock time may have to be juggled and restructured to include trajectory management within the context of the numerous tasks performed when normally carrying out the business of one's life; that is, new performances must be articulated with the old. Clock time may also have to be restructured to provide for any increase in the duration of time it now takes to accomplish any trajectory-related tasks because of current limitations in the body's capacity to perform. A combination of complicated regimen and slow movements caused by disability can poke large holes in anyone's otherwise normal schedule.

Correspondingly, changed perceptions of biographical time will reflect the foregoing. In fact, the exact parameters of temporal terms that the ill use in thinking about time depend upon what kind of illness course they (and others) predict for themselves and the types of trajectory-related situations in which they currently find themselves. For example, Fischer (1983) uses the phrase "living on borrowed time" to express the biographical time perceptions of people on kidney dialysis. Other phrases denoting perceptions of biographical time derived from our interviews include "the foreclosed future"—the future life I will no longer have; the "urgent present"—I had better hurry to accomplish what I set out to do before time runs out; "the eternal present"—life is locked into the present situation, and there seems to be no hope of change in the future; "the lost past"—the person I left behind; "the overbearing present"—a frightening or painful situation in which time seems to be standing still or passing unusually slowly.

How trajectory-related conditions alter both the body and biographical time, and therefore one's very life course, can be seen in Table 1, a simple schematic analysis done on the contents of *The Other Side of the Mountain* (Kilmont and Valens, 1975).

The schematic outline does not begin to portray the impact of the skiing accident on Jill's life. However, it gives some indication of how biographical time can be disrupted and its use changed following a major life-threatening and paralyzing accident. One can also easily see from this example how severe body failure might change the course of a life, whether the person be an Olympic hopeful or a janitor. For Jill, hopes and dreams were all wrapped up in skiing. Through her skilled and disciplined body, she hoped to achieve her dreams. When her spinal cord was severed, her dreams of the envisioned Olympic performance were shattered forever.

Changes in the Body and Body Conceptions. Jill's accident also suggests how *conceptions* of the body will change in relationship to an illness. When the body fails, body and mind that once worked in harmony to carry out a performance no longer do so. This means that an ill person must discover what body part(s) or system(s) has failed, the degree of failure, how the degree of failure might fluctuate over the course of the day, and the possibility of partial or complete recovery—all or some of which probably vary according to phase and type of trajectory. Then and only then can he or she change the nature of performances to make up for or plan around the deficits brought about by body failure.

The once-performing body becomes now the "useless body," or the familiar body becomes the "unfamiliar body," "the strange

Table 1. Schematic Analysis of the Contents of *The Other Side of the Mountain*.

Trajectory	Biography	Body	Biographical Time
Skiing accident at Olympic tryouts	Biography interrupted	Part of body feels lost, not connected	Immediate opportunity
In hospital in critical condition, medical and body	Still interrupted	Immobile and immobilized body	World closing in; biographical time suspended while clock time structured around continuous medical and body care
Third day condition improves	Suspended biography	The "no feeling body"; "body testing" to determine extent of body failure	Living in the immediate present; needs here and now; "enduring present"
Announcement of paralysis	The shattered biography; let go of dreams; mourning; loss of past and future	The paralyzed body	Collapsed time of past and future comes crashing into the present
Stable physical therapy begins; beginning comeback	The absorbed biography	New discoveries about body—how extenders and flexors work; the working body	Avoidance of the future Clock time given over to working at comeback The absorbed present
About five months postaccident trajectory projection	Biographical projection unclear: "the pending biography,"—can't be what I was before, but what will I be? No horizons visible	No conscious feeling below shoulders but developing awareness of new body sensations	Past and future now hovering over the present, with future moving in—can no longer put off the future

body," or "the puzzling body," to use the words of our respondents (see Chapter Ten and the last case in Chapter Eleven). Alterations in sensations or difficulties in moving through space will change relationships to the environment. Some people begin to see their bodies as prisons in which they are indeed contained, no longer able to make the desired contact with the environment.

Sometimes ill people's abilities to think and reflect (mind) and their abilities to physically act (body) are conceived by the ill as quite distinct entities. This usually occurs when their ability to perform physically is severely limited but their mental processes remain intact. Thus, one man in our study said there were times when he felt that neither his mind nor his body was a part of himself. His ability to function physically varied from day to day and sometimes quite drastically within a day. Some days he felt that his inability to act physically was clearly the result of his illness. At other times he wondered if the cause of his failed performance rested in his mind. (See Chapter Eleven.) Agnes de Mille (1981) (see our Chapter Eight) describes the paradox of having an unimpaired mind but now also a defective brain that has brought about bodily paralysis. (See also in Chapter Eight the cardiac case whose comeback had reached the point where he was successfully managing to write a book but was frustrated at still not being able to walk without incurring angina.)

The biographical consequences of body failure are determined in part by the degree of importance placed on the lost physical or mental functions. A pianist with arthritis, such as Byron Janis, would be more affected in his or her work than a writer with heart disease. Another example comes from a newspaper article ("Javitz' Talk to Doctors," May 12, 1984) quoting Jacob Javitz, the late senator from New York. He was in a late stage of Lou Gehrig's disease and paralyzed from the neck down. A battery-operated respirator assisted him in breathing. Yet he remained very active (with help, of course), writing papers, giving speeches, and testifying before Congress on the needs of handicapped people. He compared his adjustment to that of a famous movie star who had the same disease. The star, according to Javitz, found adjustment very difficult because his looks (performance features) and his ability to perform before others (appearance performance) were the tools of his trade. This celebrity, having lost the physical ability to carry out salient self-performance (acting) was never fully able to come to terms with his losses. The former senator, on the other hand, was still able to carry on highly important performances. For him, appearance features and appearance performances were unimportant compared with his ability to perform before and for others. A wheelchair, respirator, and other people helped him to transcend a terribly crippled body.

With some illnesses, such as stroke, there may be a blur or overlap of mental and physical processes or a loss of some combination of them. With mental illness, thought processes may be so distorted that the consequent physical functioning is impeded or deemed inappropriate. Severely depressed people often lack the energy to carry out any performance. As the wife of a schizophrenic reported, she had to tell her husband when to wear a sweater or jacket because he found it difficult to distinguish between warm and cold.

Loss of Self. When people are unable to complete actions enabling them to carry out tasks associated with various aspects of the self (whether inability to perform as a teacher or "normal" father or even to carry out the activities of daily living), then certain aspects of the self become "lost." Since the integration of these various aspects of the self forms the more inclusive self, or identity, with that loss comes an accompanying sense of loss of wholeness.

The degree to which one's identity is affected depends on the number and prominence of aspects of the self that are lost, the possibility of their recovery, the ability to discover new modes of action, the ability to "transcend" the body, and the ability to come to terms with the losses and build a new conception of oneself around the limitations or, as the ill often say, to become whole again.

Summary

Theory. To gain a deeper understanding of the actions and the experiences of the chronically ill requires a complex set of concepts and the drawing of connections among them. For this reason, this chapter addresses the interrelated themes of body, self, biography, and biographical time. The body is central to human action and a sense of self. That centrality lies in its capacity for action—its ability to act on the environment as well as be acted upon—and in the images formed of the self in the performing action. The chronically ill suffer some degree and kind of body failure, with consequent limitations of actions and a potential affecting of self-conceptions and of their sense of personal (or biographical) time. We have coined the term *biographical body conceptions (BBC)* in order to represent conceptions of self arising directly or indirectly from the body, as they evolve over a lifetime. We also use a related concept, the BBC chain, to represent the working together of those three elements.

A severe chronic illness can disturb and, metaphorically speaking, even shatter the BBC chain. Moreover, the social actions that we have called performance (before, with, for, and through others) can also be affected by the physical limitations attending chronic illness, as can the appearance of those performances in the eyes of others and the self, as well as the physical appearance of the ill person. Perceived self-failure at performing various actions that are highly important to one's sense of self can be fateful for that self (see the cases in Chapters Eight, Nine, Ten, and Eleven). Those perceived failures require the kinds of biographical processes that will be discussed in Chapter Five.

Applications. The practical implications of the material and concepts presented in this chapter include the following.

1. People who have a severe, chronic illness (or often even a mild one) cannot be regarded as merely in need of medical treatment. They are likely at one phase or another of their illness course to need counsel on deeply personal matters, and so may their spouses. Our system of health care, including the training of most types of health practitioners, is primarily organized around conceptions of illness as acute. What has been called the acute-care model of illness and treatment is pervasive, and its focus is on medical-technical interventions. Chronically ill patients need much more than medical-technical assistance, however. Correspondingly, health practitioners who work with the chronically ill—in hospitals as well as in their homes—need training in offering interventions

and counsel that will be sensitive to the kinds of problems discussed in this chapter.

2. To understand those problems it is not enough for practitioners to operate with merely commonsense concepts or even, we believe, with strictly psychological or psychiatric concepts such as stress and coping. The practitioner requires a sophisticated set of concepts allied with observer-interviewer sensitivity that will sensitize him or her to the combined psychological *and* social aspects of the chronic illness experience.

3. Central to practitioner sensitivity should be a focus on discovering for each client the meaning of his or her body—its images, appearances, perceived limitations, failures and successes in performance—and above all the body's relation to one's sense of self. "Chronic illness" connotes medical treatment; "body" should connote bodily failure or performance despite body limitations.

4. Under today's restrictive scheduling of time that can be spent professionally with the ill, it perhaps seems impractical to spell out one additional major implication of the materials presented in this chapter. We will make the point nevertheless. Effective interventions pertaining to clients' biographical concerns certainly require some listening skill, i.e., hearing with sensitivity and understanding the ill and their families. Establishing sufficient trust in oneself as a listener and possibly a potential helper is essential to allowing clients to express what they are experiencing (Strauss and others, 1984). Few of our interviews took more than a couple of hours, and the biographical themes in the interviewees' lives often became apparent in opening conversations, even before the actual interviews began. Often when people are ready to burst with anxiety, anger, frustration, and the like, one only has to listen!

5

Putting Life Back Together Again

As noted earlier, a central task of the ill is putting the BBC chain back together. This means that several positive changes must occur in the three crucial dimensions of body, self, and biographical time. Old definitions for body, self, activities, other people, interactions, events, and relationships must be replaced with new definitions, which must be sought and discovered. If there is a very successful comeback and body functioning returns, then some definitions can return more or less to what they were before. The temporal aspect of trajectory means that all of those definitions play back into action. Our interviews have shown repeatedly that what ill people discover about their body's changed capabilities gives rise to a new BBC, which then is incorporated into their sense of identity. For instance, eating without salt means eating tasteless food unless substitute flavorings are found. In turn, the latter can take on the role that salt once had. So, one can regard oneself as someone who can get along without salt and, perhaps, who can cook well with spices instead of salt.

The BBC chain is put back together through biographical work that involves four separate but overlapping *biographical processes*. Though analytically distinct, each process occurs simultaneously and feeds directly into the others. The processes are (1) *contextualizing* (incorporating the illness trajectory into biography), (2) *coming to terms* (arriving at some degree of understanding and acceptance of the biographical consequences of actual or potential failed performances), (3) *reconstituting identity* (reintegrating identity into a new conceptualization of wholeness around the limitations in performance), and (4) *recasting biography* (giving new directions to biography). Each of these processes evolves over time. Thus, coming to terms with limitations imposed by an illness takes place over time slowly and not necessarily continuously. But it is important to recognize analytically that coming to terms as a *process* rests inevitably on the biographical *work* entailed in it.

Biographical work as such is done in the service of one's biography, including its review, maintenance, repair, and alteration. Its nature is such that it must be done by those who are affected. Though others might help, only the person whose biography has been rendered discontinuous can put it back together again. The amount and type of biographical work to be done, as well as the degree to which and intensity with which it is carried out, vary in accordance with both the trajectory and the biographical contexts within which it occurs.

Trajectory phase is important too; that is, biographical work will vary, depending upon whether it is associated with acute, comeback, stable, or downward phase of trajectory. (Chapters Eight through Eleven provide illustrations.) The work will also vary with the severity of the illness and whether it is in an early or late stage. The work will vary with the degree of body failure experienced and potential or actual failed performances. Finally, it will vary according to the degree to which the biography is shattered through the impact of the body failure on each of the BBC's dimensions. This occurs through various biography-related conditions such as the number of aspects of the self lost, the meaning given to them, and the ability to find new modes of living within the limitations.

Biographical Ideational Processes

Before discussing each of the major biographical processes involved in putting back together a disrupted BBC chain, we shall note a more general conditional set of what G. H. Mead called *ideational processes.*

> Now it is by these ideational processes that we get hold
> of the conditions of future conduct as these are formed
> in the organized responses which we have formed, and
> so construct our own past in anticipation of that

future. The individual who can thus get hold of them
can further organize them through the selection of the
stimulations which call them out and can thus build
his plan of action [1932, p. 76].

In the context of this book, we shall focus on two ideational
processes: *backward and forward reviews.* They are necessary to the
biographical work done by the severely ill in putting their lives back
together.

Reviews are the reflective parts of actions and involve the use
of daydreams and various types of imagery for recapturing the past,
examining the present, and projecting into the future—all interpreted in light of the present. Reviews often serve as a basis for
future action. A person mentally rehearses or thinks through how
he or she will handle a problematic situation. For instance, one
interviewee related that he was having nightmares trying to figure
out how he was going to get up the stairs to his home after
returning from a trip. Because of Parkinson's disease his mobility
was often restricted, depending on how well his drugs were working
at a particular time. He knew he could receive assistance for getting
out of the airplane and into a taxi at the airport, but he wasn't sure
if the taxi driver would be willing or able to help him up the stairs
once he arrived at his house. Some biographical reviews, of course,
are not directly action oriented but rather function for the ill as a
way of mentally confronting and working through the key issues
with which they must come to terms, issues stemming from bodily
limitations and failed performances.

Reviews are directly related to type and phase of trajectory.
Thus, people facing certain death often think back over their lives,
putting them in order and gaining closure. Reviews are also usually
triggered by changes in trajectory and biography, by confrontations
with the illness through actual or potential failed performances,
and by interactions with others.

There are many different subtypes of reviews, all associated
with different temporal images pertaining to moments and
durations in past-present-future, as well as related to the perceived
status of one's illness. There are accounting reviews, among them
a self-assessment and evaluation of past failures and successes in

life, failures that can no longer be made right. Another type of accounting involves taking stock of strengths and weaknesses in order to plan the resources needed for the long struggle ahead. There are also single flashbacks, momentary remembrances of past events that pass through one's mind, such as those that sometimes happen when a still-conscious person is being wheeled into surgery. There are biographical replays of important biographical events, such as childhood scenes involving oneself, parents, or others. And there are future forecasts, such as projecting oneself as confined to a wheelchair in the years ahead.

There are also trajectory-related reviews. One kind is the symptoms review: looking back on the onset of symptoms and giving meaning to them in light of present knowledge. Then there are treatment reviews, in which the benefits and risks of potential treatments are weighed. There are comeback reviews, taking stock of physical recovery and assessing how far one still has to go. There are stable-trajectory reviews, wondering how much longer the illness will stay the same. There are downward-trajectory reviews, wondering how much worse symptoms can become. Here is an example of some of the reviews and how they function:

> Never before have I experienced the interconnections of past, present, and future in my life so distinctively as since the loss of my eye. Handling the present and anticipating the future have won priority, but the past has entered the picture too. Defining the loss, for example, has required the constitution of a relation-ship between now and before. "Before" and "after" surgery became like a new time in my life. I have often been tense when meeting people who knew me from "before." But the past has had an impact on the present in terms of my sickness also: there have been moments when I start dipping into the past to find an explanation for my tumor. Had I contributed to my tumor? Why had I been hit in an especially crucial part of my appearance? As a child I must have been all eyes. Later due to my eyes some nicknames were

attached to me. Why did my visually strong eye get
sick? I did not find the answers.

Reviews may consist of simple flashbacks or involve lengthy
mental rehearsals. Some occur only once; others recur repeatedly,
though their actual content may differ. Some serve a one-time
purpose, such as how is one going to get up that flight of stairs
when first returning from the hospital? However, mostly it is the
cumulative effect of varied reviews that helps the ill person to
contextualize and come more or less to terms with an illness—that
is, struggle with a perceived fate—and to reconstitute identity and
recast his or her biography.

Contextualizing

If an illness is severe, it must be incorporated into the
biography. *Contextualization* is the biographical process by which
this incorporation occurs. We can sense this process taking place in
the following sensitively nuanced sentences: "I tell myself it's just
a part of me. This lupus, like a wart, or a wrinkle. I am trying to
integrate it into my being, my self-image. But I want to integrate
it not as a blight, but as a part of me that I must accept and live
with" (quotation from an interview, two years after diagnosis,
Labrie, 1986, p. 8). The degree of contextualization can vary
tremendously. The illness may be discounted, kept separate from
the rest of a biography; it is not "part of me." If it becomes very well
integrated, then the illness and its associated work "is me," is the
major conceptualization around which one's identity revolves. For
the most part, integration lies somewhere in between: somewhat
part of biography, yet not fused with it. "My chronic illness is part
of me, but there is more of me than it."

Contextualization is a dynamic matter. Any major change in
the trajectory or biographical context that brings about a change in
the performances may correspondingly require adjustments in self,
biographical time, and body conceptions. Conditions that affect the
degree of integration of a trajectory into the total self include the
following: whether the trajectory is considered pleasant or unpleasant, is self-chosen or forced, is seen as shattering or capable of

producing growth, requires little or much work and time to manage and whether it causes much or little suffering. (See the case in Chapter Twelve, where we can see a struggle with contextualization of a forced, dreadful, shattering trajectory.)

A chronic illness precipitates an involuntary trajectory. Though people find ways of living with severe illness and the associated management work, most do not consider it desirable or particularly pleasant. Often it causes considerable physical and emotional suffering. Its management may require a great deal of vigilance and diligence. Though some are crushed by the experience and never completely recover, others are able to turn it into something that produces growth and understanding of themselves and others:

> We have been married for fifteen years and have always been close, but I think that managing the illness has drawn us even closer together. Because we are working together and because it is a whole new life-style that we have both gone into in the same way. We have had enormous growth from this, and it just wasn't one of us growing in a direction; we conquered the cancer together.

Although contextualization of the illness trajectory may begin in part with the onset of early symptoms, it does not occur in earnest until the person begins to realize its more severe implications in terms of biography. While the great intensity of effort and work usually occurs during the early months or years of the illness, the process is rarely complete and must recur each time there is a major trajectory or biographical change. For example, a young married woman with long-standing diabetes had thought very little about her illness. It was simply a part of her life, one that gave her few problems and only required minimal thought and effort to manage. However, when she became pregnant, the diabetes came into greater focus. Now she had to keep it closely monitored and under control, not only for her own health but for the safety of her developing fetus.

Contextualizing also involves discovery. It means discovering what aspects of the self have been lost temporarily or forever or on a fluctuating basis. It means discovering what aspects of the self remain and can be carried forward to provide biographical continuity. It means discovering what new aspects can be added, not necessarily to replace the old but to give new meaning to biography. (Schatzman and Olesen, 1983, refer to this new aspect of the self as the physical self.) "I received my diagnosis in late February. This is now May and I'm still paralyzed by a lot of anxiety. . . . I'm not clear on what it is that I want to do with what I think is the rest of my life . . . you know, I may want to get to know my sister better. I may want to get to know the world better. I may want to travel."

As for time, contextualizing also means discovering how to articulate illness-related tasks into the context of biographically related tasks. If the ill person can no longer perform his or her share of these tasks, then arrangements have to be made for the spouse or others to take them over and incorporate them into their own lives. Concerning the longer arc of biographical time, the ill must discover how to carry forward what remains of the past, how to live in the present, and what new paths can be used to open up the future.

For the body, contextualizing means testing and pushing it to discover the extent of its limitations. Contextualizing also means discovering the environmental conditions that can lead to body failure and thus to failed performances and then either eliminating the performances or finding new ways of performing through the use of other people and devices. A person may even be able to substitute one body part for another failed one. For example, Joni (Ereackson, 1976), left quadriplegic by a diving accident, became an accomplished artist by substituting her mouth for her hands.

Contextualizing also means conceptualizing the body as an object with limitations that must be taken into account and managed yet is still capable of various performances. For instance, one of our respondents, a woman with advanced muscular dystrophy, still manages to attend concerts and art exhibits, to hostess dinner parties, to act as a representative on her city's health council, and to serve on boards of other voluntary agencies that are of special interest to her—all from her wheelchair and with her husband's assistance.

In addition, contextualizing requires a certain degree of

coming to terms with the illness, the consequent limitations, and perhaps the prospect of death. No one chooses an illness trajectory, but having been caught up in it, one must try to learn to live with it. The only other alternatives seem to be to deny its presence, to retreat emotionally from the world, or to commit suicide. Contextualizing does *not* imply full acceptance of the illness but makes it a sufficient enough part of the self that one does what is necessary to ensure both physical and biographical survival.

For most people, integration is not an all-or-nothing matter but a process that shows some movement, usually from less to more integration, though as mentioned earlier it may also fluctuate in degree. Bodily limitations that are tolerable under one set of biographical conditions become less so under different sets and so less integrated into one's life.

Among the ill, there are wide variations in the degree of integration accomplished; these range from searing or painful nonintegration to transcendence of limitations and joyous integration. Examples of these two extremes can be found in the following cases. H. Colman (1977) tells the poignant story of her husband, who seemed to retreat from life after a second stroke. Though mentally alert he maintained very little interaction with the outside world. She struggled to give some meaning to his life, but he seemed to take very little part in this struggle. It is difficult to determine the meaning of this experience for this man because the reader is given only occasional glimpses into his private world through bits of his poetry and his wife's accounts of his depression and retreat from life. It appears from her account that he found living so painful that he pulled back almost completely into himself. For his wife, watching his biographical death was as painful as watching the physical wasting away. (See also Chapter Eleven, Case 2 of the deteriorating phase section, and Case 1 of the dying phase section. Both illustrate relative nonintegration.)

In contrast, one of our quadriplegics, despite severe physical limitations, has managed to live a full life with his wife, which includes raising children, socializing, attending school together, and having an active sexual relationship. In working out ways to carry out these activities, they have succeeded in moving beyond his seemingly actual physical disabilities. Certainly by wisely manag-

ing the otherwise difficult respective combinations of husband/
patient and wife/attendant, they have accomplished individual and
mutual biographical goals that neither could have accomplished
alone. Furthermore, they have had a good time doing it: "Caring
for him is kind of fun. It makes a relationship more attached when
you each have to give a part of yourself. I like to be needed. J. likes
to be needed. That is why we get along so well."

Coming to Terms

Coming to terms involves movement toward an understanding and acceptance of the irrevocable quality of chronic illness, of
the performance limitations accompanying it, of death, and of the
biographical consequences it brings about such as failed marriages,
lost jobs, and dependency. Like contextualizing, coming to terms
varies along a continuum ranging from nonacceptance to full
acceptance. Movement along the continuum is very closely tied with
contextualization. It is hard to speak of one type of work without
speaking of the other.

Though coming to terms involves movement through stages,
a person may move back and forth along the continuum in response
to trajectory or biographical contingencies. Even when the person
is relatively accepting, a contingency may cause him or her to grieve
again for what has been lost, though perhaps not with the original
intensity.

It is also possible once having come to terms with one set of
limitations to return to a state of nonacceptance of them. This can
happen if limitations increase or a biographical condition changes
so that the limitations become more noticeable. Then, too, one can
come to terms with certain losses and not with others, so that with
respect to the loss of various aspects of self, one can be variously
accepting of each.

The coming to terms occurs by means of confrontations
arising from potential or actual failed performances and accompanying biographical reviews. Confrontations act as identity smashers
that break or weaken the links in the BBC chain. Some confrontations are followed by reviews that either further weaken the chain
by emphasizing discontinuity of the present and future from the

past or help to foster an understanding or acceptance of the failed body performances by modulating the past and raising hope for the future.

It should be useful to outline the actual work involved in coming to terms, though of course the specifics vary. First, there is a confrontation in the form of potential or actual failed performances. This is followed by one or more reviews that may lead to denial, anger, sadness, regret, and in some cases bargaining with God or fate, while the person tries to hold onto meaningful aspects of the self. Through further self-confrontations and reviews, the person gradually realizes that these aspects of activity, of self are gone, no longer possible; in doing so, the person begins to relinquish that part of the past through a series of closure acts involving the self and others. This relinquishing involves some degree of grieving for what has been lost. With grieving may come varying degrees of depression. Eventually, one begins to realize, or realize more fully, that one can no longer live in the past but must begin to look toward the future (Becker, 1984). In embracing the future, acceptance begins; for one cannot accept unless there is hope for a better, albeit altered, future. Without hope, there is no incentive to move from letting go toward some degree of acceptance.

Hope, here, means the perception of an exit—a way out of the present situation. The future will be better: "Perhaps they can prolong my life until a cure is found." "Maybe this medication will work, and I will live to see my child graduate from high school." There may be hope that limitations will decrease, as in one's making a comeback. Or hope may be seen as freedom from fatigue, suffering, and pain, as in the release of death. It may mean that there is a life after this one.

> I tell him I dreamed that we were all at his funeral and crying. The priest said, "Why are you crying? J. is happy. He is not crying. Today is his birthday. It is his first day in the new world, the new planet he went to. You should be happy." I tell him I plan to live forever. This is only one part of our life. When we leave this one we go to another planet. . . . This is the way I try to get him to accept what is to come.

A state of no hope exists when despair arises from a perception that there is no possible exit from the present situation, that there is no escape, only the eternal present.

However, as Kübler-Ross (1969) says, acceptance does not mean a state of happiness. Acceptance means that a person has found a way of biographically accommodating to an illness through altered or changed performances, and in doing so to give meaning to life despite ongoing or progressive body failure.

Some people not only reach the stage of acceptance but go on to an even higher level, one that we call *transcendence*. Transcendence occurs when the ill have found ways to overcome their bodies so that they are able to find real joy in living (and even dying), although their performances may now be severely limited (Feldman, 1974). Life has taken on a new meaning and is in some ways better than before. Some are able to transcend their bodies through beliefs in an afterlife:

> We were telling the children how he is not afraid to die, that he is very peaceful and feels there is a purpose for his illness. My daughter said, "Gee, Mom, the way you put it, it sounds like Dad is dying for us." I said, "That is why Christ died. If your dad is willing, it makes it all worthwhile." It makes sense in the whole purpose of living and dying.

Others find that they are now able to see the world with new eyes. For the first time they keenly appreciate the beauty in nature or in people: "The loss of my eye aroused in me a new awareness of eyes in human beings. I discovered a new beauty in eyes." The dancer and choreographer Agnes de Mille has beautifully captured the essence of transcending experiences. Some months after her stroke, her past life now seemed "stale and used up" and her "new life which had begun since the stroke" was a fresh beginning. She was able to experience "things quite freshly and very colorfully, with new delights and none of the old constraints. And I was capable of growing, of learning new things. It was a feeling of freedom such as I haven't known since I was . . . five years old" (de Mille, 1981, p. 205).

Of course, some people are not able to accept their limitations. There are three dimensions of this: nonacceptance of the illness itself, of the symptoms, and of the activity limitations. Nonacceptance essentially means that there is a radical biographical discontinuity with the past and that the future and present will be always the same, or even worse than this undesirable present. In self-terms this means that biographical work is a failure. As in a case (Colman, 1977) noted earlier, the ill person cannot close the gap between past and present-future self. There is no future imagery of progress or of better times ahead to pull one through the rough periods.

Reconstituting Identity

Identity disintegration usually begins with the diagnostic announcement, when past and future come crashing into the undesirable or dreaded present. This identity shock is followed by future images of what the illness will mean in terms of biographical performances. For example: "I will be crippled." "I will no longer be able to . . ." "I might die soon." Understandably, the degree to which identity is jolted depends on the number of lost aspects of self, their saliency, and the possibility of comeback—regaining lost aspects of the self. Naturally, not all aspects of the self are lost. Most people are able to retain at least some aspects, and this continuity with the past is important for rebuilding identity. What is lost is the sense of wholeness of the self. The aim, then, is to try to regain this sense of wholeness; this is done through the process of *identity reconstitution* (Williams, 1984).

Efforts at reconstitution may not result in complete reintegration of identity. Also, because of illness contingencies, a person can stop short of or die before successful reintegration is achieved. Moreover, some measure of disintegration may recur if a confrontation precipitates an identity-smashing review. In addition, to proceed toward reintegration, there must be at every step a corresponding letting go, grieving for what has been lost, and closure. Meanwhile, the person is always moving toward a new self, a better self, even a transcendent self.

This reintegration involves three major steps: (1) defining

and redefining identity, (2) refocusing direction, and (3) integrating identity. Each step is aimed at keeping important aspects of the self in focus and active, pulling in new aspects, and discovering other new and unsuspected aspects. Depending on the combined biographical and trajectory context in which the steps take place, some can take longer than others, involve more struggle, and involve more interactions between the ill person and other people. (Chapter Eight provides a good illustration of this.) And, again, biographical reviews are central to reconstitution. Reviews follow the crucial confrontations, and through them one works out who one was, now is, and could have been or could possibly be in the future.

Defining and Redefining of Identity. Identity reconstitution is difficult to describe because the steps are overlapping and progressions are often followed by regressions. For analytical purposes, we have broken it down in the following manner. As already noted, reconstitution can begin with the diagnostic announcement, which precipitates questioning: "Who am I? What does this mean in terms of my life?" From there, the defining and redefining of identity begin.

Defining and redefining take place in at least two ways. The first includes refamiliarization with the body through testing limitations and sometimes by fighting them—in the form of attempted performances. "What can I do? What can't I do?" "For how long will I be able to?" Or "How long before I am able to?" Testing and fighting are often accompanied by anger and depression as performances fail or are not fully realized. One must let go, grieve, and achieve closure on lost aspects of the self before one can move on: "I went through the whole shot that paras and quads go through—blame everybody, the rebellion, the deep depression. Then I finally came to realize that nobody gives a damn and it is up to you whether you do anything or not. You have to fend for yourself." With each testing and retesting the process may begin again.

The second way of defining and redefining the self involves a values reorientation, the establishment of new priorities about what is important in life. For example, a recently injured quadriplegic who still had some upper body movement told us he could, perhaps with considerable therapy and effort, learn to carry out for himself the activities of daily living. However, the eventual performance of these activities would really take considerable time and energy. Instead, he had chosen to turn over those activities to his wife, as difficult as it was to yield them (especially those concerned with his body care) so that he could carry out a more important job—to counsel other patients with spinal cord injuries.

Refocusing Direction. The next step in reconstitution is refocusing direction. Biographical reviews done forward and backward and identity boosters in the form of successful performances help a person move on to this refocusing. Its consequence is the knitting of biographical continuity, which takes place through an essential continuation of performance even though the latter has been rendered problematic by body failure. This may mean modifying, altering, or changing the nature of performances.

The refocusing of direction occurs in several ways: (1) by giving new importance to old and still intact activities; (2) by shifting the importance of action from body to mind or mind to body, depending on which has been more impaired by body failure; (3) by substituting new activities for old; and (4) by using devices or changed body parts to carry out activities. This means that when preillness performances become problematic, they are followed by new ones that substitute for the old, however flawed or different these new ones are. Some, if successful, are central to identity reconstitution as performance validators and thus identity validators, too.

Here is an example: Mr. G., a quadriplegic, says that he and his wife loved to dance before his devastating accident. Part of his identity reconstitution involved learning to dance in his electric wheelchair, which he does with gusto in the middle of public dance floors. He even does "wheelies" and spins around. For him, dancing involves a performance for the self; it is something he likes to do for his own self-enjoyment. He is also doing it for his wife. Because he does it in a public place, it involves a performance before others, which he also enjoys. Moreover, it is a mutual performance, each spouse coordinating steps or actions in response to the other. Mr. G. is not concerned about the appearance of his performance before others except to show them that he too can partake of public activities and have a good time. Nor is he shy about his performance features—others seeing him in a wheelchair while he is dancing. The activity acts as a performance validation for him.

Another example involving another quadriplegic demonstrates how performances can also be carried out through others. This man had become so closely identified with his wife that he often volunteered to do activities (for example, cooking) when in reality she would have to carry them out because he was physically incapable of doing so. His wife had become his hands and legs, and he carried out performances important to himself through her.

Reintegrating Identity. Through continued validation of each successful performance—however altered, changed, or flawed the actual performance—the ill person begins once more to achieve a sense of identity integration, a feeling of wholeness. Nevertheless, one cannot validate performance and identity by oneself; part of the process necessarily entails receiving validation from others. For instance, a model, Lenor Madruga (1979), who had lost her hip and leg through surgery for cancer, achieved a large measure of integration through a series of validated performances not only for herself but also for, before, and with others. In her performances, she was not only concerned about performance appearance but also about her appearance features. Her performances included being able to do the family cooking, though this involved hobbling around on one leg or on crutches, returning to a satisfying sexual relationship with her husband, driving, putting on talent shows, looking over the farm with her husband, caring for her children, riding a horse and a three-wheel bike, dancing, and modeling. Contributing to this reintegration, which involved femininity as well as body function, was her general presentation of self through body handling and the use of clothing, as well as her willpower in searching out and obtaining a "shapely and lifelike" artificial leg and then using it skillfully.

Other people are also crucial in the reintegration process by engineering performances to be done by the ill person so that they will be successful and by mitigating the ill person's failed performances. Much of this identity work involves various levels of awareness between the participating parties. For example, F. and K. carry on a mutual pretense concerning his public speaking performances. They are both aware that he shakes when speaking.

Yet when reviewing a presentation together, neither mentions his inability to control the shaking. Rather, they focus on the successful part of the performance: what he said, how he said it, and the audience's reception of it. On the other hand, others can be brutally open; even spouses occasionally shatter already fragile identities: "After three or four months of my going in and out of the hospital, my wife told me that she was sick and tired of living with a cripple and hoped that she would never see a wheelchair again and left me. I will always remember that."

L. plays an elaborate game of closed awareness. After her husband was forced to retire from his job because of a severe cardiac condition, he became very depressed. L. attributed this to the loss of his feelings of importance and a need to be associated with his former job. So she set about devising ways to make him feel needed and important by coming up with all sorts of odd jobs around the house that she pretended she could no longer do without his assistance. If he was aware of her game, he made no mention of it.

Though a comeback may be far from easy, each important successful performance helps to put identity, in fact the whole BBC chain, back together. In downward trajectories—where indicators are getting worse—the performance failures, symptoms, and tests give negative feedback that affects the BBC chain. Some declining people withdraw into themselves or commit suicide. Yet others manage to keep their identities intact and go on with their lives. What keeps these declining people from totally despairing and falling apart emotionally?

Some conditions that help to keep people going include the following. There are fluctuations in the worsening of their disease, and sometimes there are remissions and days of feeling relatively well. Being able to continue with one's work at least to some extent is very helpful. Moments of joy can temporarily render the illness relatively unimportant. Success derived from activities, or simply the busyness of routine life can help. It also helps if there is no betrayal through word or act by others about one's bodily condition, appearance, or performances. A number of strategies can help: for example, changing the salience of what is important in life. There are also helpful personal philosophies, such as, "it is God's will," or "I just take things one day at a time," or "I take things as they come." Perceived success in slowing down or overcoming the illness by careful management is helpful. Some who are dying spend their remaining days searching for cures among traditional as well as less traditional modes of medicine. Then, too, there is hope that around the next corner lies a cure, or at least a means of slowing down the debilitation or death process. An intense and deep commitment to oneself and others can keep one going, too. Some people evince a tenacity for life—a strong desire to live and willingness to do what is necessary to live, until they simply wear out or the illness gets the better of them. For others, life is miserable, but there is no alternative that they can conceive of except the final release from it.

A long-running play and movie, *Whose Life Is It Anyway?* reflects this process as it occurred with a sculptor who was paralyzed from the neck down after an automobile accident. The play portrays the time from his first awareness of his condition until his final decision to stop the life-support system because he can see no way to reconstitute his life into a meaningful whole given the extent of his injuries. He comes to terms with his condition as is manifested by his decision to discontinue the supportive treatments that enable his broken body to go on living.

Thus, when conditions change or strategies fail, the BBC chain breaks; if it is not repaired, the break can be followed by the feeling that life is no longer worth living. At this point, people give up and let themselves die. But those who are able to move beyond acceptance of the body and bodily limitations are able to let go of life when the time comes primarily because they have come to terms, contextualized, and reconstituted their identities, in other words, put the BBC chain back together and kept it together. Even though there are periods of nonacceptance, they do not last, and hope or another conditional situation arises to pull these people through. As Mrs. Birch Bayh said, she had finally found a physician who would walk a road of hope with her. Her two previous physicians had used language that tore her down.

Recasting Biography

A fourth type of biographical process is actually taking place simultaneously with the others: *the recasting of biography*. This involves arriving at a biographical scheme that will give direction to the future biography. Two major conditional processes are necessary for arriving at such a biographical scheme. One is what we shall call crystallization. The other is having control over the trajectory.

Crystallization. Crystallization is the realization of what body failure means for one's biography. This realization may evolve slowly or come as a sudden insight. An instance of the latter is the experience of Jonathan Nasaw—paralyzed in the lower half of his body from an automobile accident—who, when he first encountered a reserved parking spot for the handicapped, suddenly realized: "The sign, I don't know, crystallized things for me, crystallized all Cripple Willie's rantings down to a little cold hard place inside me that said—This is it" (1975, p. 210).

Crystallization is based on perceptions of performance, whether present or potential. It can occur over and over again whenever a self-image *de*crystallizes. In turn, the latter is brought about by precipitating conditions in the form of blocked or failed performances followed by trajectory and biographical *re*viewing and *fore*casting: "This is what I was; this is now what I will be." Not all confrontations and reviews necessarily lead to decrystallization, for a review following confrontation may simply lead to the conclusion that nothing much has changed or to some rearrangement of resources or division of labor to ensure that nothing much has changed. Nevertheless, a review is necessary for decrystallization to occur.

Crystallization is a two-phase process. In the first phase, one realizes what performances are no longer possible now or in the future. (As we shall see amply in later chapters, this realization is closely tied to trajectory phase.) Once these limitations are realized, there follows a second phase during which biography is projected forward in light of those limitations.

However, when decrystallization occurs, a *re*crystallization need not necessarily follow. It fails to take place when trajectory and biographical projections are put off until a later date. This happens when one recognizes that the possibility or potential extent of limitation reversals is still unknown or still too painful to think about.

A double image of the potential impact of one's illness on biography is possible with illnesses such as terminal cancer, where remissions and temporary reversals of symptoms (but not of the disease itself) occur. One image pertains to the disease: a projection to death. The other image pertains to the symptoms: there is a temporary reversal so one does not know what performances (and when and for how long) are possible. This ambiguity affects the crystallization process.

Control over Trajectory. The second necessary condition for recasting a biography is having some degree of *control over trajectory*. Otherwise, one cannot open up and plan the future in terms of biography. Having this control understandably requires both a clear trajectory projection and a trajectory scheme. In turn, achieving control over biography creates a context that also facilitates control over trajectory. Optimum management exists when each is in a state of relational equilibrium. Since any number of contingencies may arise to disrupt this equilibrium, the building and maintaining of this state require both sound trajectory and biographical schemes. These are derived through clear trajectory and biographical projections and are carried out through performance of both trajectory and biographically related *work*.

Summary

Theory. In Chapter Four we discussed the interrelationships of body, conceptions of self, and biographical time and how they are linked to form the BBC chain. Then we suggested how the chain can be disturbed by failed performances brought about by a failed body. In the present chapter we have addressed what the ill do—indeed, have to do—in order to put the BBC chain back together again.

The chain can be mended by means of four basic interrelated biographical processes and associated biographical work. These processes are (1) contextualizing (incorporating the illness trajectory into one's biography), (2) coming to terms (arriving at some degree of understanding and acceptance of the biographical consequences of actual or potential failed performances), (3) identity reconstitution (reintegrating identity into a new conceptualization of wholeness around the limitations of performance), and (4) biographical recasting (giving new directions to one's biography).

Central to all of these biographical processes are the ideational processes. These consist essentially of backward and forward reviews, which are the reflective parts of actions and involve the use of various types of images for recapturing the past, examining the present, and projecting into the future.

Each of the major biographical processes is related to trajectory phase and type, and certain conditions can further or hinder accomplishment of the associated biographical work. Since each of the biographical processes is complex and takes place over time, each consists of various steps or aspects.

Applications. Some far-reaching implications flow from the identification of the biographical processes, their associated work, and their components.

1. Chronic illness is incurable; that is, it persists over a lifetime. It follows that even if the illness is not unduly severe, biographical consequences can occur over that same lifetime. In grappling with such consequences, the ill do the types of biographical work outlined in this chapter. Any person giving counsel or aid to the ill and their families should understand the complexity of this work and who is doing it.

2. Furthermore, the practitioner needs to locate *where* the ill person is in terms of the biographical process and the work he or she is doing. Is her work now principally related to coming to terms, or has she moved on to engaging in more identity reconstitution or biographical recasting, or has a recent event thrown her back from one of the latter work types into intense coming to terms again with the consequences of the new development? Part of assessing the ill person's location is to comprehend which aspect or step is most relevant at the given period of time, for instance, which phase of crystallization is going on?

3. A practitioner needs to be especially sensitive to clients' trajectory phases in relation to their current biographical work. A client who has long been stable will now be doing different types of biographical work (or the same types differently) when he or she moves into the beginning of a deteriorating phase or has recently

suffered an acute setback but is in the beginning of an upward path that it is hoped will end in stabilization again. What the ill and their families can profit from by way of practitioner interventions is closely tied to where they are in terms of the link between trajectory phase and the allied biographical work. We do not merely mean that they profit from appropriate counsel or therapy for their biographical problems; even more drastically, the ill and their families may simply need more, or fewer, of the usual medical-nursing aspects of interventions if offered in a manner appropriate to their current biographical status.

6

Balancing the Tasks of Everyday Life, Medical Care, and Personal Accommodation to the Illness

The chronically ill go to hospitals primarily during acute phases of their illnesses; or, if they are more or less permanently incapacitated and without sufficient familial resources for custodial care, then they will be found in long-term care facilities. But the majority of the chronically ill live at home, where they attempt to manage their illnesses—often with the help of advanced medical technology (drugs, medical machinery, procedures). At the same time, they must carry on with other aspects of their lives. Management of an illness, unless it is unobtrusive, is not usually accomplished in the home without some degree of difficulty and a great deal of work on the part of all who live therein.

This chapter will explore the details of why that is so. It will also extend the conceptual linking of trajectory and biography, begun in previous pages, through the concept of *work*. This work takes place within the context of everyday living, which necessarily places constraints on the attempts of the principal characters in the illness drama to manage the dual problem of the illness *and* its effect on living. This is at the heart of what trajectory management in the home is all about, profoundly affecting what the final illness and biographical outcomes will be. For this reason, we shall be focusing on what the range of work at home consists of, the problems arising out of the context of daily living that constrain the work, and the efforts couples put forth to carry out the multiple types of work within those constraints.

Lines of Work: Illness-Related, Biographical, Everyday Life

Trajectory management at home implies at least two major lines of work that must be carried out: *illness-related work* and *biographical work*. From preceding chapters, we know that illness and its associated work can greatly affect the biographies and biographical work of the ill. (Indeed, the ill can scarcely escape some degree of biographical work unless their illnesses are relatively unobtrusive.) Of course, biographical processes and the entailed biographical work can in turn affect the illness work and so potentially the illness course itself.

A third vitally important line of work is *everyday-life work.* Not only can its performance, whether effective or not, affect each of the other major lines of work, but as we shall see below, they in turn may affect it. Biographical phasing, for instance, such as often accompanies someone's moving into a demanding new job or losing a treasured old one, can have consequences for the amount of time, energy, and enthusiasm put into daily tasks just as inability to perform those daily tasks well or at all, because of illness, can be devastating to one's self-conception. Thus illness-related, biographical, and everyday-life considerations and work are inextricably linked and reciprocally interactive.

Each line of work is made up of different types of work. For instance, illness-related work consists of regimen work, crisis prevention and handling, symptom management, and diagnostic-related work. Everyday-life work encompasses the daily round of tasks that helps keep a household going. It includes housekeeping and repairing, occupational work, marital work, child rearing, recreation, and activities such as eating. Associated with each type of work are interactions with spouse, children, friends, health professionals, and others in the gathering and dispersing of information, expressions of concern, caring, or anger, and the division of tasks. Together the three major types of work make up what Strauss, Fagerhaugh, Suczek, and Wiener (1985) call the total arc of work to be accomplished over any specific period of time.

Of course, each type of work consists of clusters of tasks that must be sequenced between and within other types of work. For example, regimen work for a respiratory condition may include taking medications four times a day and performing respiratory hygiene three times a day. If the purpose of one of the prescribed medications is to liquefy secretions, then it should be taken before the respiratory hygiene in order to increase its effectiveness. And the respiratory hygiene must be fit into the daily routine of going to work, running errands, cleaning house, and cooking meals.

The work, whether in the service of illness or everyday-life management, is performed under conditions that can vary anywhere from routine to crisis. Treating insulin shock is an example of a crisis situation, whereas administering the morning insulin injection soon becomes a routine task. Since trajectories and everyday lives can differ from day to day, the total range of work to be performed each day can vary in amount, degree of difficulty, amount of time taken, and the consistency with which it must be done. Overall, then, there is a great deal of variation in the total types of work to be done for each line of work and also in the properties of that work. One usually goes to work each day, prepares perhaps two to three meals daily, yet vacuums only once a week. Medications may be taken three times daily, whereas physical therapy may be required only three times a week. Some tasks, such as exercise, may be flexible; others, such as taking one's heart medication, are not. Still others require a great deal of attention to detail and busywork, whereas some can be done simply and by rote, requiring very little time and energy.

Moreover, each time the illness state, everyday-life, or biographical conditions change, there may be a corresponding change in the type and nature of one or another line of work. For instance, after a comeback from a stroke, one may still need to take medications for hypertension but no longer need frequent occupational, speech, or physical therapy sessions. With improvement and extra time, the person may be able to take on more of the household chores or return to a job. On the other hand, when a trajectory such as arthritis is in an active period, a person may be required to spend

time each morning just slowly and painfully moving the stiff joints
to loosen them sufficiently to perform the most basic of life's daily
activities, such as dressing and eating breakfast. As one woman put
it: "I get my coffee sitting on the edge of the bed. Then I take my
pills and begin to move all my muscles, while my husband listens
to the groans." Then, too, other tasks that are part of occupation
or household managing or both may now take longer because of
pain and stiffness and because they must now be done in perhaps
more tolerable but less efficient ways (Wiener, 1975a).

The Management Context

Discussion of the management context centers around two
main structural conditions that impact upon the trajectory
management process. The meaning of this is captured by the terms
structure in process and *reciprocal impact*.

Structure in Process. The term *structure in process* implies
that the structure under which management takes place is a
fluctuating and changing one (Strauss, 1969; Glaser and Strauss,
1968). The consequences of such change for work performance are
multifold and as such call for a close scrutiny of the various
dimensions underlying that structure.

A home is organized around the concept of family living.
Unlike hospitals that are designed for efficient care of the ill en
masse, each home is individualized to meet the needs and suit the
tastes of those who live there. When someone acquires a chronic
illness, his or her relationship to the home—its physical, social, and
emotional structure—can change, sometimes slightly but sometimes drastically, depending upon the nature of the home and the
type and phasing of the trajectory. For instance, if there are stairs
to climb to the bedroom and bathroom areas and the ill person loses
his or her capacity to climb stairs, then a dining room may have to
be converted into a bedroom and a closet turned into a bathroom.
If the ill person has difficulty in walking, carpets may have to be
removed, furniture rearranged, and handrails added in bathrooms
and hallways. If the ill person is confined to a wheelchair, doors
may have to be widened, bathrooms remodeled, and ramps built to
accommodate it. If quiet and rest are essential to recovery during or

after acute episodes, the activities of children and others may be constrained or redirected. And household furniture may give way to a hospital bed, commode, lift, and other trajectory-related equipment. A once adequate living space may seem crowded and confining as the process of trajectory management is added to the other functions of a home.

With every major change in trajectory phasing, different structural aspects of the home are brought into play to meet the changing needs of trajectory management. With each change in the nature of the trajectory, the nature of the relationship of the ill person and others to the structure of the home changes correspondingly. For example, as a cardiac or stroke patient recovers, he or she may again be able to climb the stairs to the bedroom or bathroom but may still require a space downstairs into which to retreat when overcome with fatigue.

It is important to emphasize that illness work takes place within the context of everyday-life work. The management of everyday living, like the management of an illness trajectory, requires that certain tasks be carried out through a complex division of labor. While tasks such as housekeeping, earning a living, and caring for children can be held in abeyance while a person is hospitalized, these tasks can be held off or shunted onto others for only so long. Once the ill person returns home, temporary arrangements must give way to permanent ones and new ways of performance discovered and rediscovered with each major change in performance ability.

Furthermore, the amount of daily work to be done in the home increases, at times significantly, as trajectory-related work is integrated into and around the work of everyday living. Bed linen may have to be changed daily, special meals prepared, and frequent trips made to health care facilities. Meanwhile, the overall amount of work to be performed may increase, and the ability of the ill person to participate in the usual shared division of labor may decrease, shifting the responsibility for work onto the other family members.

Moreover, since everyday life is never at a standstill, the work involved in its management is always moving, changing. Even the most routine and repetitious of everyday tasks can vary in terms of the manner and timing in which and by whom they are performed. Also, since biographies change over time, such change is accompanied by a change in the structure of everyday life. Tasks change not only in nature; their number may also increase or decrease with a marriage, the birth of a child, a new job, or retirement.

In examining the structural context of illness management in the home, one must not ignore the nature of an illness trajectory and its associated work. The types and nature of work associated with any trajectory vary with the type and severity of the illness and the shape that the trajectory takes as it passes through various phases. With each trajectory phase (comeback, stable, etc.), different tasks are required for its management and different resources are necessary to perform those tasks.

An illness course may be routine or problematic and thus too its management. A person may have a single illness or multiple illnesses, giving rise to single or multiple trajectories. While managing one illness may be complicated, think of how much more complicated the management of two or more illnesses can be. This is especially true because drugs tend to interact and sometimes cause severe and unanticipated complications, and physical incapacity from one illness may interfere with the management of another. It is hard to give oneself an insulin injection if one's dominant arm is paralyzed from a stroke. Moreover, some people are prone to crisis or complications, making management that much more complex. And when illness changes bring about sudden upward or downward turns in a trajectory, the routines of household managing and illness managing can be thrown into disarray, further complicating trajectory management.

Even relatively stable trajectories can become unstabilized to some degree under certain conditions. For instance, a quadriplegic with a high-level injury may develop severe respiratory complications if he or she catches a cold or the flu from a family member or friend because of a decreased capacity to cough and expel mucus from the lungs. Hot smoggy weather may increase breathing difficulties in those with decreased lung capacities. Pregnancy can complicate the management of diabetes by increasing the need for insulin while at the same time making episodes of hypoglycemia more likely. Each change in illness conditions not only brings about changes in illness management but also affects the management of everyday life.

What structure in process adds up to is that the conditions under which trajectory management takes place in the home are to some degree *always* changing over time. Sometimes the change is radical; at other times it is very subtle and almost imperceptible unless viewed from the longer perspective of time. We do not mean to imply, however, that the illness or everyday life is in a constant state of flux. There are often long periods of relative stability. Yet even during the most routine and stable periods of an illness or everyday life, variations and fluctuations can influence the management of either.

Even slight changes in the routines of everyday life can have important consequences for trajectory management. Changes in the timing and content of a meal can be disastrous for the diabetic, who must keep a balance between food intake and insulin injections, and social life. Dinner at a restaurant or in the home of a caring but unknowing friend can overextend the sodium limit of a person on a low-sodium diet. An exciting and stimulating discussion in the morning can severely limit the energy available to a cardiac patient for teaching a class in the afternoon. Of course, the ideal context for trajectory management would be a controlled environment in which change and contingencies could be minimized. This is a difficult ideal to realize.

Reciprocal Impact. Another major contextual feature of trajectory management is *reciprocal impact:* the interaction between the illness status and the ill person's biography. The reciprocal impact, in turn, affects the directions taken by the total trajectory and tends to control it. For example, it is not unusual for a severe disability or illness to bring about all sorts of consequences to biography, some small and some large. The writer Cornelius Ryan stated the matter this way:

> There is a communications breakdown between my mind and my hand. Is it me or is it the book that's stalling out? I have to get some straight answers about my health. . . . I think if I could put cancer behind me I could come to grips with the book research. . . . The

monotony of not being able to write is terrible. But the
constant fear of cancer which inhibits my ability to
work is becoming unbearable. . . . It even invades my
sleep. The other night I sat bolt upright in bed. I
heard Neligan say that the operation hadn't worked.
It was seconds before I realized I'd had a nightmare.
(Ryan and Ryan, 1979, p. 276)

Conversely, it is not unusual for biography to have an impact
on steps taken to manage the illness and so ultimately on the status
of the illness (de Mille, 1981; Madruga, 1979). Consider the
following:

I have been praying lately, something I don't think I
consciously did for years. I want time to finish this
book. There is so little else I can do for Katie and the
kids. It is so very hard to accept the fact that my sexual
desires are now nonexistent and harder, still, to know
that my manhood is eroding away each time I take a
female hormone. If I didn't have the book and the
family I don't think I would have taken the estrogen
at all after Willet told me the cancer had invaded the
bones. If I'd been alone, with no commitments, I
would have allowed the disease to take over. (Ryan
and Ryan, 1979, p. 292)

Reciprocal impact of illness and biography is ongoing. It is
not limited to an initial impact at the onset of an illness. Thus any
change in the status of an illness can lead to consequences that will
have implications for trajectory management of the illness or daily
life or biographical concerns. For instance, a man may be able to
return to his old job after the first heart attack but find after the
second that his job is no longer waiting for him. This is what
happened to J. "The next heart attack was two years after the first.
They let me know, after I had recovered sufficiently, that I would
be put out to pasture." As a result, J. had to come to terms with the
loss of his job, rearrange his finances, and find new ways of
achieving fulfillment and occupying his time.

While changes in illness status often have a strong impact on biography, biographical changes can strongly affect management of illness and so illness itself. For instance, pregnancy in a diabetic woman may provide just the incentive to motivate her to keep her blood sugar within acceptable limits, something she had found difficult to do earlier because of competitive desires that derived from her biography at the time. Now it is important for her to safeguard the health of her fetus and live long enough to see the child grow up.

Although the relationship between illness and biography is reciprocal, it is not necessarily mutual. The consequences of one for the other are not necessarily felt at the same time and to the same degree. Rather, they may be felt immediately. The impact can vary in intensity or permanency, and the impact of one may be beneficial or detrimental to the course or management of the other. Finally, though the consequences of illness management are felt primarily by the ill person, biographical consequences may also be experienced by the spouse and other family members.

When an illness is out of control because of an acute or crisis situation, everyday life tends to be disrupted (Bury, 1982; Dingwall, 1976) Control over everyday life may also be lost unless considerable effort is exerted to keep it. Similarly, when biography is out of control—as in a crisis brought about by divorce, the death of a loved one, the loss of a job then considerable effort must be directed at illness management and daily life to keep them from going out of control. At such a time it is not unusual for symptoms to increase, complications to develop, the progression of a downward trajectory to accelerate, or a reversal in comeback to occur as a result of stress associated with biographically related problems or crisis (Isaac, 1974).

Summarizing the Management Context. In summary, what makes the structural context under which trajectory management takes place so important are its implications for the work of managing. Structure in process means that there are changes and fluctuations in the course of the illness, everyday life, and biography. Fluctuation and change signal the creation of a new set of management conditions. Reciprocal impact indicates that changes in the illness or biography or daily life, or actions taken to manage

one or another of these, can have consequences for each and every
person involved. These consequences also create a change in the
management conditions for them. While some changes in conditions can be anticipated and planned for, others are quite unexpected. Expected or not, these changes influence the number and
type of tasks to be performed, who performs them and when, and
what resources will be needed for their performances and the
potential success of management outcomes (Freidson, 1976);
Strauss, 1985).

Relative Equilibrium

> Just because you are a diabetic doesn't mean
> that you don't like to sleep in on weekends. Usually,
> I just alter my schedule. I have one schedule for during
> the week and another for weekends. My insulin dosage
> for weekends is different because of a difference in
> schedule. You just have to work it out according to
> what your life-style is. If you work with it, it is easy
> enough. You just have to feel and adjust. You have to
> continue living. You can't make the world go around
> depending upon how much insulin you have taken.
> Life goes on. Like I wouldn't go out to a restaurant
> and gorge myself without taking an additional shot.

How do people continue to hold onto life despite illness and
the demands of its management? A clue may be found in the
quotation above. They seem to balance illness demands against
demands on everyday life and biographical concerns and then come
up with an action plan that will satisfy all three sets of demands.
(This is what trajectory management is all about.)

Trying to satisfy all of the demands is like walking on a
tightrope (Charmaz, 1983). Some sort of relative equilibrium must
be maintained among illness, biography, and daily life, in terms of
effort and other resources (time, energy, money). Unless a relative
balance is maintained, effort and resources may be usurped in the
management of one task, leaving little or none for the management
of the other tasks. If all of one's effort, time, energy, and money is

absorbed in the process of illness management, what happens to the quality of one's life?

Nevertheless, any equilibrium achieved is relative. The ratio of effort and resources appropriated among illness, biography, and everyday-life management can vary considerably in accordance with the various management needs. For example, an illness may be completely out of control in the sense that treatment is no longer effective in containing its progress; death in the near future is inevitable. Yet pain and energy depletion are sufficiently amenable to control to enable the completion of biographical closure and give meaning to life in one's remaining days. That is, a relative balance exists between effort and resources expended in the management of the trajectory (pain and energy control) and what is now comple-tion of important biographical work (closure)—even though the ratio may be weighted more heavily on one side than the other, depending on how difficult the pain is to control and how strong the individual's need is to complete closure and with whom.

This ratio work may be subject to temporary or permanent changes because of the progressive nature of chronic illness and biography and the variability of everyday life. With a change in the phasing of trajectory or biography or when complications occur in everyday life, effort and resources may be shifted from one or another, thus disrupting the balance among them. And when control is regained, the balance may restabilize at a higher or lower level of the person's functioning than was previously the case.

Up to this point, our discussion of illness management in the home has been theoretical. Now it seems appropriate to move to the data that show the preceding concepts in action.

A Case Example

The story of Paul and Clara's illness management is told from her perspective, for Paul had died some months before from renal disease. (Clara is a nurse; her husband was a high school teacher.) This story illustrates how one couple lived with and managed an illness, how their lives went on around it, and how they attempted to maintain some quality of life as the illness plunged into a downward spiral. (See Chapter Ten.) The story also sets the stage for the discussion to follow, a discussion of trajectory management in action.

In reading this story, take note of the following points: (1) the *phasing* and miniphasing of the trajectory as the illness moves progressively downward and the changes that the trajectory phasing and associated management bring to mutual and individual biographies and the couple's everyday life; (2) all of the family members' *hard work* in maintaining some control over and in shaping the nature of their everyday lives and biographies despite a loss of control over the illness, and in turn how these efforts affect the illness management; (3) the various *types of work* involved in the management of both illness and everyday life and how the nature of the work changes in response to the illness, biographical phasing, and everyday occurrences; (4) the manner in which the *work is divided* among the family members and yet how the unified efforts of all of them (as well as various outside resources such as physician, visiting nurse, and friends) are required to complete the total range of the work to be performed; (5) the *coordination of effort* and people necessary at each phase of the illness to accomplish the various types of work, and what happens when coordination fails to take place.

Stable Trajectory. Clara knew Paul was a diabetic when she married him. He looked healthy and played basketball. Not until they were married did she find out that the diabetes would affect their lives. "Everything was planned so that his routine wouldn't get too disrupted, particularly with eating and insulin."

The couple had three normal children, who liked to roughhouse and fight, especially in the late afternoon between four and six o'clock. While such activity is hard on a healthy man after a long day at work, it was especially hard on Paul because of the fatigue and low blood sugar he experienced at this time of day. His intolerance to family activities during these hours became the family joke.

Traveling by car had its moments of difficulty too. Long trips were especially hard on Clara because Paul wanted to drive without taking periodic breaks. Clara was concerned about hypoglycemic reactions. Eventually, she did take over the driving. "I started thinking that if I didn't take over we could all be killed."

At first Paul was resentful, but "I told him it just wasn't worth the risk. I guess at first it was a blow to his manhood. The driving was a weight on me, but I chose it. Then, too, the children were able to help out with it."

According to Clara, Paul had little difficulty following his diabetic regimen. For the most part he showed considerable self-control. "I think that is the frustrating part. He did try for the most part to follow the regimen and still the darn thing marched on."

In time, the diabetes increasingly intruded into their lives. It reached a point where Paul could no longer feel the impending signs of hypoglycemia. To compensate, he would try to anticipate these reactions and plan around them. If he knew that he had to work late, he would have a late lunch. But sometimes he would become so absorbed in what he was doing that he would forget to eat and something would happen.

Occasionally, Paul worked late at school. "If he was late coming home from work or something, I would worry that he had hit a telephone pole. His insulin reactions were usually between 5:00 and 6:00 P.M. The average man you would simply say was working late, but I knew that Paul had to eat or he would be in trouble."

One day he fell and hit his head. Though his temple was swollen, the doctor didn't think much of it. About two weeks later, Paul's blood sugar dropped and he had a seizure that "scared the wits out of everybody." The doctor said it was related to an electrolyte imbalance in the brain. Fatigue and low blood sugar knocked Paul over the threshold. Clara noticed that after this he began to lose confidence in his ability to go places except the high school alone. He no longer had that inner confidence that nothing would happen. The doctor told her at this time that Paul would never be an old man with her. "I got angry with the doctor because Paul looked so healthy. I felt the diabetes could still be kept under control."

Clara says that Paul never really accepted the epilepsy. It frightened him and hurt his self-image. He feared that he might die if he had a seizure and no one was around. He talked about death. He even dreamed of it. As a precaution, Clara taught the children how to protect their dad. During a seizure they could do very little for Paul. But once he regained consciousness, they were able to comfort him and provide him with the nurturing that he needed to overcome the depression that would inevitably follow.

Once he stepped on a staple near a swimming pool. Because of the state of his neuropathy, he didn't realize the staple went into his foot, which became infected. The surgeons wanted to amputate it. Paul refused. The doctors became upset because they didn't feel he was facing reality. Finally, he changed doctors. It took ten weeks, but they managed to save his foot. At this point, Clara decided to go back to school. "I realized that I wasn't going to have him for very long. His body reacted so violently to the infection."

Following the foot infection, Paul's blood pressure became elevated. The doctors attributed this to kidney damage he sustained as a result of the antibiotic therapy he underwent to control the infection in his foot. Clara feels that "probably by this time his cells were so susceptible to problems that the added assault of the drug put him on a downward course."

Paul continued teaching after the hypertension was diagnosed. The illness appeared to be stabilized. Then one day three or four years following the onset of the hypertension, Clara received a call from a mother of one of the boys at the school. She told Clara that her son had seen Paul staggering in the hall. What appeared to be an unrelated incident was, in fact, related to complications of the illness. The incident occurred late in the afternoon. While carrying a briefcase full of papers and books, Paul had to climb some steps to get to his office. The climb exhausted him. Because of nerve damage to his legs, the fatigue caused him to lose his balance while walking and he kept bumping against the wall. This was the first visible sign that his kidneys were failing.

Clara was mortified by the phone call but felt she couldn't tell Paul about it. Then when his colleagues began to tell her that Paul appeared more tired than before, Clara suggested that he see his doctor. A friend of Paul's reinforced her suggestion. This seemed to verify to both Clara and Paul that the situation was changing with regard to his illness. When Paul went to the doctor, his creatine and BUN were found to be elevated.

At about this same time, Clara noticed the beginning of impotence in her husband. Paul, she says, had always been a very loving husband, but sex became more and more of an effort for him. He was simply too tired. This to her was another important sign of change.

A kidney transplant was indicated, but because a pressure sore on Paul's foot would not heal, the transplant was delayed. In the meantime, he was placed on a special diet to keep the progress of the kidney disease under control. Clara says the combination of the antihypertensive and kidney diet regimen just about broke up their marriage. The doctor put Paul on a low-sodium, low-potassium diet. These added restrictions to the diet that Paul was already on because of the diabetes began to frustrate him. Many of the fruits and vegetables that he had formerly eaten as part of his diabetic diet were restricted because of their potassium content. "A 2200-calorie diabetic diet is not hard to live with, but when you are on an antihypertensive and kidney regimen also, you don't know what to eat. Normally, they put kidney patients on suckers and Popsicles to keep up their energy, but he couldn't have that because of the diabetes."

What bothered Clara most about this period was that the doctors accused Paul of not adhering to his regimen whenever his electrolyte level was out of balance. The nephrologist would scold him for drinking too much or for eating fruit. "It got to be a real guilt trip. The doctors couldn't accept the fact that it was the disease that was going out of control. They said it was because he was not adhering to his dietary regimen, when in fact he was making a valiant effort."

Paul was oriented toward living. When things went wrong, he was more hopeful than Clara. He would be delighted each time his doctors proposed a new procedure like a shunt or kidney transplant. He saw this as a new lease on life. It was Paul's brother who gave him a kidney. The children wanted to give their dad one of their own, but he would not allow them to do so. He felt that they had too much life ahead of them. Paul saw the transplant as hope for a better future, but Clara was not so exuberant. The doctor told her it might only buy one year of life, and that is what it did. She knew but Paul didn't know about the possibilities of failure until well after the transplant failed. She didn't want him to be told too soon because she felt it would destroy the little hope he had left.

Finally, when she knew that Paul was entertaining the thought of another transplant, she had the doctor tell him. The doctor told Paul that they would try to maintain as much quality of life as they could but that he would have to be on dialysis for the rest of his life. His body simply could not stand the assault of another surgery.

Clara says there were times when Paul would become depressed—a hopeless sense of no end to the suffering would come over him. Usually, it would occur when he became too tired to keep going. However, it never lasted long. He had a good sense of humor and a sharp mind. He would use cynical humor to cope with it. When people came to visit, he didn't like them to concentrate only on his illness. He loved to have them talk about their own lives, even if it was the trouble they were having with their teenagers. Sometimes, when the children knew he was depressed they would call and say, "Let's go out and eat." When Clara noticed Paul was quiet, she would ask what was bothering him. He was open about what he was thinking.

Toward the end, it became more and more difficult to maintain any quality to his life because of the dietary restrictions and increasing body failure. Sometimes when they went out to eat, Paul would order an omelette and a side order of pancakes or even a Reuben sandwich. Clara comments on these occasions:

> I would just cringe and say he shouldn't. I thought, where do I shut up? I don't know. Perhaps if he hadn't done this he could have had another couple more years of life, but I doubt it had much effect. He did it so seldom. I could see the other side. I know how much trouble I have losing weight. I think it had to do with control. He would get so mad at the doctor he wanted to say, "Oh, screw you. I've done all I can; my body isn't acting right. I am going to enjoy a few things in the time I have left."

Paul drank copious amounts of liquids all his life; suddenly the doctors told him he couldn't have liquids. He was angry about that.

We really ran into trouble then. I would bring him a quarter cup of coffee in the morning, and he would say, "For Christ sake, you may as well not give me anything." I would become angry at this because I was worried about the overload on his heart. I told him I wasn't the one laying down the rules. His body was the one dictating a lot of this stuff. I didn't know how to handle it, so I would internalize it. He would become angry and then very quiet.

Finally, Clara talked about Paul's behavior with the visiting nurse. The nurse pointed out that Paul was a grown man and could make his own decisions. He knew it was a strain on his heart.

The doctor would say, "I don't understand Paul; he is very bright, but he doesn't seem to understand physiology." I replied, "I don't think the problem is that he doesn't understand. The problem is just that he has chosen not to. It is too much of a compromise for him. He has compromised every avenue in his life and is no longer willing to do so." Paul was taking thirty-eight pills a day after the transplant. How can you take that many pills with only a sip of water?

At this time, it seemed that every time we turned around we were arguing about something. For a while I bought into what the doctor said. But then I got tired of hearing the doctor scold. I knew that Paul did not abuse things. The doctor perceived it as an insult to his practice.

Throughout the illness Paul insisted that Clara continue working. Every day she would leave with him the phone numbers where she could be reached if there was an emergency. She said she tried to put out of her mind what was going on for the eight hours she was at work. Much of the time she was not successful. Every night while driving home she hoped and prayed she would find Paul in good shape when she arrived and that things would go well that evening.

Throughout those painful last years, it was important to
Clara that her husband not feel that he was a burden to the family.
Sometimes he would say to them that he was a stone around their
necks. When he said this, she would look at him and say, "No, we
love you too much to feel that you are a burden. You are an
important part of our life even if you are sick." The kids would tell
him that too.

Often Clara and the children organized activities for Paul.
One such instance was taking him to his thirtieth class reunion.
Whenever they considered an activity, they had to plan around the
dialysis schedule and take into consideration how he would feel.
Their daughter helped to make the arrangements for the reunion.
The daughter and her husband accompanied Clara and Paul to the
reunion. It took the combined effort of all to carry it off. Without
the help of the family, Clara says,

> I would not have been able to pull off as many things
> as I did. To make it work you have to plan ahead and
> make it be like it is going to be wonderful, and it is
> because you do so much planning. [They did all this
> without telling him.] If I ever gave a clue that it was
> too much of an effort or if I showed how tired I was,
> he would say, "Oh, I am so sick of this whole thing."
> So I knew that I could never let him know that I was
> too tired to go someplace or do something. Sometimes
> I became so tired that I wished he, just once, would
> take care of me.

Paul did do things such as take care of the finances when he
felt well enough, but he didn't have the energy to do much. He
couldn't do things such as battle with the insurance company and
arrange for his disability. The arguing was just too much for him.
He wanted to "throw in the sponge. But you can't if you need that
$1100 dollars a month for expenses. It meant getting a lawyer and
going through a hassle. He was too tired to do those things so I
found myself having to be much more forceful in those things than
I wanted to be. He had to forfeit a lot of his position in the family,
but none of us ever looked upon him as a weakling because of that."

Paul tried to make concessions in when and how his care was given so that Clara had some flexibility. On Sunday he would tell her to go to church. He would have his breakfast and bath later. He gave a lot because of his sense of humor and their conversations. He always asked about her day. He told her when the meals were good. Before he became ill, he helped her with the housework and grocery shopping. It bothered him that he could no longer help around the house. He felt Clara worked too hard. She knew it bothered him, and it was helpful to her that he did not expect her to be and do all things. He enjoyed having her sit next to him in the family room while he watched television. When she couldn't be with him, she would have one of the children sit with him. It would take a lot of the pressure off her.

After the kidney transplant, Paul lost the use of his legs. The high creatine levels hurt the nerve endings. That just about did him in psychologically. He would try to go ahead and do things, but his legs would not do what he wanted them to do. He would trip on the carpet. Clara would awaken at night to hear him crash on the bathroom floor. When she asked him why he didn't call her, he said that he wanted to do it by himself. When he found at last that he had no choice, it didn't bother him as much to ask for her assistance.

During the last few months of his life, Paul had a suprapubic catheter. That was another blow to him. After the transplant, the doctors ordered intermittent catherization to prevent a backup of urine into the newly transplanted kidney. Because of Paul's low resistance to infection and the frequent catherizations, he developed a pseudomonad infection. "We found out afterward that frequent catherization is not necessary." From that time on, Paul became cynical about the medical profession. He told them that he had lived in spite of them. He felt that the only reason he was able to keep his body intact was that he argued with the doctors.

Paul's care at home in those final months became more and more complicated. After the catheter was inserted, he had unbelievable pain in his penis from the catheter because of the infection. The pain was controlled with Demerol injections. Once the catheter was inserted, he had to have three sterile dressing changes a day. Bars were inserted in the bathroom so that he could get on and off the toilet, and a Swedish shower was installed so that he would not have to have a bed bath. He went for dialysis every other day. The family used a chart to plan who was to take him to dialysis and who would pick him up. They also charted the days the nurse would be there. While it was Paul's suggestion that a nurse come a couple of days a week to conserve Clara's energy, it was hard on him to have a stranger putting him in the shower.

Clara normally began her day at 4:30 A.M. She dressed for work, then woke Paul and got him ready. They had the daily routine systematized so that he would be at the hospital for his dialysis at 8:00 A.M. It was the responsibility of their youngest son to drive in the morning. The other children helped by picking Paul up when the dialysis was finished.

The dialysis created a new kind of structure for all of them, and there were moments of resentment among the family members as a result. They felt tied to routine: "You couldn't say to hell with it; it had to be done." There were times when Clara wished they had the finances to afford more help. Sometimes at the end of the day, she barely had the energy left to get Paul into bed.

Toward the end, Clara began to choose very carefully whom she would invite to visit because of the strain that being with people placed on Paul. At times, she had to make up excuses about why a particular person could not come. Paul felt his life was now too short to waste energy on people he didn't want to see or enjoy. He began to pull more and more into the family and close friends. The children always came by.

Clara felt closed in at times. Relief was provided by three of Paul's close friends, who asked what they could do to help. She asked them to come by on Tuesdays and Thursdays from three to five o'clock so that she might have a break. Sometimes she was able to attend a concert or movie at night. Friends occasionally stopped by with food. Clara welcomed these gifts since she no longer had the time to bake. Looking back on those last few months, she says she had probably reached her limits. She could not have taken much more. But at the time, she didn't realize how much it was taking out of her. She pulled through it by saying to herself, "If he can take it, I certainly can."

Finally, Paul began to evince signs of heart failure. One night Clara noticed he had difficulty breathing. Paul assured her that all would be fine after he had his dialysis in the morning. He died of a cardiac arrest at four that morning.

As this case shows, even under the routine conditions of illness and everyday life, but even more so during critical periods of the illness, a tug-of-war goes on among the management needs of illness, everyday life, and biography. A person will follow a regimen, keep a doctor's appointment, and undergo needed surgery, but he or she will also fight to maintain at least a little bit of normalcy in life—like that morning cup of coffee. Maintaining a state of relational equilibrium regardless of the struggle is not easy. There is a tendency toward an instability of the balance. Next we shall examine why.

The Interaction of Structure and Process

From attempts to control an illness and maintain some quality of life within the home context, there flows a set of consequences. These consequences can be thought of as outcomes arising from the interaction between structure (context) and process (management). Each consequence is capable of upsetting the relative balance among the major lines of work. Unfortunately, the consequences rarely occur alone. Rather, the occurrence of one tends to lead to the occurrence of the others. Thus what we often see is the combined impact of all the consequences working in unison to create conditions tending more toward instability than relative equilibrium.

Competition for Resources. One consequence is the competition for resources among the three lines of work. (*Competition* is ordinarily thought of as an interaction among persons or organizations, but we employ the term here to mean an interaction among illness-related, biographical, and everyday-life work.) Resources include manpower, equipment, and other forms of technology, energy, and space (Gerson, 1976).

More specifically, by *resources* we mean the money to buy drugs, equipment, and the latest technology. We mean a spouse or child to provide physical and emotional sustenance to the ill person and, in turn, someone to sustain the spouse so that he or she can continue to sustain the ill partner. And we mean occasional psychological and sexual counseling by professionals. We mean also the availability of equipment such as a hospital bed and space for that bed. Other resources include someone to drive an ill person to a medical facility for treatment; enough time and energy to perform a complicated regimen, such as tube feeding three or four times a day; and the knowledge and skill to carry out procedures such as suctionings, bladder irrigations, and catheter insertions at home.

The number and type of resources needed vary with the type, degree of difficulty, amount, and consistency of the work to be done. The more severe the illness and the greater the physical disability, the greater the number of resources needed to keep the illness under control and to provide for the physical, social, and biographical needs of the ill person. The same holds true for everyday life. The more complicated the household—for instance, the presence of young children and illness or infirmity in the spouse—the more resources are needed to keep everyday life under control. At times, as during an acute illness period, backstopping is needed to supplement home efforts. This includes friends, visiting nurses, and the hospital itself.

Underlying this discussion is the implication that resources are available to match the needs. In truth, however, the resources are often inadequate. This leads to a competition among the lines of work so that priorities must be established to determine how the limited resources will be distributed. The ill person or couple must decide where their time, energy, money, and so forth will go. Sometimes the illness and its management are given priority; sometimes daily life or biographical concerns are. Inevitably, one or another is shortchanged. Ultimately, all are affected by that situation, the resource because one set of consequences unfortunately has a way of becoming a condition for still another set. If not interrupted, the chaining of consequences can continue until almost every aspect of life is affected.

Competition for resources is most likely to occur when the need for resources is high, as when the illness is severe but the proportional availability of resources is low. For example, many of the women in our study were the sole caretakers of husbands, not through choice but because they simply did not have money to hire outside help. Mrs. J tells us what this means for her: "My doctor said to me, you have to be careful because you have a bad back. I do. All I would have to do is sneeze out of line and I would be down. I can't afford to have help. They don't tell you how to cope with it, how you are going to afford to hire somebody to come in. I have to do it."

These women lack the finances for several reasons. Outside help is expensive. Many of the couples are retired and living on fixed incomes. Often the husband, who was the sole or main source of financial support, is no longer able to work, or is working in a considerably lower level position than he was before the illness, or the well spouse has had to quit her job in order to be able to take care of her husband. Many couples are living on Social Security supplemented by small savings. The cost of food, rent, clothing, utilities, and medications and other health-related items uses up whatever money they have. Sometimes, even when state aid is available to hire an attendant, couples find the amount of money allotted is insufficient to hire and keep qualified people. In fact, according to McCready (1984), one of the problems faced by people with spinal cord injuries is the hiring and keeping of attendants because of the hard work and poor pay.

Sometimes, even when attendant aid is possible, a couple will choose to have the spouse provide for the caretaking needs of her mate not only because she is consistently available but because the couple need extra money to survive or resent the intrusion on their privacy. State aid does not provide payment to a wife for furnishing the same care as an attendant. To get around this, some couples make arrangements with an attendant; the wife does the work, and the attendant claims to do it. The attendant then turns over to the couple the money he or she receives from the state. In fact, couples devise all sorts of ingenious strategies to increase their financial allotment.

> I get $824 a month. You learn to play a game with the
> workers about what you need in the way of medical
> care. You have to lie or you get the least. I tell them
> I need help with brushing my teeth, everything. They
> pay $270 a month for an attendant, and you have to

put out $200 in addition out of your pocket. It costs
me $325 a month for rent and utilities. That doesn't
leave me much for food and a quad needs a lot of
protein. To save money I hired my spouse.

Medicare does pay a fixed amount for care in a nursing
home, but it does not provide payment to the spouse for home care.
This means that the wife or husband works for nothing and that
many other costs, such as payment for occasional visiting nurses,
are out-of-pocket costs unless the couple can prove that the ill
person is in need of acute medical care. To continue to receive
benefits, a couple must go on state aid. That means selling their
home and giving up other assets they may have. The total financial
and emotional costs of illness are often difficult for the uninitiated
to imagine. Illness can rapidly drain away money that a couple had
kept in reserve to live on in their final years. More than one spouse
in our study expressed considerable concern about the loss of
savings and wondered what would happen after all the savings had
been used up in caring for the sick partner.

Not only does illness drain away money, but it can also drain
energy. As Clara said, she had reached the limits of her tolerance in
terms of energy, though she didn't realize it at the time. True,
programs are available to provide relief for the caretaking spouse.
In California, the Veterans Medical Centers have respite programs.
There are centers for the elderly, where for a moderate fee a van will
pick up the ill in the morning and deliver them to their homes in
the late afternoon. There are visiting nurses. Children sometimes
come to help. But most of these (except the respite program) do not
provide twenty-four hour coverage as the caretaking spouse must
do. The latter does not have a diet kitchen in which to prepare the
ill mate's special diets or a housekeeping department to wash dirty
bed linen or get time off for holidays and vacations. The responsibility is his or hers twenty-four hours a day, seven days a week. The
caretaking spouse does not even have the consolation of knowing,
as does a new mother, that his or her charge will in a few years grow
up and become independent. The future includes only more of the
same.

Unbalanced Work Loads. Another potential consequence of

illness management in the home is unbalanced work loads, or what some refer to as a lack of equity in the distribution of tasks. Whether the partners' division of labor is based on traditional or more modern forms of task allocation is not the important issue here; the issue is the degree of decreased abilities of the ill. When the ill mate can no longer perform his or her share of the work, then somebody has to take up the slack. That somebody is usually the spouse, unless he or she is unable or unwilling to do so. This means that a husband, in addition to holding a regular outside job, may now have to take over the grocery shopping, cooking, and other household chores. In addition, a spouse is often called upon to assist the ill partner in the most personal and basic of self-care tasks. For example, a husband may have to get out of bed in the middle of the night to help his arthritic wife onto a bedpan because she is unable to walk to the bathroom.,

While some tasks, such as cleaning a bed made wet or dirty by the ill mate, are simply unpleasant, others make the well partner feel inadequate: "I was almost paranoid about getting up on the roof when he wanted me to do something with the antenna. I was scared half to death. I was frustrated with myself because I wasn't a man." On the other hand, it is just as frustrating and difficult for the ill to relinquish to another person their self-care or the tasks once considered part of their domain.

Much of the time, couples are able to work out a new division of labor, depending on the type of illness and trajectory phasing, to keep work loads more evenly balanced. Often ill mates take on alternative tasks, such as dusting, peeling vegetables, or driving children to appointments, to lighten their partner's work load. Other strategies include flexibility in the timing of tasks, the differentiation of genuine needs from the less crucial wants, and provision for the occasional relief from the work so that couples can socialize together or the spouses can have time away to renew themselves. Without such strategies, spouse fatigue, illness, frustration, and resentment begin to build up. In time, even the most committed spouses will discover that they can no longer carry the load. "We used to talk that some day I might have to put him in a nursing home. Then last October [after twenty-four years], I realized that I just couldn't handle it anymore. I had had it. Making the decision was the hard part. I went through a lot of grieving with that. It would have been much easier just to lose him completely."

Sometimes keeping the work load within the limits of tolerance is a matter of setting priorities among the total range of tasks to be performed and eliminating those that do not seem to be essential or that can be deferred or done by others. Occasionally, ill mates will push the boundaries of their limitations and discover abilities to perform certain tasks, thus lightening their partner's work load.

Work loads tend to peak during acute phases of illness or when complications develop in the illness, daily life, or personal life. At such times, the work load increases while the performance ability on the part of the ill person stays the same or decreases. It is not unusual for a spouse to feel overloaded under these conditions. Often, however, overload is the result of the culmination of an unbalanced work load that continues year after year. The point at which overload occurs varies, depending upon level of tolerance and opportunities for relief from the work.

Among the conditions leading to overload are the following: unbalanced work loads that continue for some time with little opportunity for relief from task; the addition of new and demanding types of regimens or other forms of trajectory or biographical work; decreased performance ability by the ill due to progressive downward trajectories; decreased performance ability of the well partner due to illness, age, or injury.

Disruption of Work Flow. While the work of management can eventually become routine in varying degrees, the routines are often intruded upon by contingencies flowing from the nature of illness and daily life that disrupt the normal flow of work. Such disruptions may be minor or extensive, temporary or permanent, and they may occur frequently or infrequently. Minor, infrequent, and temporary disruptions can usually be accommodated without undue difficulty and routines reestablished as soon as the underlying cause is resolved. But even temporary disruptions can cause management to become problematic. For instance, it is difficult for a diabetic to adhere to a specified caloric intake during the holiday season or adhere to meal schedules while traveling. Similarly, it is difficult for a spouse with the flu to awaken every two hours during the night to turn her quadriplegic husband.

Genuine crises can also interfere with work flow because the work then shifts from routine to critical. However, unless the crisis is prolonged or allowed to progress into a downward cycle, it too passes and routines can be reestablished. When the disruption is permanent or extensive, as after new acute episodes or downward spirals of illness, then new work patterns must be established. That means repeating the cycle of routinization by determining what tasks are to be done, how, and by whom. The couple must also reacquire task competency; and rediscovering the problems, they must work out their solutions all over again. When permanent and extensive disruption takes on the added dimension of frequency, one can readily see why frustration, stress, strain, fatigue, and gaps in the total work occur. There is no routine to hold onto, and this necessitates a constant expenditure of time, energy, and perhaps money and manpower. Sooner or later resources are depleted.

Conditional Motivation. Money, prestige, and satisfaction are the usual conditions motivating work, at least in most occupations. However, illness management in the home is not a usual kind of work, and money and prestige are not the usual motivations for it. Rather, motivation rests on another set of conditions: namely, having trajectory and biographical schemes, hope, and commitment.

As noted in Chapter Three, to do trajectory work persistently one must have a projection of what lies ahead and some idea of how to get there—a trajectory scheme. Visualizing the course of the illness and some of the attendant medical work is usually the physician's task. But the patient and spouse will have to discover all that is really entailed in carrying it out on a day-to-day basis when it has the potential of interfering with the family's life. But just as important is a biographical scheme, for one must wish to live, even if just long enough to achieve closure. That means carrying out such trajectory-related tasks as making a will and saying good-bye. And having a biographical scheme means that to some extent individuals must have come to terms to some degree with their illness, their limitations, and the potential outcome of the illness.

Hope is another condition for work performance. According to Miller (1984), hope is a powerful resource inspiring individuals to action. Trajectory and biographical schemes are useless unless one feels that with the performance of certain necessary tasks, those schemes are attainable. Thus, without the hope that chemotherapy will cure or at least provide relief from pain or other symptoms, there is no reason to undergo this potentially debilitating therapy. Without hope that one will someday walk again, there is no reason for a stroke sufferer to undergo fatiguing and often painful physical therapy.

Commitment (Becker and Geer, 1960; Charmaz, 1983) is yet another important condition. Here commitment implies carrying out trajectory and biographical schemes, as well as the daily work—and for spouses to do so for each other. Interestingly, it is not always love in the traditional sense that sustains spouses' commitments to carrying out the tasks necessary to fulfill their trajectory and biographical schemes. Many times a spouse's love, at least in the romantic sense, has been lost over the course of time, and it is a strong sense of duty or obligation that underlies the work performance. For instance, one woman in our study took back her sick husband after being separated from him for ten years and cared for him until his death.

Nevertheless, because of the long-term nature of chronic illness and the juggling that must take place to carry out the work of its management in the home, it is difficult to keep motivation high unless there is some payoff. For example, some illnesses, such as Alzheimer's disease, some cases of stroke, and mental illness, bring about drastic personality changes. In caring for the sufferer, the well partner finds that the caretaking activities require continuous output, while the other can give very little or nothing in return. The love between them dissipates through lack of reciprocity, and commitment turns to duty. Finally, the well mate becomes so overwhelmed by the work demands that the sense of duty or obligation breaks down. In the end, he or she frequently seeks out custodial care for the spouse, though often with feelings of guilt and a sense of having abandoned the other.

Maintaining biographical projections and updated schemes is problematic in the face of much uncertainty. How can one plan when one has only a vague definition of what the future will bring? Will I (or my partner) come back? How far? How much longer do I (or my partner) have to live? How disabled will I (or my partner) become? Will there be a flare-up of the disease or complications? If so, when? What will bring them on? Why continue with the work when there seems to be no gain?

The Domino Effect. The many consequences flowing from the interaction of structure and process entailed in illness management are like dominoes that lean serially one against the other. If one falls, it causes the next to fall and so on until they all fall. Similarly, if the downward spiral of consequence is not interrupted, it can lead to a loss of control over management outcomes. Competition for resources, unbalanced work loads, disruption of work flows, and decreased motivation lead to fatigue, overwork, overload, episodes of acute illness, resentment, anger, and widening of the marital gap. These consequences may eventually lead to a loss of the delicate equilibrium of trajectory management. Its loss in turn may lead to work deficits or gaps in one or another major type of work. This may lead to a loss of control over illness and/or everyday life. If the illness work is not done, then one cannot expect the illness to remain under control. And if there is neither the time nor the energy necessary for keeping a marriage alive and the partners growing together, then the marriage too will crumble.

The key element in the downward spiral of loss of control over management consequences is that the consequences keep ricocheting off one another, bouncing back and forth until the relative balance of trajectory management is so upset that it leads to major gaps in the work and to irreversible loss of control over illness or daily life or both. The only means of preventing the irreversibility of a downward spiral is to check it in its early stages. The longer it continues, the more difficult it is to reverse the consequences.

How, then, can one keep the consequences in check and maintain a state of relative equilibrium under conditions tending to produce instability? That is not an easy matter at best, but the more severe, complicated, or changing the illness or daily routine, the more difficult it is to keep those fateful consequences under control.

Management in Process

Maintaining a state of relative equilibrium requires a type of management that we shall call *management in process*. This method of management involves strategies and techniques for control that can be adjusted and changed in response to any unexpected contingencies that arise. Management in process, like any method of management, necessitates an understanding of tasks, planning and coordination of these tasks, anticipation of problems, a resource pool to draw from, and a motivated work force. However, it differs from other methods of management in how basic *work processes* are carried out—that is, work is always carried out with an emphasis on adaptation to change. These work processes include (1) calculating resources, (2) maintaining fluid boundaries in the division of labor, (3) planning and coordinating the total work, and (4) sustaining oneself and each other.

Calculating Resources. When competition for resources exists, maintaining a relative balance in the distribution and utilization of resources among illness, biography, and everyday-life work involves continual calculation of resources. This work process can be broken down into four steps. The first involves calculating the degree of need within each line of work. This means legitimating or authenticating the claim by demonstrating the type and degree of need. It also means assigning priorities to needs in terms of their immediacy and importance. From this, one can estimate what resources are needed, for what uses, when, for how long, and so forth.

The second step is to calculate the degree of availability of resources that may be apportioned among the lines of work. Resources can vary in their degree of adequacy. In calculating adequacy, one must consider attrition, exhaustion, conservation, and how resources can be combined, recombined, or simplified. One must consider how utilizing a given type of resource allows amplification of other resources—for example, how a medication or technological resource can raise energy levels or improve one's ability to perform, thereby increasing the self as a resource, decreasing the need for others as resources, and increasing others' time and energy for the accomplishment of other tasks. Calculating the availability of resources, however, may also involve a search for resources not immediately available. (Many people turn out to be extremely "resourceful" in discovering resources that they would not have dreamed existed had they not been forced by their worsened circumstances to find them among friends and public and private services.)

Matching need with availability is the third step. When the demand meets the availability, a match exists. In such a match, the problem becomes one of building, maintaining, and renewing the resource pool. The relevant issues then become the degree of resource deficit and whether needed resources can somehow be acquired, recruited, or trained to fill in the gaps. That means looking at options, establishing priorities, juggling resources, channeling from one line to another, calling on backstopping agents, and negotiating various agreements. In making decisions about resource utilization when resources are scarce or lacking, one needs to consider the following: ethics, in this context the quality of life and the right to live or die; legislation that supports programs for the disabled; availability of Social Security and other third-party payment systems; community programs; the structural makeup of the home environment; and the state of technology.

The fourth step in the work process of calculating resources is allocating resources among lines of work according to need. Resources are moved into and out of the work arena in accordance with the demands. Moving resources flexibly increases maximum efficiency and prevents depletion of the resource pool.

Maintaining Fluid Boundaries in the Division of Labor. Tasks in the home are divided by many different means: according to tradition, efficiency, physical ability, desire, safety, availability, and so forth. Then, too, there are daily variations in those divisions, depending on conditions such as boredom, fatigue, acute illness, vacations, and biographical phasing. When illness work is added to everyday work, it not only creates new work demands but brings about a situation calling for more variation and fluidity in how tasks are divided among family members. As needs attending the illness change or performance ability increases or decreases, major shifts will be required in who does what illness or everyday tasks, and when, and how.

In terms of the division of labor the following conditions exist. First, there is a clear understanding and acceptance of how the tasks are divided, not only during routine circumstances but also when conditions vary. Second, there is a perceived mutuality between the partners, a perception that each is doing a fair share or all that each is capable of doing under the existing conditions. Hence work loads are as balanced as possible. In extreme cases of disability, perceived mutuality may be difficult to maintain. However, some active involvement of the ill or disabled person and some degree of reciprocity, even if only a thank-you, help to maintain the perception of mutuality.

A third condition in the division of labor is that there is follow-through with task performance. Here we get into the issues of responsibility and the taking on and letting go of tasks, as well as the power to determine who does what tasks and whether and how well those tasks are accomplished. A fourth condition is that there is flexibility in who does what tasks and when. Being flexible means shifting with daily cycles such as fatigue, acute illness, and fluctuation in trajectory. But being flexible also means being alert to the limits of one's tolerance and the possibility of overload, and then being able to reallocate tasks.

Of central importance in the division of labor is how the allocation of tasks is established and the work performed, how shifting is brought about, how disagreements arise and are settled, how power struggles and the issue of responsibility are handled (Strauss, 1985, in press). Because of the complexity with which these issues are worked out in interaction, we will discuss them more fully in Chapter Seven.

Articulating the Total Work. Any endeavor requires planning and coordination if the work is to proceed smoothly and to completion. We shall refer to this as the *articulation of work,* the term used by Strauss (1985) to denote the planning and coordination necessary to operationalize *any* arc of work. Articulation of illness and everyday-life work takes place at three levels. The first is at the task level. Each type of work is made up of bundles of tasks that occur sequentially or simultaneously. For example, insulin must be drawn out of the vial and into the syringe before it can be administered.

The second level of articulation occurs among lines of work. They must be planned for and coordinated around one another if gaps or omissions are to be avoided in any of them. Early morning urine testing and insulin administration have to be worked into the daily routine of getting up and dressed for work. Sometimes priorities have to be established about what task or type of work is given preference. For instance, the urine should be checked before the insulin is injected, and the insulin should be injected before breakfast is eaten.

The third level of articulation is the level of resources. Time, people, equipment, space, and so forth must all be planned for and coordinated between tasks and lines of work. If regimen work calls for two people working together, as in percussion to induce coughing, but no one is available to do the percussing because the spouse is away working (or angry at the ill mate or too busy with other concerns), then although the coughing must occur anyhow it might not be as effective in getting up the phlegm as it would have been had it been preceded by percussion.

Since the working conditions may not always be routine, keeping lines of work going calls for constantly assessing the status of these conditions. For effective management, this assessment should be followed by a rearticulation of the plan as based on identified need. For example, during a crisis it becomes important to assess the intensity, amount, and complexity of work; the amount and types of resource necessary to manage the situation; and how other types of work will be affected by this shift to crisis action. After this assessment, tasks should be prioritized, resources rechanneled, other aspects of life temporarily put on hold until the crisis is resolved.

If one asks a couple how they manage to keep some balance between the illness and their lives and at the same time keep both under control, they usually cannot answer precisely. Yet when various couples' stories are analyzed, one can see that managing an illness at home is very similar to operationalizing work in a factory. It too involves a set of organizational and coordinating tactics aimed at keeping the work flow smooth and eliminating gaps in the total range of work.

These tactics include the following:

1. Making arrangements, as with a laboratory, to have blood drawn for testing twice a week, or month, etc.

2. Securing, allocating, and maintaining resources, such as money for an attendant or respite care.

3. Managing time, including its planning, scheduling, pacing, fitting together; and juggling tasks, such as timing one's vacation and chemotherapy treatment so that the peak benefits of the chemotherapy are reached while major side effects will have passed by the time of the vacation.

4. Establishing routines by scheduling tasks, equipment, and people; by familiarizing oneself with the work; and by streamlining the work to eliminate busywork.

5. Doing information work, including networking, scouting out, coaching and training, providing and clarifying instructions, distinguishing between needs and wants, and searching for people, places, and necessary things—for instance, calling a restaurant ahead of time to find out whether it can accommodate a person on crutches or in a wheelchair.

6. Tending to details, such as filling out forms for Social Security or insurance payments.

7. Making choices among options—"Do I want to undergo this form of treatment?"

8. Prioritizing and reprioritizing tasks—sometimes the illness work is given priority and sometimes one's daily life.

9. Devising—coming up with new or modified ways of performing the work or with devices to assist in work performance, such as placing railings in the hallway to assist with walking after a stroke.

10. Troubleshooting—being on the lookout for potential problems and complications such as overload, recognizing one's own and others' limitations, preventing or handling situations of conflict.

11. Distributing tasks, responsibility, and rewards among the work force, and distributing equipment and other resources between two lines of work.

12. Monitoring work performance and work flow: Are regimens being followed? Is there time for recreation and other forms of renewal work? If not, why not?

Sustaining Oneself and Each Other. As we have noted, if people are to continue to put forth effort to do requisite or desired work, there must be some perceived payoff to motivate them. However, sometimes the payoff is not apparent, as in a progressively downhill illness. No matter how hard one works at controlling it, the illness continues downward. (See Chapters Ten and Eleven.) The salient feature of sustaining oneself and one's partner is that partners keep themselves and each other going *despite* conditions such as overwork, decreased confidence, increased dependency, and lost dreams. Why is this so?

Couples sustain an individual as well as a common definition of the situation, that is, a trajectory and biographical projection and scheme. They sustain hope. They sustain commitment to each other and to themselves and to the work. Finally, they sustain within themselves and each other cherished identities.

Arriving at and maintaining a mutual trajectory and biographical projection and scheme require that couples share the same level and types of knowledge and information, not only about the illness but also about their needs, wants, and expectations. This calls for open commitment. If one partner holds back relevant information from the other, it is nearly impossible to work out mutual visions about the illness or life or to make and carry out the plans by which to achieve those visions.

Talk, talking about, and talking through are all required to keep the lines of information flowing, to set and clarify goals, to negotiate divisions of labor, and to resolve conflict. Also required are individual and mutual priority setting and a willingness to revise and update both their vision of the future and their plans whenever a major change in illness or their lives occurs. Sustaining hope means that the partners help each other to realize their mutual visions and to believe their goals are attainable. There are options to choose from; there is an "exit" from the situation: the possibility of cure, diminished pain, a better future, even relief in the form of death.

Sustaining commitment to each other means keeping the relationship going. This includes taking time out for marital work and finding ways to enjoy intimacy with or without sexual relations. Sustaining commitment to the work is knowing when to take on or relinquish tasks and when the boundaries of tolerance have been reached. It also includes giving the other person space and time away from daily work to pursue individual goals and to do other types of renewal work.

Sustaining cherished identities is a form of sentimental work (Strauss, Fagerhaugh, Suczek, and Wiener, 1985). This is accomplished by making the other person feel important through sentimental acts such as encouraging participation in family decision making and child disciplining. It is also accomplished by letting the other person know that he or she is needed and loved despite the illness and its limitations, that even limited contributions are important, and that his or her work is appreciated.

The unifying thread in each of the preceding work processes is interaction, which is absolutely necessary to implementation. Without interaction there can be no securing and allocation of resources, no division of labor or articulation of tasks, no sustaining of oneself and one's partner. In Chapter Seven we will explore in detail the interactions that form the bases for actions taken to carry out trajectory and everyday-life work.

Summary

Theory. This chapter links trajectory and biography and also operationalizes trajectory through discussion of several concepts: lines of work, structure in process, reciprocal impact, relative equilibrium, and work processes. The three lines of work—illness, biography, and everyday life—can be divided into subtypes, and the performance of any one of these types of work can impact upon the performance of the other two. We call this interaction among the three lines of work reciprocal impact, and we have shown that it is especially common between illness work and everyday-life work. We coined the term *structural process* to underline that the context in which illness management takes place not only fluctuates but also evolves. In addition, unforeseen contingencies affect all three lines of work.

Consequently, it is difficult for couples to juggle all the different types of work and keep some sense of balance between illness management, biography, and everyday life. The balance is one of relative equilibrium, with the weight shifting more toward one type or the other, depending upon the illness, biography, or everyday-life circumstances that are in play. Interaction between the structural context under which management occurs and the management process itself leads to a set of consequences that can be conceptualized as (1) competition among lines of work for the human and other resources that are available for management, (2) unbalanced work loads in which one marital partner carries the greater share of the responsibility for work performance, (3) disruption of the management routines because of contingencies, and (4) motivation that is conditional upon the partners' sustaining common trajectory and biographical schemes, hope, and commitment.

The downward spiral that so often results when the three lines of work become unbalanced is characterized by such factors as declining motivation, resource depletion, overload, and mental and physical exhaustion of the work participants. The prevention of this situation calls for a type of management called management in process.

Management in process indicates a fluid approach toward management. It suggests that effective management should shift and change in response to changes in the structural conditions brought about by illness, biography, and everyday life. This type of management can be achieved through skillful use of the work processes, that is, through calculating resources, maintaining fluid boundaries in the division of labor, articulating the total work, and sustaining oneself and one's partner.

Applications. The foregoing theoretical points have two important practical implications. First, practitioners should assess each case situation for competition among lines of work for resources, unbalanced work loads, conditions that tend to disrupt the established routines, and the factors upon which motivation to continue the work is contingent. This means that several questions will have to be asked: What types of work—illness, biographical, and everyday life—are called for in *this* phase of illness? What are the resources, human, financial, technological, etc., available with which to perform this work? Who is doing what types of work and for how long, and is one partner carrying the major share of the work load? If so, with what consequences? Have routines been established for work performance? What are the major contingencies that disrupt those routines? What are the bottom-line conditions necessary for each partner to continue the work?

Once these and similar questions have been answered, the practitioner can then help a couple to establish a style of management, through use of the work processes, that is responsive to their particular set of conditions. This means calculating what resources are needed by the partners at this particular trajectory point and at the same time projecting what they might need in the future, and then trying to match their needs with the resources that are available to them. Where there are gaps, the couple can be assisted in filling those gaps through referrals, counseling, teaching, and so forth. Practitioners should also help to establish a division of labor that shifts according to each partner's physical/mental status and when signs of overload begin to show up in one partner; if the latter occurs, the practitioner should then find resources to relieve some of the work burden. Such resources might include home health aides, respite and day-care programs, and helpful devices. Furthermore, practitioners should help the couple to be alert to the need for finding new ways of doing things when the situation changes— for example, establishing priorities among tasks and deleting those that are either not really necessary or no longer helpful, monitoring work flow, and watching and planning for future problems. Finally, the practitioner can help the couple to establish communication patterns through which they can arrive at mutual trajectory projections and schemes, share cherished identities, and explore what is needed for oneself—and from the other—to maintain motivation.

7

Working Together to Manage Illness

Wanda had a mastectomy of her right breast. She conscientiously returned to her surgeon for follow-up appointments over the next year. When the surgeon discovered a lump in her other breast, she had a biopsy. It turned out to be negative. Later, when still another lump was discovered and turned out to be negative, the surgeon suggested another mastectomy (to be followed by implants) to reduce Wanda's anxiety regarding the possible recurrence of cancer. His suggestion greatly upset her. She could see herself being "whittled away piece by piece" and feared that some day another malignancy might be discovered somewhere else. She decided to take control of her illness management, and for the next few weeks spent much time talking to people and doing library research on cancer therapies. Finally, she chose a regimen that involved adherence to a diet consisting of organic foods, freshly made liver juice, and carrot juice.

Wanda's husband, Bill, was very supportive. As part of the therapy, Wanda was supposed to get plenty of rest and be free from stress. Though Bill worked every day from nine to five, he did all the shopping for the organic food, helped to make the liver juice on weekends, and did most of the cooking. Wanda found it difficult to make the juice, so she hired a woman a couple of hours daily to help with this and other household tasks. This freed the couple from some chores and allowed them more time together. According to Bill, much of their life revolved around the regimen for the first year or so. To help themselves cope with the daily demands, the couple, both artists, collaborated and put on "couple shows."

127

Always close, Wanda and Bill felt that working together so intensely to manage the illness and other aspects of their lives drew them even closer together; they "needed each other for support."

The regimen was both expensive and time consuming because it required the purchase of sizable quantities of liver and the laborious grinding of it by hand to extract the juice. Nevertheless, the couple believed they were fortunate to have the resources to follow through with the therapy, the purpose of which was to rid Wanda's body of toxins and rebuild its natural abilities and defenses. Others whom they met were not so fortunate in having the necessary resources to carry out this regimen. What made the regimen possible for Wanda and Bill was that they had each other for support, Bill's steady income, their comfortable and properly equipped home, their art, the friends who remained constant, their memories of their travels together, and their planning of future travels and art projects. They also lived in an area where the required foods were readily available. As a result of their efforts, Wanda felt she was on her way to becoming healthy again, and Bill felt that he was healthier as a result of the therapy because it forced him to eat more nutritiously.

From the foregoing description, one can see that a good deal of work is going on: regimen-related work, occupational income-producing and mutual interest work, and household work. Wanda and Bill also give a great deal of emotional support to each other. One central question concerning such work is how couples are able to carry out so many kinds of work given the constraints they often face when a chronic illness is involved. That is, how does all the work get done?

A quick analysis of the situation described above shows that the couple have many resources and have developed a collaborative work pattern. In addition, the work is carried out through the essential work processes: a division of labor; articulation (coordinating time and energy between the types of work, making arrangements, setting up routines, and so forth); resource calculation and management (their use of money, his time, her time, and outside help); and the sustaining of oneself and one's partner (their shared interest in art and their continued support of each other).

There is yet another facet of work performance without

which work could not go on: *interaction*. Here there is an aligning of one person's actions with the other's. Implementing the work through the work processes requires ultimately that the couple's actions (and those of other workers) fit together. Interaction acts like *a pivot around which the work processes—the means by which work is carried out—revolve.* Through interaction a division of labor is worked out and maintained. Through interaction tasks are operationalized and coordinated. Through interaction resources are acquired, allocated, and maintained. And through interaction the work necessary to sustain oneself and one's partner is identified and takes place.

To use an analogy, one might say that work, work processes, and interaction are like a bicycle wheel. The tire on the outside represents the work, the spokes represent the work processes, and the hub represents the interaction. They all function together to create the balance and pattern of motion that keeps a bicycle going.

The focus of this final theoretical chapter is on *work performance:* how types of work, work processes, and interaction all function together in achieving this performance. We shall address the issue primarily through an extended case analysis. However, first it is necessary to provide a framework for analyzing what will be described; otherwise, the case would consist of sheer description—interesting perhaps but not very enlightening. The framework is a further extension of the one that we have been building cumulatively throughout this book.

We shall be addressing directly a key issue in the sociology of work. Ordinarily, it is assumed that work is carried out through a division of labor, by having adequate resources, using voluntary or involuntary (hired or coerced) workers, and so forth, and that work performance is completed efficiently or not, with a greater or lesser degree of work satisfaction. If, however, one considers more closely the matter of exactly *how* work can be carried out—that is, the social mechanisms or processes involved—then it should become evident that such an approach settles for too simple an analysis of what is a relatively complex phenomenon. This issue is of direct relevance to understanding trajectory management. Because work is a central aspect of that management, it cannot be understood without a clear picture of how work actually takes place.

Work Processes

We shall begin with some general properties of work processes. (See Chapter Six for their specifics.) First, work processes tend to be mutually affecting. The degree of presence or absence of one has repercussions for the others. For instance, if outside human resources are minimal or lacking and the ill person can perform very little work, then the burden of work is shifted to the spouse. If overloaded, the spouse may find it difficult to articulate all three lines of work, performing only those that must or can be done. Furthermore, since such a large portion of the resources is being spent to sustain life on a basic level, few resources may be left over for higher levels of biographically related work so important in keeping oneself, one's partner, and the marital relationship going under the long-term accumulation of work load, stresses, and strains that accompany chronic illness.

Second, the work processes depend for their existence not only on individual but also on collective work or interaction. Though certain tasks or even types of work may be performed by one partner, it takes the efforts of both partners working together to accomplish the combined everyday, biography, and illness work.

Third, the work processes must all be present in each situation to some degree if the work is to go on. For example, it is hard to imagine how Wanda could follow her regimen without all four work processes being operative.

Fourth, one or another work process is usually more prominent than the others at any given time. Sometimes the emphasis is on the division of tasks, or on their articulation, or on calculating the degree of need against the availability of resources, or on discerning what type of work is needed to sustain oneself or the other person.

One last point, a proviso: while these work processes are the most important in this study of spouses' work, it may well be that in other work situations the same or different work processes emerge as more important.

Interaction and Alignment

Hardly any form of work can proceed without interaction. Even solitary acts such as writing a book usually involve self-interaction in the form of thinking through ideas and reviewing and criticizing what one has written. Furthermore, they often involve brainstorming and talking over ideas with others. Even seemingly solitary work such as housework necessitates that homemakers not only communicate with themselves in planning and organizing their activities but have countless daily interactions with others: the children, the grocer, the banker.

In speaking of interaction in regard to work we mean more than the fact that people communicate. What we are referring to is the process by which people mutually align their actions toward the performance of some form of work through self-communication and communication with other people.

In approaching this topic we draw on the writings of the American pragmatists John Dewey (1921) and George H. Mead (1934). In general, they assert that (1) interaction is a condition for people's actions but in no strict deterministic sense, (2) during interaction, each person is constantly interpreting the actions of others, (3) each person is also using this information as the basis for his or her action, and (4) as a result, each person's stance toward action undergoes transformation in response to the actions of others as the interaction moves along. Another sociologist, E. C. Hughes, refers to interaction as something that stands at the heart of work since without it the formulation of a collective division of labor could not take place (1971, p. 34).

Putting together these two conceptions with our own findings, we have come to define *alignment* as a process by which actors fit together their respective work-related actions by means of self-interaction and interaction with others. By fitting their actions together, actors are able to carry out the division of labor, the resource calculating, the discerning of what types of work are needed to sustain oneself and others, and the total articulation of work.

Before looking more closely at alignment, we shall note that the structural conditions deriving from illness, biography, and everyday life, along with the broader macro conditions, together greatly affect how efficiently, effectively, and quickly (and even with what mood) the work can be carried out. They also determine where the work will break down along the way, stutter, and perhaps pick up again. The conditions give changes in coloration to whatever degree of alignment is attained, for as they change they call for new adjustments and a refitting of actions.

Alignment, Misalignment, Disalignment, and Realignment. Alignment is made up of two phases. First, there is the *interactive phase* (self and other), in which agreements about the division of labor, articulation, resource calculation, and identification of type of work needed to sustain take place. Second, there is the *implementation phase,* in which agreements that have been worked out through interaction are implemented. During either phase, the alignment may break down. People make agreements or fail to make agreements during the interactive phase, or they make agreements but break them during the implementation phase. The consequences affect not only the quantity and quality of the work but enter as conditions that affect the next interactional sequence.

Alignment may range during either phase anywhere from 0 to 100 percent, the former percentage representing complete overall *misalignment.* We shall use the term *disalignment* to refer specifically to the perception of an actor about a failure to make or keep an agreement regarding the performance of work. Disalignment may occur at any level of the work—the arc, one or more lines of work, types of work, subtypes, or task clusters. It may be perceived by only one party or by all of the parties involved. And although it usually centers around the division of labor, disalignment may occur for any of the various work processes. While disalignment may be reversed, the longer it continues and the higher the level of work for which the disalignment exists, the more likely it is to lead to greater and greater disalignment.

Realignment refers to the process by which new agreements are reached regarding work performance. Before realignment can occur, one or both participants must be aware that there is some degree of disalignment between them. Once this is perceived, there must follow a process of assessing the degree of disalignment, of determining how fast it is happening, of trying to determine its causes and what can be done about them. These tasks may be accomplished by various interactants by means of face-to-phase interaction or self-interaction followed by some action or a trial phase to determine whether the solutions work. (Participants usually talk it over, but sometimes the perceiver of disalignment may simply reach a conclusion as to course and act on it.) As mentioned above, structural conditions will affect whether disalignment can be brought back into alignment.

With regard to realignment, we might ask the following questions. What actor(s) initiates the proposed solution? What are the strategies for bringing it about? What are the sequences of actions once it gets under way? What consequences result if realignment is brought about? If it fails to take place?

The process of alignment brings into play the mental phases of action with all of its imagery (a playing out of scenarios and self-interaction that precedes or follows performance). That imagery also enters the overt action itself. Furthermore, much of the imagery and self-interaction relates not only to one's actions but also concerns the other person's and then one's own actions in terms of that other person's.

As for the misalignment in general, which pervades the whole relationship between or among the interactants: its causes are varied. They include external contingencies. These may range from small to large, such as those associated with changes in the illness or biography. Or contingencies may be internal: associated for instance with power struggles in the relationship and with misunderstandings and misperceptions. Misalignment may be unnoted, it may vary in scope, and its effects may be cumulative rather than immediate. What is important is whether or not misalignment is recognized by one or both spouses and whether or not they attempt to bring their actions back into better alignment. If the couple recognizes its situation of misalignment, then we call it disalignment. Also important is the self-interaction as well as the mutual interaction that takes place as the partners alone and together try to figure out what is going on and how the situation can be changed and then try to reach agreements.

A Structural Interactional Stance. To supplement the discussion of the alignment process, we need to keep in mind that the theoretical stance taken in this book is a structural interactional one. It is both structural and interactional because the two are combined to form a single perspective that will be useful in addressing issues about alignment. This builds on previous work (Strauss, 1978) that points out that two sets of conditions constitute a negotiation context that affects the cluster of acts pertaining to any process of negotiating. One set includes the broader political-socioeconomic conditions such as those that lie behind the American judicial system. The other set includes conditions that are more closely tied to the actual negotiation itself, for example, the stakes that each negotiator considers and reconsiders and how he or she makes decisions, along with each participant's awareness of those stakes, and so forth. These two sets of conditions affect the negotiation process; but the negotiation's outcome in turn feeds back into these two sets of conditions to enter into the next negotiation context.

In our book, however, the emphasis is on action in the form of work performance. The structural components of this work context have been identified in Chapters Three, Four, and Five. There we discussed illness, biography, and everyday life and how the three combine to create the types and quantity of work to be performed and also create conditions under which that work takes place. The present chapter expands upon that description of structure by showing how interaction *enters* into and *combines* with those structural conditions to create a work context. Our central concept of trajectory is used to order and organize all of the work-related action that takes place within that context. The context then illuminates the heart of action by showing how interaction becomes the means by which work performance is carried out. Hence structure and interaction are intertwined. This intertwining will become increasingly clear as this chapter moves along. But first it will be useful to describe some properties of interaction as they pertain to our specific materials.

Properties of Interaction. Recollect, first of all, that interaction allows spouses to make more or less firm agreements about the what, how, and where of work that will be carried out through the work processes. Second, each spouse brings to the interaction an interactional stance. This stance is derived in part from relevant structural conditions. Among these are the spouses' degree of knowledge about the illness, the number and types of selves "contained" in their respective biographies and how these are affected by the degree of body failure, the degree to which the partners have come to terms with the illness and limitations, their biographical projections, and the complexity of their respective and mutual everyday lives. During the actual interaction, the interactional stances may remain the same or change, depending on each person's degree of awareness of where the other is coming from, his or her interpretations of cues given off by the other, and the responses to overt and covert actions taken by the other. Thus the interactional stance of each partner is evolving throughout the interactional sequence. Here agreements are either reached or not reached, and alignment or realignment either does or does not occur.

A third property of interaction is its developmental nature. Is it proceeding forward, or is it interrupted, abandoned, changed in midstream? Who initiates it, keeps it going, or changes it, and why? And fourth, there are questions pertaining to the partners' respective assessments concerning the implementation of agreements. Does the division of labor take place as agreed upon? How are resources acquired, maintained, and allocated? Are the agreed upon tasks completed to the degree that together the spouses are able to complete all of the work necessary to sustain oneself, the spouse, and the relationship? How are the various types of work articulated within and among the lines of work, and who assumes responsibility for this complex set of tasks?

Apropos of all of this, we need to ask also about the consequences flowing from the respective courses of action that are taken. In speaking of consequences we are not only addressing the immediate ones but also the "looming potential" ones (Schuetze, 1981), that is, the future ones that might result should the present set of structural and interactional conditions continue or intensify in their negative impacts. Stance defined, we are now ready to move into a description of our specific framework for addressing work performance.

Interactional System and Conditional Matrix

Our framework is an interactional system because it allows examination of a series of evolving interactions involved in a work performance situation as the interactional flow passes from one phase to the next. This interactional system possesses certain other characteristics. First, it is made up of interrelated levels, each level representing a set of conditions. Shortly, we will represent these levels diagrammatically by means of inclusive circles, a bit like Chinese boxes, one within the other. Second, this system moves both inward toward the center, to the smallest circle (or level), and outward away from the center. Third, each level feeds into the next in some defined manner as it moves inward and outward in a cyclical loopwise fashion. Fourth, the consequences from action may come back to impact upon the present set of conditions either to help maintain or to change those conditions. Hence, the consequences enter into the set of conditions that make up the context leading into the next phase of the interaction between the spouses. More than that, these consequences may spill over to become part of the conditions affecting a related or unrelated work performance situation.

Diagrammatically, this interactional system can be represented as a matrix diagram. Although one of its significant features is, of course, that it allows us to follow the course of an interaction as it moves through its various phases, nevertheless this movement is very difficult to convey in a single diagram. Keep in mind, then, that the conditional matrix presented here represents only one phase of the total interactional development. It is a cross-sectional slice of the evolving interaction. (See Figure 5.)

The matrix represents an action scheme for denoting (1) the conditions, (2) work-related actions and interactions (strategies), and (3) consequences involved in work performance with the problematic situations encountered by the interactants as individuals as well as participants who are sharing in the interaction. Here those situations pertain to a couple's life that is complicated by the fact that one or both partners have at least one chronic illness. In explaining this matrix we shall move from the outer large circle inward, for each level acts as a set of cumulative conditions bearing on the next level.

The outer circle represents what are often called the macro conditions. These are the political-socioeconomic conditions that exist at any time during the interactional evolution. For a couple,

Figure 5. Transactional System Between Spouses.

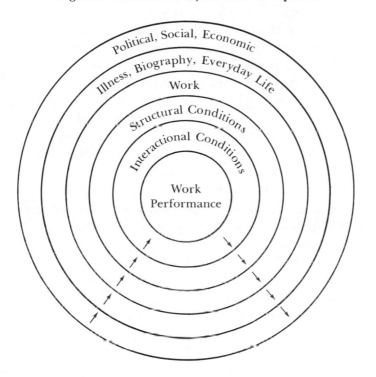

these include health-related legislation, the number and types of resources available within a community, and the state of medical technology.

In the next circle we find a set of conditions that bears more directly on work performance. These are the illness, biography, and everyday life. Together they combine to create the management situation. (See Chapter Four.) Illness includes type, degree of severity, and the disease course that it ultimately follows. Biography includes such items as body, degree of body failure, and the biographical processes by which the shattered BBC is put back together. (See Chapter Three.) Included under everyday life are occupation, marital and parental status, and friendships. The two central features of this management situation are reciprocal impact and structure in process.

Work makes up the next circle or level of our matrix. From

the combination of illness, biography, and everyday work comes the arc of work that in the couple's case can be broken down into the three major lines of work and their various subtypes. This is the work that must be identified and performed by the spouses if each line of work is to be managed. Next, there is a structural context. This emerges out of attempts to maintain control over trajectory, biography, and everyday life under conditions of reciprocal impact and structure in process. The structural context includes the work processes and (in our study) the concomitant tendency toward competition for resources, unbalanced work loads, disruption in the work flow, and conditional motivation.

At the next level, that of the various work processes, interaction per se enters the matrix, for, work processes cannot be accomplished without some degree of self-interaction or interaction with one's partner.

Next come the interactional conditions. These arise from the interactional stance taken by each spouse. Remember here that the spouses' stances are constantly evolving in response to the interaction itself and as the conditions from previous levels of the matrix change.

In the next circle we find an interactional context. This context involves the degree of alignment as perceived by each interactant at either the agreement-making or agreement-implementing phase of interaction.

Moving on, we reach the developmental aspects of the interaction. Here we find interactive strategies taken by the interactants during each phase of interaction, either to bring about or carry out their agreements. Should those agreements fail to take place or be carried out, then counteractions will be taken.

Finally, in the center circle we find work performance per se and the degree to which it takes place. Flowing from work performance as represented in the diagram by arrows, we find the consequences that arise from whether or not and how that work takes place. In turn, these consequences bounce back through the different levels of the matrix to affect, in varying degree, each level. Thus they become conditions entering into the next phase of the action related to work performance.

Case Analysis

*Introductory Comments.*We now have a set of related concepts that together allow analysis of how work is organized and accomplished through performance of various types of work and their related tasks. In our study, this performance is aimed at managing the three major lines of work. The entailed interaction has several major characteristics. First, the participants are engaged in work-related action. Second, to some degree their actions are aligned. Third, the alignment is of some duration. If anything occurs to interfere with that alignment, the resulting disalignment affects the work processes and therefore the performance of various types of work. Disalignment has two kinds of consequences that relate ultimately to the transaction itself: consequences for its development of the transaction, and consequences that impact on the illness, biography, or everyday-life course. The consequences may be proximate (close in time to the transaction) or distant (pertaining to the long-range future). Consequences that are both severe in impact and long-range in time have been poignantly referred to, as noted earlier, as a "looming potential" (Schuetze, 1981).

In analyzing the case below, we shall examine various transactions between spouses. These transactions represent episodes in the management of illness, biography, everyday life, or their combination. The general structural context will be presented first to provide a background and enhance an understanding of the transactions. Thereafter, this context will not be repeated in our analysis of each interactional episode except where it seems especially pertinent. The immediate focus here, of course, will be on the type of work in which the couple are involved, the work process(es) by which they are attempting to carry out that work, the development of the interaction, the degree of alignment of their actions, and some of the consequences that result.

Though the transactions between the spouses reported in their interviews occurred over a period of about two years, these are not necessarily sequential or related except in a broad sense. Each episode is presented as the respondents told it to us. Keep in mind that what is significant in terms of ultimate outcome to illness, biography, and everyday life is not each individual episode but the cumulative effect of the episodes.

The case we are about to present is complex. Each partner suffers from a chronic illness: one illness manifests itself by physical symptoms, whereas the other's are behavioral. But their underlying causes are difficult to pinpoint—are they due to illness, to the drugs given to control the illness, some other physical or biographical problem, or a combination of these? Also, because both illnesses have different manifestations, the partners are not always able to be resources for each other, and their division of labor reflects this. Yet their illnesses increase their total amount of work, while at the same time their performance abilities decrease. Thus both must put forth tremendous effort and undergo inner turmoil in attempting to carry out the work through the work processes. Yet because of illness or biographical reasons they often fail in their efforts. The resulting physical and emotional strain placed on their respective lives and on their marital relationship is evident.

First, we shall give a general overview of the case. From this, the reader can fill in the structural components of the matrix. Next, portions of each interview will be presented along with an analytical interpretation of each excerpt in terms of the type of work being performed, the individual and interactional strategies used by the partners to carry out this work by means of the work processes, a discussion of the interaction in terms of the degree of alignment of their efforts, and the consequences, both immediate and looming, that result.

The focus of the work-related problems presented by each respondent is different. This is not only because their illnesses differ but also because of frequent differences between their respective perceptions of the problems and how much each should partake in the management of his or her own and the other's illness management. We see Tom doing his own trajectory, biographical, and everyday-related work as well as a share of Helen's. And we see just the reverse. When alignment exists in the widest sense, we see all the lines of work getting done somehow. The couple are fitting their lines of work together to get the job done, even though the interaction itself may be characterized by some degree of conflict.

Where disalignment exists, we see the perception by one or the other that some type of work is not being accomplished.

Background Information. Helen and Tom got married when they were in their late twenties. At the time of our study they had been married for two years. Helen is a writer and part-time college teacher, and Tom is a freelance consultant and does most of his work at home. Helen has suffered for fifteen years with migraine headaches. Until recently their cause was unknown, but now the cause is believed to be related to an immune deficiency disease. From time to time a poor balance in Helen's cells, as a result of the immune deficiency, finally leads to brain swelling and then symptoms of headache, wild anger coming out of nowhere, personality distortion, spaciness, and disorientation.

For eleven years Helen's headaches were controlled with some form of ergot, to which she had an extreme chemical sensitivity. This drug in combination with certain foods, unpurified water, and polluted air caused a toxic overload that her body, because of the immune deficiency, could not handle. As a consequence she was getting sicker and sicker.

Two years ago Helen switched the timing of her drug to smaller, daily prophylactic dosages. This compounded her symptoms. "I thought I was mentally ill and so did Tom. I was paranoid, really hostile, weepy, volatile, and had impulses to dance on tabletops. I had self-destructive and bizarre impulses." Realizing that something was drastically wrong, Helen renegotiated her medication dosage.

About a year ago, her behavioral symptoms became so bad that she had to taper off the drug. This brought about a severe headache, the pain of which was so intense that she wanted to die. After three months, Helen was off all drugs and felt "terrific." She even lost some weight. However, she did not yet feel ready to return to writing. She kept busy around the house, doing things that required very little intellectual activity.

Helen returned to her teaching position and started to feel sicker and sicker as the severe headaches began again. She reluctantly returned to taking drugs because she was "going crazy from the pain." Her bizarre behavior returned. She tried another drug, which seemed to control the headaches and decrease her behavioral manifestations. This worked for about three months, and she was able to finish her thesis. Gradually, the psychotic-like behavior returned, and she thought, "Perhaps it's not the drugs, but I am really nuts." She began to get belligerent at faculty meetings and abrasive with students and to feel physically sick. At about this time, she and Tom went away for the weekend. What was supposed to be a great romantic interlude turned out to be a disaster. "I was complaining nonstop about everything. I didn't know where this new personality had emerged from and I didn't like it much. Tom certainly didn't."

Soon she was showing her serious psychotic-like behavior again. Her doctor told her to discontinue all drugs. Once again she had a severe headache, which continued on and off for two months. She was treated with morphine injections and oxygen. During this time, "I was too sick to be left alone in the house because I would throw up so violently that I could pass out and hit my head falling down. I couldn't get anything done in my life, and I was desperately clutchy and fearful."

Tom, who had been doing research on Helen's illness, suggested she might have food allergies. "So I promised him I would not eat sugar, chocolate, and coffee. And for two months I would not eat them in front of him. That was my compromise. Meanwhile I was eating them addictively. What I didn't know until I was hospitalized was that I was allergic to them as chemicals." Then, not knowing where to turn, she read a book Tom had given her. Seeing the relationship between what the book said and her symptoms, she went to see the doctor whom Tom had been urging her to see. All of her symptoms fit the description of immune deficiency disease, and it was decided that she should be hospitalized for the testing.

Characterizing herself, Helen says of this time:

> At this point I was ready to check out. I had been through two periods of status migranosis form of the disease. I sat down with Tom and said, "I am seriously considering checking out. I promise I won't just leave a suicide note and do it. I promise we will sit down and talk it out. It will be a rational decision. I cannot

continue to live this way. I do not have a meaningful
life, I do not have work, I am not going to wind up
with any friends. It is a serious question to me why
you are hanging around. I am not much fun to be
with." I figured I had not tried everything yet, and I
thought going to the hospital and having the testing
would give me some breathing space while I figured
out what the hell I wanted to do.

In the hospital Helen experienced the typical three to four
days of withdrawal symptoms. Then she started feeling much better.
But even then she had bouts of irrational behavior. The most
difficult part of all of this was that nobody understood her or could
give her an explanation for her behavior. She had been told over and
over again that she was a hypochondriac. It was difficult because
her behavior was inconsistent with her perceptions of herself: "My
irrational hostile, volatile, difficult behavior doesn't jibe with my
sense of self. I see myself as a real good person. I am kind to people.
I look out for and do what I can for them."

Tom's chronic condition was of more recent origin. A month
after he and Helen were married, they were in an accident. While
they were walking arm in arm down the street, an automobile struck
Helen in the knee and sent her flying into the air. Tom grabbed her
and yanked her out of the way of the car. He took the brunt of
Helen's fall. As a consequence, he sustained permanent back and
neck injuries from which he suffers flare-ups of pain. Sometimes the
pain is so severe that it causes physical incapacitation.

As Helen says:

From a month or so after the time we began to live
together one of us has been in crisis or we both have
been in crisis. If you think it is hard for one person to
be ill in a relationship, it is unbelievable when both
are. Because if you are both sick, it is like you barely
have the resources to manage for yourself, but then
you have to do double service for the other person.
Essentially, we take care of each other. I try to run
errands for him. Tom gets himself in trouble trying to

do nice things for people. He has very little elasticity
left. Some of it is protective for me because I don't
want him to get wiped out. Then not only can he not
help me out, but he can't help himself out and I have
to help him out. And I can barely keep it together for
me. There is a lot of self-interest in that, or selfishness,
whichever way you want to look at it. But it is real.

With this background in mind, we now present excerpts
from the interviews. Since each spouse is dealing mainly with a
different set of problems, their respective verbalizations about these
will be presented separately. Each excerpt covers some type of work
in which the couple are engaged. Some scenarios represent the
phase of actual interaction or action; some deal with the mental
aspects of interaction or action during either the preactive planning
phase or the postactive review phase.

As mentioned previously, an analysis will accompany each
excerpt from the interviews. This analysis will be centered around
how work gets done or not done. More specifically, we will look at
(1) the actions used to carry out the work processes, (2) whether the
actions are in or out of alignment, (3) the structural and interactional conditions that deter or enhance alignment, (4) how the
couple try to bring their actions back into alignment when
disalignment exists, (5) what they do if they cannot bring their
actions into alignment, and (6) some consequences of all of this. As
will become evident from the interviews, the spouses may be
operating at any one or more levels of the conditions as outlined in
our matrix diagram during any one phase of the action/interaction,
and the level at which they are operating may vary with the phase
of the action/interaction. Whenever two people are interacting, they
sometimes operate from different levels; this helps to explain why
sometimes they are able to fit their actions together and sometimes
they are not. What happens during the actual interaction (that is,
whether or not they are able and willing to respond to cues put forth
by the other) is crucial to determining the state and degree of
alignment and therefore how well and to what degree work
performance takes place. Each interview excerpt given below is
designed to illustrate a different point.

Interview Quotation (Helen). I cannot walk downstairs to the garage area, where Tom has an office set up, or the basement because the walls are so damp and full of mold. . . . Tom can't carry the garbage cans. Until I went to the hospital, I did all the heavy stuff. I did all the carrying of things back and forth like the laundry and the garbage. Now I am not supposed to go down there. What do we do?

Analysis. Here we see Helen thinking (the mental phase of action) about a problem: how will the very simple everyday tasks of carrying out the garbage and doing the laundry be articulated? Before her hospitalization these were, of necessity, her tasks in the division of labor. The issue here is one of resources (physical ability), and Helen is calculating the need for but the lack of them. Helen is supposed to stay out of contaminated environments, and Tom is not supposed to lift anything. Realignment through a shift in the division of labor is not, at least now, a realistic alternative. Yet the work must go on, and so Helen does it. In terms of the personal consequences: "Each thing that each of us does is at some physical cost. Every accommodation that we make to the other is at some physical cost." In terms of the long-term interactional consequences (to their alignment), there is not yet extreme disalignment, but the illness blocks realignment that would otherwise be possible through a renegotiation of the division of labor.

Interview Quotation (Helen). One of the things I get crazy about in my relationship with Tom is that, for whatever reason, I am the person that handles the money. I guess it is partly because some of the money is from my family, partly because he doesn't have a very good business sense. I also make more money than he does. I hate that. I get frustrated and crazy when he doesn't do what minimally needs to be done. The fact that we have two illnesses means that we are spending a whole lot of money. My medical bills have been phenomenal. Tom's a good typist, but it hurts

him to do much typing, so he sends it out. His illness
forces him to do things in the least economical way.
He uses a cab instead of the bus, goes to a closer Xerox
place near us that costs more, and doesn't return
broken objects because of the time involved. I spend
all the time it takes to deal with things that need to
be done to get more money like doctors' letters to get
special P. G. and E. rates. I go to the hospital and the
letter arrives, and Tom lets it sit on the desk. He
doesn't deal with it, and it makes me feel crazy. I get
real upset about it. On the other hand, Tom needs to
do what he does in order to survive. . . . The worst of
it is that he simply doesn't do things that need to be
done. If they don't get done, it means that I feel I have
to do them since somebody has to. So in addition to
doing those things I have to deal with, I feel that I
have to clean up the mess that he leaves, bills that
don't get paid, etc. He just isn't coordinated about
those things. And if I didn't have a chronic illness and
he didn't have a chronic illness, we wouldn't have to
run each other's errands so often. It means whoever is
home has to pay bills.

Analysis. Here Helen is talking mainly about money
management. Two analytically related and important points are
brought out in this episode. One relates to the division of labor.
Helen tells us about the conditions that brought about their usual
division of labor with regard to this task. Basically, it was arrived
at by default because a large part of the money that they draw on
comes from Helen's inheritance, and besides she sees herself as more
adept at handling money. But just as important in terms of
alignment is that Tom is unwilling to take on this task, referring
it back to Helen—even during the period of her hospitalization.
Form Helen's perspective, Tom did not then make a shift in the
division of labor, therefore realigning his actions to meet her
inability to perform. Though Helen may not call it such, what we
have in this situation is her perception of disalignment. How she
handles it in order to articulate work performance is reluctantly to

do the work herself. This leads us to the question of how long the disalignment can continue before serious consequences result. What tactics will Helen then take to bring about realignment in terms of the money management?

At the root of the couple's disalignment stands the competition for resources, along with a perception of an unequal distribution of work load. One of these resources is money, which must be managed carefully. However, impinging upon that careful management are the illness-related conditions. The cost of managing their symptoms creates a resource drain, and decisions have to be made about where money will be spent and how it can be conserved. In addition, there is competition for time and energy. Both partners have limited amounts of these because of their illnesses. Conservation again becomes important. The questions here are as follows: With a competition for limited resources, where will they be used? And how can the division of labor be renegotiated so that the tasks are distributed more equitably? In an attempt to bring about alignment, Helen proffers the tasks, but Tom does not accept. To keep the work going, Helen takes up the slack.

Of course, behind each partner's position concerning the division of tasks there are reasons arising from conditional motivating considerations. While Tom's motivations are not clear, Helen's are clearer and are concerned with the calculation and use of resources. First of all, we see that she is the one who must pay the bills and therefore make the money stretch. Here the outermost level of our matrix is at work: just how far a given amount of money will stretch in our society. Then we move down to the second matrix level and see biographical considerations entering in: to waste money is inconsistent with Helen's frugal background. We can also see illness and biographical considerations at work, for Helen perceives that she must carry the full weight of the responsibility for task performance regardless of her whereabouts or ability. Having to take up the slack, which includes cleaning up the mess left over from the disruption of the work flow during her hospitalization, means that more of her time and energy must be given over to the task of money management, leaving less for other types of work. The conditions influencing Helen's perception of the situation become even clearer in the next excerpt, in which some conditions behind Tom's stand on the division of labor also begin to emerge.

> *Interview Quotation (Helen).* I am compulsive about details, which is a response to my need to have something in my life work right when everything else is a mess. Tom needs to do the least amount of anything stressful to get through. So our illness needs actually provoke each other unmercifully. He needs to be unstressed, and I blow up. Not so much because of the pain, though there is an incredible amount, but because the swelling of the brain tissue makes you nuts. There is a noticeable difference. I have two personalities. One is even-tempered and rational, kind, organized, self-assured, competent, professional! The other is "don't fuck with me, just don't fuck with me." The latter tends to erupt around household management things. Because of Tom's illness he can barely manage to get his work done. But I see that no matter what, his professional work gets done. This makes me childishly jealous. I am too busy picking up. To live in a house, you have to pay taxes, call the electric company, and so forth. Tom will look at his work and say, "I am sorry, I can't do that this week. I am sorry I can't do that this month." It drives me crazy because someone has to do it. So it falls on me and I am already having a lot of trouble getting my own work done. I see it in terms of professional competitiveness. I am joyful for him and I think his work is important. I also see that his work gets done at what I perceive is my expense. Some things have to get done so that you are sheltered and fed. And because of the illness we both have things that must be done that are peculiar to the illness like special pillows. . . . There is twice or three times as much running around and chores as there would be otherwise.

Analysis. Here we see that illness enters into the situation as a condition not only by increasing the total amount of work to be performed but also by limiting the amount of physical ability and energy available to do that work. Biographical conditions enter into the situation too. They influence the calculation of resources in terms of oneself and the other person and also the interaction flowing from Helen's tactics to bring the division of everyday work back into alignment.

While Tom's and Helen's biographical projections for themselves and each other may be similar, nevertheless because of limited time and energy, there is a difference of opinion on how these resources should be spent. Their prioritizing of tasks differs. Tom manages to articulate his biographical work by putting off everyday tasks. Helen in articulating the everyday work puts off her biographical work. These conditions create a situation in which there is a competition for resources, a perception of an unbalanced work load, a disruption in the flow of work, and perhaps some reassessing of conditional motivation. Under these conditions it is difficult to maintain a sense of balance over the distribution of resources and therefore over performance of the three main lines of work. Helen, when reflecting upon this situation, feels overloaded with everyday tasks, frustrated, and envious of Tom because she has little time or energy to put into her important biographical work. She has a very definite perception of disalignment. The part that Tom plays in the division of labor and how Helen feels about this can be seen in the next excerpt.

> *Interview Quotation (Helen).* But what Tom does—well he blows up when I blow up, or he gets sulky or whatever, as any normal person would do, but he has a lot of compassion. He has helped me to understand my own symptoms. He has researched my illness and found the doctor who finally was able to diagnose what was the matter with me. He is not real good at handling things; that is not his style. Plus he is so physically uncomfortable when he gets up in the morning, so stiff and hurts so bad that he doesn't want to be touched. I think the thing that I feel the worst about in this relationship is the consequences of my

illness that make it hard on him in a way that I feel is real painful. I have said to him, "Look, I would have left you if you were half as disagreeable as I am." Though for long periods of time I am just fine. Last night Tom came home in a terrible mood. Though I only eat foods that are on my diet, I made an elaborate dinner for him. It helped. It was like he needed to be taken care of, and I can finally do something. I feel that with this illness I have to do so much more of my share at everything just to not be so far behind. If I did all the paperwork and money earning for the rest of my life, is that going to even things out when he has to live with me as I am? Sometimes I feel that the nice things I do don't count either because I am already so far down. I have fucked up so much, my national debt is so big, there is no way to erase it.

Analysis. In her reflections on herself and the work, Helen perceives that while the work is unbalanced in the sense that the burden of everyday work is on her and weighs upon her, in essence not she but Tom is carrying much of the brunt of illness (hers as well as his) and relationship work. Therefore, she feels that she must not only carry the weight of the everyday work but also perform other tasks such as cooking a nice meal to repay the considerable resource debt she feels she owes him. Thus, we see quite specifically how reflection upon her own and Tom's actions affects her future actions and task performance. The next excerpt deals with interaction and how the spouses attempt to work out their problems.

Interview Quotation (Helen). Tom is more of a putter-offer than I am. "Let's talk tomorrow, three days from now. It is not a good day. I don't want to talk now." I blow up. We do finally sit down and say, "Okay, what is not working? What can we do to make it work? What do you need from me? What can I give you? What is your bottom line? What can't you tolerate from me? What do you need as a promise, a

guarantee?'' Tom needs me to promise not to yell.
When I yell, he literally cringes and it hurts his neck.
I have made an agreement with him: "All right I
won't yell, if every time I try to talk in a rational way
about what is bothering me that you won't say that I
am whining or lecturing. I blow up because whenever
I try to talk about what is bothering me you don't hear
me. We made an agreement.'' We try real hard to keep
those agreements. We don't always keep them but we
make them.

   I am a laundry list keeper. I think that this is
one of the major problems in our relationship. I don't
know if Tom forgives more than I do, but I tend to
keep some kind of record in my head of the ways in
which I have felt hurt. That is terrifically destructive
to any relationship. However, I work real hard at
figuring out what it is that I am doing that is fucked
up, where I am not being responsible. Tom and I have
made an agreement that if he says to me "you are
rushing," I will stop. Sometimes I say, "I may be
rushing, but I don't care, you are still being a shit."
That is it. We end the discussion. We won't talk about
whatever it is I am upset about until my eyes are back
to normal. I will go and look at myself in the mirror.
When my eyes are out to there, it is real clear to me
that I am not dealing with stuff in a way.

   I am not a total monster. I don't yell and scream
all the time. Perhaps once a day I raise my voice. He
comes from a family where nobody yells. Making the
[no-yelling] agreement has made a big difference. For
example, he doesn't like to feel that he is monitoring
me and that I am not an adult responsible for her own
actions. Having to monitor me is a big bind for him.
I feel that there are a whole lot of times that I am
chemically out of control. He says, "Well if I accept
that, believe that, then I am a caretaker. We do not
have a peer relationship." I say that is not true. We
haven't worked that one out yet. What I want him to

acknowledge is that I am doing the absolute best that
I can and that I am not always responsible for my
behavior. We are both willing to say that often I am
not responsible for my feelings, that my feelings are
often irrational and chemically caused. I am trying to
get to the point that even though I feel like blowing
up, I recognize that there are consequences and stop
doing it.

Analysis. This quotation brings out several major points
directly pertinent to our theoretical analysis of the alignment
processes. First, we see how the couple attempt to maintain
alignment during interaction. In this case, interaction pertains to
the spouses' attempts to realign their work efforts, especially in
terms of the everyday types of work and Helen's symptom management. Second, to articulate the interactional alignment Helen and
Tom have set up agreements about how each should behave. Third,
impinging upon that alignment are conditions (both illness and
biographically related) that break it down. Fourth, we see what each
is asking of the other and therefore the perspectives each is asking
the other to bring into the interaction. Fifth, even though tactics
have been established to keep the interaction in alignment,
sometimes the alignment breaks down, and so other tactics have
been mutually established to attain some degree of realignment.
Because Helen's symptoms as manifested in her behavior are part
of the reason for the disalignment, Tom usually initiates the tactics
to bring about realignment. In turn, Helen must pick up and
respond favorably to those tactics if realignment is actually to occur.
Sixth, again we can see how the prephase and postphase are part
of the action/interaction itself. The action/interaction brings about
reflection, and that reflection becomes part of the set of conditions
entering into behavior during the next interactional sequence.
Seventh, the consequences of action/interaction in any of its phases
have an impact (biographical or illness) on the actors themselves,
on the action/interactional sequence, and on alignment. Other
interactional agreements that the couple have worked out can be
seen in the next quotation.

Interview Quotation (Helen). It turned out there was a logical explanation for everything, but before that I was accumulating evidence that I was bizarre. So I was very defensive about his perception that I was behaving peculiarly around our friends. There was more covering up of symptoms in front of friends than in front of Tom. Tom sniffed things out very fast. My driving (I do most of it as he doesn't care to drive much) was one of the first things to go because I would be disoriented and my vision was affected by the medication. Tom . . . would just say that he felt like driving. I knew it was because he felt I was disoriented. As long as he didn't say anything, I was all right. If he said anything, I would get belligerent about it. We had a lot of tacit agreements.

Another area where we worked things out was around friends. What he would do is cue me that I was being weird. . . . He would quietly cue me that I was being speedy and needed to be quieter. We formalized that. I wanted that because I knew that I was out of control. Tom would sometimes try to get my attention to monitor what I ate at a party. Sometimes I don't like the cuing. Most of the time I don't like it when it is happening, but I am almost always grateful for it afterward. . . . He has a tremendous amount of power in that if he says that I am rushing, then I will stop. He has never abused that power. Because he has never abused that power, I trust him.

Analysis. We see here how the couple have achieved alignment in several subtypes of work and the conditions contributing to it. The alignment can exist for some subtypes of work and tasks while not existing for others. In these situations, the partners have articulated the work by establishing a formalized set of interactional cues based on a division of labor; one acts as a monitor and cue giver, and the other acts as a respondent. By such means they are able to control Helen's symptoms and carry out the work of driving and of maintaining relationships with friends.

Thus, these means help to relax both partners, because they are self-sustaining and relationship-sustaining. However, this alignment is built upon a set of conditions, and these are part of the perspectives that each partner brings to the interaction. Hence, a change in any of these conditions could throw the interaction and its subsequent action out of alignment. Just as important is what transpires within the interaction itself, the cues given and the other person's response at the time—to accept or reject them—and then the other's response to that acceptance or rejection, and so forth as the interaction proceeds. Consequently, even a well thought out and planned for interaction may not always proceed according to plan. Each participant's response to the other's actions in the end determines how the interaction will ultimately turn out.

Interview Quotation (Helen). I tend to see me as the really ill one. Not that I don't think he has a real illness that gives him a lot of pain, but he doesn't need emotional caretaking in the same way that I do. He needs somebody to make sure he doesn't exert himself, to empty the garbage, to ask, "Tell me about your work?" The emotional caretaking he needs is for me to be quiet and calm and perceptive and interested in his work. Sometimes I get threatened by his work, because I am going through a time where I have no intellectual interest whatsoever. I can't do my own. . . .

The emotional sustaining I do of him is to shut off my own needs, which are overly plentiful, and to tune into what will make him feel relaxed, like being cooked for. I run interference for him about phone calls. I know who he doesn't want to talk to or see. Though it is a task I don't particularly relish, putting people off, I have learned to lie and say that he is not home and take a message. I see him as a genius whose genius has to be protected. I see him as someone who is so physically handicapped that he has maybe two or three hours to work on a good day. So his time is very precious, and I protect his time. I try to protect it by not taking too much of it myself. I definitely protect it by not letting other people make unreasonable demands on him. He feels like he should put himself out for other people because other people do that for him, but when he does, it is always at a physical cost. Sometimes I get jealous because I see him do a physical errand that I know he wouldn't do for me. He needs a support system that is bigger than me and so that is not a rational feeling. I was not the type of person that I have become in the process of this illness. It is my hope that if I am better that I will feel less pressured, less desperate, less volatile.

Analysis. We again see all four work processes functioning as Helen outlines how she willingly articulates acting as a resource for Tom (through a division of labor in which she performs acts that help to sustain his biographical work). We also see how she feels about the work, about herself, and about her reactions to Tom and what he does. All of this acts as a set of conditions for the interactional/action sequence that follows. Though Helen puts forth a great deal of effort to sustain Tom because he in turn does so much to sustain her, she does *not* perceive disalignment with regard to this work—mostly biographical—as she does with regard to everyday work.

Interview Quotation (Helen). After I got my Phd D., I wanted a party and I wanted Tom to do it. He didn't want to. I didn't realize that it was because of his illness and at the time he was feeling over-whelmed. He didn't have the energy to do it. I was hurt for a long time. He finally explained it was the illness, but it was almost too late for it not to hurt. He doesn't verbalize 90 percent of what is illness-related behavior for him, and I verbalize 200 percent. I verbalize to a tedious excess, and he does not verbalize enough. . . . You feel bewildered and hurt because the other is not coming through. He does not come through because he can't. If I knew it at the time, it

would take care of 95 percent of the hurt, but he
doesn't always verbalize.

Analysis. This excerpt shows how interaction—or more
precisely, aligned interaction—stands at the heart of work where
each interactant is coming from the same interactional perspective,
or where, if they are not coming from it, at least their perspectives
are brought together during the interaction itself. Here Tom failed
to perform an important type of biographical work for Helen.
Though body failure and illness-related conditions were impinging
on Tom's failure to do this work, according to Helen, these reasons
were never made clear. Thus each person carried a different
perspective into the interaction. Furthermore, not until much later
were their perspectives realigned. In the meantime, the consequence
was Helen's hurt.

> *Interview Quotation (Helen).* The number of
> practical things that have to be done when you have
> a chronic illness becomes almost overwhelming. Even
> if I had a normal person's energy, it would take the
> energy of three people to take care of all the other
> complicated things that have to be done. Tom has very
> important, high-level, sophisticated management
> skills, like not telling everyone how sick I have been
> because of the implication it may have, like for my
> getting a job. But he fucks up on the little stuff. In the
> long run what he does is very important. What I do
> for him is endless amounts of little stuff. . . . If he
> could work eight hours a day, I would not protect him
> in the way that I do. There is no question that I
> wouldn't. He does a lot of emotional shit work; I do
> a lot of physical shit work. Neither one of us would
> do as much for the other if we weren't both ill.

Analysis. This excerpt summarizes the tremendous impact of
chronic illness on a person's daily life and how that impact
multiplies when both partners are afflicted. It also shows how the
nature of the work to be done differs according to the respective

symptoms and how the partners work out a division of labor in which each does what is necessary to sustain the other. In other words, an overall alignment is worked out according to each partner's perceived respective needs and abilities.

> *Interview Quotation (Tom).* Probably the key role that I have played through all of this is a kind of monitoring in terms of the psychological stuff. Is she acting crazy? And if she is, is it because she is reacting against something in the world, is it the drug, or is it some sort of physiologic condition? If it is one of these, then I am in some sort of position to try to calm her down. I try to let her know what is going on from my view. Like sometimes she will have time distortion, and it will take her a half hour to go from one room to another, get dressed, or one thing or another. When this happens I say "hurry up, hurry up," then I realize that she is spacing out. Then I say, "Oops, you are doing the time thing. Do you realize that twenty minutes have gone by?" She will say, "No, you're kidding" and look at her watch. Sometimes I help the world to go by more slowly for her and in a more orderly way. Sometimes that just means explaining things to her and making sure that things go smoothly, that there isn't a lot of confusion.

Analysis. This excerpt shows the inner dialogue (self-interaction) that often occurs during an action sequence, especially when that action is problematic rather than routine. As a result, Tom performs symptom management work for Helen. He articulates this work through such tactics as reorienting and making the world go more slowly for her and by preceding that action with an analysis of what conditions might be operating to cause her behavior. From his analysis the tactics to manage the symptoms emerge.

> *Interview Quotation (Tom).* There is a heavy moral responsibility about a thing when one person has

to judge the psychological status of another at any given time, especially when it is a fluctuating entity. I don't know if I am making the right decision. For instance, I don't know if she is just really pissed off at me about something, and I say, "You are nuts at the moment." I have to be sure of myself, that I am not taking advantage of where she is at. I try to be real careful about that, but it still goes against my moral grain to do it at all. Part of me feels that someone should be responsible for his or her actions no matter what. The other is saying, "Okay, she is going through this." It doesn't mean that she should get exemption for her behavior. Yet on a practical basis I continue to make adjustments for it because it is easier to do it than to not. Adjustments in the sense that she gets really volatile. At that point I have a choice to make allowances for her behavior, to say, "You are being a total asshole and I do not choose to interact with you at the moment." Well, if I did that each time that she was volatile, our relationship would be in shambles. So contrary to this moral feeling that I have, I make excuses for her on the basis of her condition. . . .

We have talked about it. I think that she relies on more of a physiological explanation of her behavior than I am comfortable with. She says, "My brain swells; that is why I yell at you." I say, "That may be so, but you have a choice in how you react or not react, the degree to which you say that you have a choice in how you react."

Analysis. Additional analytic issues lie behind Tom's words. First of all, we can see the issue of spouses' different stances that lead to the possibility of discrepant actions. Erving Goffman (1974) refers to this as *misframing,* a useful term. However Goffman is typically focused in his writings on the mechanics of interaction—what makes it flow smoothly or allows it to be disrupted—and rarely on interactional process beyond single episodes or on evolving relationships between the actors themselves. Second, these different stances have consequences for a succession of interactions and so for the evolving relationships between the spouses. Again, these particular excerpts refer to the central interactional issue of alignment and disalignment.

Here Tom is assessing and making judgments on his own action as well as on Helen's. His judgments are profoundly affected by the uncertain medical diagnosis of Helen's disease. The diagnosis is imprecise and nonspecific for any given action. Helen herself cannot always be sure why she has acted "crazily," either because she is physiologically awry at the moment or just uncertain about what is making her act as she is. As for Tom, sometimes he is quite uncertain whether a given inappropriate action by Helen is due to her physiology or her personality. So his choices are either to act as if indeed he does know that it is physiological (telling himself that he must be patient) or to be pragmatic (telling himself that life must go on or else their marriage cannot go on). Helen's inability to be self-reflective during episodes of interaction when she is physiologically awry is followed in the postinteraction phase, as we saw earlier, by self-reflection concerning either her physiological disturbance or her craziness. Then the couple may talk together about the entire episode. They may discuss their situation in anticipation of a similar episode occurring in the future. Tom, as is indicated in the preceding excerpts, may bring up the subject after a prior interaction. Thus, the before and after reflections of both spouses enter into succeeding interactions, also affecting the evolving relationships between them.

Tom's words also provide insight into the relationship between two levels of alignment: the more general level dealing with the actual work performance through the work processes, and the narrower aspect of alignment dealing with interaction through which the work processes are carried out or worked out. During interaction, agreements are made or not made. During the ensuing action, made agreements are either carried out or not carried out according to the standards of quantity and quality set forth in the agreements. In this particular situation, alignment did not occur at either level of alignment. The spouses' respective tactics and countertactics are as follows: Tom proffers the task; Helen rejects it. Then Tom aligns himself with her response by making adjustments and excuses, that is by doing the necessary symptom management work. Clearly underlying their respective positions are illness, biographical, and other structural conditions that bear upon the interactional stance each takes toward the situation.

> *Interview Quotation (Tom).* We have an agreement that if I say, "You are flooding right now," she will stop. That is the agreement. It doesn't always hold. I don't always agree with her and then we get into a fight. Then it escalates. So while that is the verbalized agreement and she tries to be good about it, it doesn't always work. . . . Sometimes I try to defuse the situation, quiet her down and not let her get more disoriented. In that case I end up swallowing a lot of my anger. I end up sitting on it at the moment because for me to express my irritation or resentment at that moment would not work very well. I just hold it in and try to talk about it later when we can do so rationally.

Analysis. Though agreements are made and become the conditions brought to the interaction/action, again the responses that each partner makes during these interactions can change their potential course. To prevent escalation of the argument and Helen's irrational behavior, Tom must take an interactional stance that is the opposite of Helen's. Fitting his actions with Helen's in this and similar instances means that regardless of how angry he is, he must swallow that anger or sit on it until Helen is willing and able to sit down and talk things through rationally.

> *Interview Quotation (Tom).* There is the public-private thing in our relationship. She is not like that all of the time; it is just that sometimes she gets like that. In private it doesn't happen as often. I am always placed in the situation with friends of saying that she really is not like that at home. It is just when she gets around a lot of people and has a lot of input coming in that she gets kind of nuts. She doesn't

realize what is happening. . . . Sometimes people would choose to battle it out with her, getting into sort of severe arguments. . . . I would have these images flash in my mind, the entire evening of Helen and someone else screaming at the top of their lungs and I would be sitting there saying, "Oh, no!" It wasn't just argument, though that was a large part of it, but there was just [her] being a little bit off. I would be the only one who could tell, perhaps a little bit too much talk or loud laughter. I could tell that it would mean that later she would be even worse. I think in a way I become hypersensitive because other people would say, "She is fine. Don't worry about it, we will tell her if something is not right."

Analysis. Images of past behavior enter into the present, in this case as a flashback, to influence one's perception of the situation and the direction of any actions taken. Because Tom knows that Helen's behavior tends to escalate in public (her interactional behavior is out of alignment with the people with whom she is interacting), he is constantly assessing her behavior in terms of its alignment with other people's behavior, then forecasting how she will behave, and planning how he will bring her behavior back into alignment should she go too far. This is symptom management work, but it revolves around biographical types of situations—mainly being with their friends and in activity groups. Much of what happens in public, of course, depends on how other people interpret and react to Helen's behavior—the interactions they carry out with her, whether they get into arguments with her or simply ignore the behavior. As Tom says, one of the conditions that makes him so intent on assessing her behavior is that he has now become hypersensitive to what other people say.

Interview Quotation (Tom). In company, I try to signal to her or say quietly to her in the kitchen, "Slow down, you are behaving irrationally." Because she is feeling irrational, she says, "What do you mean

I am being irrational!" in a loud voice and everyone looks. We have tried very hard to develop a set of signals to use in company, where I would sort of set a signal with my hand so she would not react like that. None of them really work very well, and her behavior has really alienated a lot of my friends. If the setting can absorb her behavior like when it is an open rowdy sort of gathering, then it is okay, but at a small dinner party it is not great.

Analysis. Here Tom tells us about the agreements he and Helen have made to keep her behavior aligned with social situations and explains how they fail. To articulate management of Helen's symptoms they have a set of interactional signals. However, the nature of Helen's symptoms at any given time influences how she responds to the signals and therefore whether or not she acts to bring her behavior into alignment. Tom can signal Helen, but only Helen can control her own behavior.

Interview Quotation (Tom). I think the reciprocity thing is very important. There are a lot of things that she is doing for me. It is not all just give, give, give. Her behavior is also intermittent. . . . A week, several days can go by without any symptoms. At those times you forget, and the image that you hold in your mind is that of a healthy person. At all times, you carry a certain image of a person, and my image of Helen is not of Helen sick but of Helen well. Also I have been increasingly involved in my work and she has tried to be in hers, and that helps. . . . I am a temperamental person and unusual in lots of ways. I am not a real conformist, and Helen has a lot of tolerance for that sort of thing. That combined with her support and loyalty keeps the marital relationship going.

Analysis. In assessing the degree of the couple's overall alignment, as reflected in this excerpt, we can observe many conditions that come into play as we move up and down our matrix diagram. First of all, Helen's erratic behavior is only intermittent. Second, even during difficult times, Tom carries within him the image of Helen as well. Third, much of the work they do for each other is mutually sustaining. Fourth, both have their own careers they can turn to for psychological sustenance. The consequence of this, of course, is to motivate them to continue the work, which in turn keeps their lives and their relationship going.

This case history illustrates the centrality of interaction—or our specialized usage of it in terms of alignment—with respect to work performance. Alignment pertains to the continued adjustments that people must make in fitting their actions to the actions of others in order for work performance—whether it be trajectory, everyday, or biographical work—to take place. The case also demonstrates how important types of biographical and everyday work may fail to occur because of temporary misalignment or more drastic misalignment. Finally, the case illustrates how the different levels of conditions come into play to influence each person's responses during an interactional sequence.

This couple's struggles to bring about, maintain, and realize their actions so that the three major levels of work can take place are clearly visible. Our readers will probably not be surprised to learn that the overwhelming amount of work brought about by Helen's and Tom's chronic conditions plus the problems they encountered in carrying out the three lines of work under the conditions vividly shown in the foregoing sequence of interview excerpts finally led Helen and Tom reluctantly to dissolve their marital relationship.

Summary

Theory. This chapter concludes the theoretical portion of the book. In it we introduce the concept of interaction, emphasizing the interactional alignment process that takes place during work performance. We then link interaction and alignment with the other major concepts discussed in earlier theoretical chapters, namely, illness, biography, everyday work, lines of work, work types, and work processes. When linked, these concepts form a model that furthers understanding of what happens in work-related interactions, that is, how work gets done through alignment of actions around the work processes within a given context of conditions. This occurs at each phase of the interaction and encompasses how the consequences of each phase become part of the situational context and therefore conditions for each succeeding interactional phase. It occurs because conditions for subsequent interactions involve the same or different types of work as the trajectory moves along in time. When viewed in this manner, interaction is broken down analytically into preinteraction, interaction, and postinteraction phases, with the first and third phases constituting self-reflection. Each completed phase is a stepping stone to the next phase of work-related action, always within an evolving structural context. We use a "conditional matrix" to illustrate the complex analytic nature of the contexts within which the ill and their partners do their trajectory management.

Applications. What are some practical implications of this way of conceptualizing and studying the microdynamics of how the ill and their partners actually carry out this necessary work—or stumble or fail in their attempts?

1. It is not enough for practitioners merely to assess a family's resources, motivation, intelligence, medical knowledge, and so forth. Equally important is the gaining of information of their joint, or collective, work style: How do they actually and usually work together or in some measure fail to do this? What goes into their particular modes of working things out, both routinely and when contingencies arise?

2. Also important is an assessment and understanding of the several sets of conditions (the matrix) that affect a couple's working together. If they are working together effectively, then the tendency is for everyone—the practitioners included—to take this for granted. But just why, under what sets of conditions, is this joint effort possible? One needs to assess and understand (and put into the record) why the couple work so well together. When there is a change in the illness course, even for the better, then the micrody-

namics of their joint work may well be affected. Each trajectory phase, in fact, brings its own hazards.

3. When a couple is having major alignment difficulties, it is especially crucial that the alignment process be carefully scrutinized for its strengths as well as its more obvious weaknesses. How can the strengths be built upon and what additional changes are really feasible given specific probable recalcitrant conditions? What new conditions and interactional means can be offered to the partners that *they* can understand and that *they* can agree to *and* implement? Practitioners whose well-intentioned interventions disregard the specifics of the alignment process will unquestionably fail.

We turn now to the substantive portion of our book to demonstrate how our theory illuminates the various types of trajectory phases. (It may be useful first to review the section on trajectory shapes and phases in Chapter Three.)

PART TWO

Managing Chronic Illness

We have reached an important juncture in this book. Our basic theoretical approach to understanding a number of salient and striking accompaniments of chronic illness has been presented. The next set of issues to be addressed pertains to the differing fates of those who suffer from chronic illness. Although each person is likely to be struggling with the same general problems, the specific forms in which those problems occur will vary if only because illnesses vary. And so, of course, do people's circumstances: their material resources; their relationships with health professionals, spouses, children, and other relatives; and their own inner resources and self-commitments. How, then, can we analytically capture both the commonalities and diversities of their experiences?

One way of bringing some order to our understanding of the great diversity of experience is to think of different types of trajectory shapes, classified in accordance with their direction: upward, stable, unstable, and downward. Those directional courses pertain to all chronic illness. Of course, combinations of them are frequent. Thus a comeback, as noted earlier, can turn downward, a progressive downward course can have long plateaus, and a stabilized illness may have ups and downs in symptomology and, indeed, in the disease course even though it eventually turns radically upward or downward.

Illness itself comprises a background condition for whether a particular sufferer experiences a sense of deterioration or a sense of comeback or at least a holding steady. Yet physical condition is only one crucial condition among other potential ones that tell us what is happening or has happened to the chronically ill. Recall that trajectory rather than illness is the key tool for conceptualizing

167

the work and experiences of the ill and their associates and also for conceptualizing changes in their lives. The phases of work, biography, and interaction they proceed through are trajectory phases, *not* merely physical or physiological or medical-treatment phases.

In fact, it is worth emphasizing—and the following chapters will illustrate the point amply—that the ill see and react to physical condition mainly in terms of symptoms. Although physicians tend to think in terms of disease, the ill vividly experience the intrusion of symptoms into their lives. Indeed, body failure comes down to just that as a practical, everyday matter. (Except in downward trajectories, when thinking ahead to their potential or looming deaths, the ill may also imagine vividly what is happening inside of themselves, for example, cancer eating up their organs.)

So in discussing *trajectory phases,* we shall again be referring to trajectory issues. The questions here for each type of phase include the following: What are the different types of work? How do they get done? How do the central work processes and interactional developments enter into getting the work done? What are the biographical processes that accompany and affect those matters? By viewing those questions through four different sets of lenses, which correspond to the major trajectory phases, we can hope to bring some order to the confusing welter of variation in the experience and fate of those who undergo those phases at home.

In short, the main theoretical concepts running through the preceding chapters (work and trajectory) will now be joined with an intensive scrutiny of trajectory phases: the work and experiences involved in each. As the descriptions and theoretical commentary cumulate, chapter by chapter, we shall see how the experiences deriving from the illness and attempts to manage it are often poignant and, alas, sometimes devastating. They are also subtle and ultimately immensely complex.

For instance, the comeback phase is not merely a time of physical recovery. Even recognizing that it has psychological accompaniments is scarcely to do justice to the complexity of any first-time comeback from a severely acute period, let alone to understand what is involved in recurrent comebacks after repeated setbacks. In Chapter Eight we note how a comeback can represent a complex uphill journey back to a satisfying, workable life within the boundaries imposed by actual and perceived physical (and possibly mental) limitations. A comeback involves the regaining of prominent aspects of the self lost because of illness or injury. Comebacks can have varying properties. They may be difficult or easy, marked by visible indicators of progress or ambiguous ones; they may be partial or lead to complete physical recovery (although often with at least partly altered selves); and if they are lengthy, they may go through subphases. Virtually all comebacks carry a complex set of questions for the ill: How far back will I come? How long will it take? Can my own actions affect the speed and degree of comeback? If so, which actions and how much?

The properties and impacts of stable phases of illness are quite different. In Chapter Nine we emphasize particularly that the usual medical perspective on stability—that careful adherence to a regimen and the proper conditions of life are the chief instruments of maintaining stability—is far too physiological in its thrust. This purely medical view also greatly oversimplifies the truly vast amount of work and ingenuity of work relationships that goes into keeping many illnesses stabilized. It also underestimates the juggling of what can be very complicated life considerations. In a sense, the view that stabilization depends on faithful adherence to regimens and the proper life conditions simply obscures all the complexities of action required in meeting those prescribed requirements. The information in Chapter Nine spells out in considerable detail what those complexities really entail.

Unstable phases are among the most anguishing for the ill, as we discuss in Chapter Ten. In essence, everything is more or less out of control: first, the illness course (which may not even be accurately or completely diagnosed), then the symptoms (none or only some of which may be controllable, and only for a time), and understandably, the conditions of living and of personal action. Instability may, of course, mean that there are different degrees of severity and that they may vary in duration. But the impact of instability (unless it is merely brief) is also potentially devastating for self-conceptions. This is because instability can profoundly affect what one can and cannot accomplish.

Finally, there are varieties of downward (deteriorating and

dying) phases, as examined in Chapter Eleven. Obviously, many people who have suffered from these phases, or lived with people who have passed through them, understand the phases very well. So do health practitioners. Yet if we ask what "understanding them very well" means, we can see that this means primarily in a descriptive sense. Conceptualizations of even the general patterns of deterioration or dying, let alone their variations, are not very powerful in an explanatory sense. *Coping, adjustment,* and *stress* are terms that seem to us, again, as either obscuring very complex biographical processes and work processes or as missing many of the interactional and sociological aspects of what is happening during downward trajectory phases. In Chapter Eleven we attempt to fill in some of the conceptual gaps in what are probably the most written about (by lay people, health professionals, and behavioral scientists) periods of illness. Undoubtedly, we too have failed to do justice to these very complex and varied phases. Our main contribution is the sharp reminder that no downward trajectory— unless it is very short—is devoid of combinations of other phases: of comebacks (however brief or incomplete), of unstable periods, or of stable plateaus. Indeed, it is the uncertainty of the combinations and especially of the repeated plateaus that are succeeded by increasingly lower levels of physical and sometimes mental functioning that provide some of the major problems of those who are passing through these aspects of trajectory.

In Chapter Twelve we depart from the examination of trajectory types and turn to look more generally at the experiences and actions of the spouses of the ill (some of whom are ill themselves) regardless of what phases their ill mates are passing through. Understandably, the degree of stress and strain of living with an ill partner varies considerably, depending on a host of relevant conditions. We detail some of the most important conditions but are mainly concerned with their impacts, letting the spouses speak more or less for themselves. We do present case studies that illustrate, for instance, the great emotional drain that can be experienced even when little or no physical caretaking is involved. We also illustrate how spouses' work and its impact on the well mate vary by trajectory phase, how the well mate may also have a great deal of biographical work to do, and how the impact is not necessarily all negative. On the other hand, we show that in every marital situation there is a "looming potential" for the physical or emotional breakdown of either the well spouse or the marital relationship.

With this variation and complexity in mind, the chapters to follow should fall into place as part of the total landscape through which any given person's illness course may take him or her.

8

Comeback Phases:
Recovering from Illness

    This chapter is organized around a set of case histories whose narratives include short analytical prefaces and asides, as well as reminders or references to various theoretical points discussed previously. We begin by discussing general features of comeback. We go on to present several cases, each emphasizing different features of comebacks.

    Why are we using cases in this and the following chapters as the primary vehicle for organizing analyses of trajectory phases? Cases can give a relatively vivid sense and deep *understanding* of the speaker or writer. Using several cases also brings out *variations* as well as *similarities* of the general pattern. We have selected the cases not simply for their dramatic effect but because they highlight the patternings of specific theoretical points bearing on the different aspects of work and inner biographical processes as a person struggles with an illness-precipitated fate. Because Chapters Nine through Twelve follow the same format, the case presentation is intended to serve a third function: to *contrast* and yet bring out *similarities* among the main types of trajectory phase.

    Several different kinds of comeback experiences are covered in this chapter. The first case is composed of separate interviews with a husband who has very recently become a paraplegic and with his wife as the couple struggle to understand what has happened to their lives and to comprehend what they will and can become in the face of his disaster. Our analytical emphasis is on their individual and joint biographical work and the actual interplay of that work in overt action. The second case concerns a moderately severe cardiac condition and emphasizes matters such as body imagery, body-mind distinctions, rehabilitation strategies, trials and tests, improved bodily condition and performance of varing degree as well as plateaus of varying duration, interactional phases, and the spouse's agentry and own biographical phasing. Our third case is about Agnes de Mille, the celebrated dancer. It illustrates especially the trajectory and biographical phasing, the types of trajectory work, work processes, relations with health professionals and kin, and the crucial relationships with her life's work and audiences for that work—in her case, dancing and choreography.

These cases have been selected on theoretical grounds (Strauss and Glaser, 1970). The theoretical points are specified from time to time with the intent of adding to the reader's own experiences and knowledge. We have attempted to avoid interfering unduly with either the narrative flow itself or the reader's own thought processes.

Theoretical Considerations

Nature of Comebacks. A comeback represents an uphill journey back to a satisfying, workable life within the boundaries imposed by physical and possibly mental limitations. It involves the attempt to regain salient aspects of oneself that have been lost because of illness or injury. However, when an illness such as a myocardial infarction occurs, or a disabling condition such as a spinal cord injury is suffered, then immediate attention is usually focused upon medical management, prevention of physical crises, and survival. The concerns of physician, family, and affected person, if conscious, center around necessary illness work and immediate questions about the illness or disability. What course will this illness or disability take in the proximate future? What work is necessary to pull the person through? What will be the residual effects, if any? Because the focus is on the illness or disability, biographical concerns are temporarily relegated to secondary status. Once the immediate crisis period is over and the fitness condition is stabilized, then biographical issues come into play; these include new issues if the body failure is at all severe and seemingly permanent. Once the moratorium is lifted, the ill person tries to contextualize the illness or disability into his or her life and begins to ask questions such as these: How did it happen? What does it mean in terms of my future? How will I manage to integrate the illness or disability and all the work that it involves into my life?

The comeback may be partial or complete, depending on the nature of the illness or injury and the degree of body or mind failure and also on specific features of one's biography. Comeback may be easy or difficult, marked by visible indicators of progress or ambiguous ones. It involves phases, often discernable to the ill but certainly discernable to the researcher if the data are sufficiently detailed. Comeback may move slowly or quickly along a course until the ultimate comeback potential is reached; or it may be arrested for a time or forever at any subphase along the way; or it may reverse or improve and then stabilize temporarily or permanently.

In medical language, comeback is commonly referred to as *rehabilitation*. This term focuses primary attention on the physical aspects of "recovery." To get a more complete picture of what is involved in a comeback, one must consider at least three general processes: (1) *mending*, the process of physical healing, which broadly speaking means getting better; (2) *stretching of physical limitations*, pushing the body to the boundaries of its current limitations and thereby increasing body performance as well as possibly hastening or improving its mending; and (3) *reknitting*, or putting the biography back together again, around the boundaries of residual body and social performance limitations. These three processes may occur simultaneously or one by one. One or another may be in focus at any particular time.

Conditions for Comebacks. Embarking upon and making continued progress along the comeback trail after a major or first acute episode requires the presence of certain conditions that not only act as precursors but continually come into play throughout the comeback trajectory. Among these conditions are the following:

1. The possibility of physical recovery, though just how far one can come back physically is limited by the degree of bodily injury.
2. The belief that the parts of the self that are lost have been

salient aspects of that self and therefore it is worth working to regain them, whether in the same or different form.

3. Crystallization or a clear realization of the future, followed by mobilization to provide the impetus to embark on the comeback path; and, should decrystallization occur, recrystallization and remobilization in order to keep the comeback process moving.

4. A comeback initiator (usually the physician but occasionally another person) who devises the initial trajectory scheme and sets the ill person upon the comeback trail (Becker and Kaufman, 1983).

5. A tailored fit between the comeback scheme and the individual, both medically and biographically.

6. A pool of resources, including people, environment, health personnel, finances, and objects to draw upon to support the comeback process.

7. A willingness to do the requisite work of management (Kaufman and Becker, 1986; Rosenberg, 1980, p. 179).

8. A comeback articulator who coordinates both the various types of work involved in comeback and the workers' efforts.

9. Teamwork by both the ill person and other comeback workers, each one moving in and out of the comeback work and undertaking specific tasks according to the trajectory and biographical phasing and the type of work to be done.

10. Realistic future goals to work toward.

11. The ability not to be permanently discouraged, depressed, or crushed by setbacks, long plateaus with little upward movement, or generally slow progress.

12. The ability to be flexible, to compromise, devise, and use the imagination.

13. Periodic indicators of progress.

Basic Questions of Comebacks. Usually a comeback poses a series of additional questions. They are thoroughly infused with considerations of body performance, self-performance, and biographical time (see Chapters Four and Five). A list of these questions should also be useful for understanding the cases in this chapter.

1. Given the present medical status after initial crisis, how reversible is this illness or disability? (The future may again be like the past if the illness or disability is reversible and so not like the present.)

2. How far back will or can I come? All, much, some, a little of the way? And with regard to which of my activities? (How fast will I come back, whether part way, most of the way, or all the way? How quickly will the future be identical with or at least somewhat like my past? Does the future, like the present, stay this way for a long, medium, or short time?)

3. How long will I remain on the present plateau, this "stuck present," before moving upward? Is this a permanent plateau from which I will never progress any more? How soon will I really know? (Will this present-present be permanent so that I have no future—except perhaps in terms of reversibility—other than the present-present?)

4. Is this setback—reversibility—if not permanent going to last for a short, medium, or long time? (And will I be losing time in any event?)

5. Is this setback permanent, my comeback finished? (Will the future be just like the present?)

6. Can my own actions affect the comeback? In amount or rate? Or is that all just dependent on fate? More specifically, what actions will improve the chances of comeback? Following the regimen, praying, what? How much of this must I do, and for how long?

7. What about fluctuations, hourly or daily or weekly, in my actual functioning? For instance, no matter how far I come back, at whatever level of performance, I might fluctuate (do fluctuate even now) in capacity. How much of that will remain and be part of my daily living? And when will I know for sure?

Case 1: A Paraplegic and His Wife—Initial Months of Comeback

Some kinds of body injury, such as characterize the situation of paraplegics and quadriplegics, typically are relatively intractable to much physical improvement and precipitate enormous physical, interactional, and biographical problems. The physical ones involve not merely the loss of ability to move limbs but also the potential and actual misfunctioning of physiological systems. After the accident, paraplegics and quadriplegics are usually physiologically out of balance and psychologically stunned. Eventually, however, the body does begin to mend to some extent in the sense of physiological stabilization. If paraplegics and quadriplegics can summon sufficient motivation, they can get started on the comeback trail through intensive rehabilitation work.

With a spinal cord injury, one can only come back as far as the new body limitations will allow. Some people come back more than others because they work hard and successfully at rehabilitation. In such cases comeback does not mean physical recovery but the ability to perform: the injured become more or less independent in their bodily performances and self-performances. Among the injured, there is tremendous variation in comeback, depending on the amount and location of injury, on their motivation to engage in strenuous rehabilitation work, and on their motivation to stretch their imagined performance limits. For example, many quadriplegics are able to drive their cars but need special equipment and the will to drive. Similarly, they cannot reach above them to objects on shelves, but if sufficiently motivated, they can use sticks to bring the objects down, or unashamedly ask others to reach for the objects, or rearrange their rooms so that objects are within their reach.

If physiological mending and rehabilitation are essential ingredients in the comeback of paraplegics and quadriplegics, those ingredients are nonetheless overshadowed by the reknitting process. Imagine what the world seems to hold in store for someone who has abruptly and permanently lost the use of his or her lower body or all limbs. Immediately after the incapacitating accident, the future is plunged into gloom and seems absolutely impossible to imagine living in. Yet the injured must live if they can face that situation. Some cannot. We once encountered a relatively young woman in a nursing home, a stroke victim, who after the stroke had simply given up, not believing that any comeback was possible. Apparently no one was able to motivate her sufficiently to begin the reknitting process so essential to the comeback. Indeed, reknitting outweighs the other two processes, especially during the early phases when the will to live is the first prerequisite to the rehabilitation work that will be so important when the injured return home.

The first case concerns a paraplegic husband, Peter, and his staunchly supportive and intelligent wife, Mary, both in their mid forties. Both are doing the biographical work necessary for Peter's embarking on the long comeback trail. Excerpts from their separate interviews, arranged so that they are addressing generally the same issues or events, will be presented. Each partner is talking about two months after Peter's gravely incapacitating injury. We can almost literally hear him trying to sort out his own and Mary's options, trying to decide what their future life is going to be—can sensibly be hoped to be. He goes through a list of activities noting those that he can still do and those that he can no longer do and gives us biographical-review imagery pertaining to both the future and the past. Peter talks about working out in imagination what the future can and will and might mean to his wife and his relations with her and gives his biographical scheme for handling that too.

Mary's words supplement and amplify our understanding of the conditional motivation, resource calculation, rearrangement of the division of labor, and articulation work (both of a trajectory and biographical kind) that are necessary to get started on a successful comeback course. Her functioning in those work processes is crucial to Peter's undertaking the long climb back to some sort of normal life. They both see that very clearly and enunciate it explicity and graphically. Peter particularly can be seen in the beginning phases of coming to terms with his actual and probable limitations and therefore with an altered life as he trades off what is at least bearable or possibly even as good or better than before.

Mary begins her interview by explaining that immediately after her husband's accident, the physician told them that there was virtually no chance that he would ever walk again. "But there is," she believes, "still a little bit of hope" that he someday will. "I believe that doctors know a lot about everything, but their word is not the end." Mary continues:

> Looking back on the next two months, I kept a lot
> from him and I normally don't do that. I am very
> proud of myself because I am a big crybaby and still

I have never cried in front of him. I tried not to because he loves me very much and I knew if he knew how badly I felt that would have made him feel worse because he felt bad because everything he had worked so hard for he could see going down the tubes. He said a couple of times he didn't know if he could have stood it if he had seen me cry. So I think that that has helped. He would not have to worry about us. He could just take care of himself. . . . I didn't know and the average person doesn't know, but when you are injured you have no muscle control from here on down and so you are like a newborn baby. He has to learn to sit up again. Every little thing is such an accomplishment. . . .

At first I didn't cry at all but tried to support him, when he would ask what they were going to do. "Everything is going to be fine." At first he had a period of orneriness. He didn't want to do therapy. I talked with the doctor and therapist to see if it would be okay if I would push him to get up and ready for therapy. I decided then I can't baby him; he is going to have to face reality. I just felt that it was about time that he had some of the responsibility. His mind isn't injured and he can handle that. If I think he is acting like a brat, I tell him. I argue with him just like he was at home.

And now Peter:

Having her around helps me feel manly and gives me security. You do get down. It helps strengthen me. When she is around, I can't weaken and for her it is probably the same way. I know it really helped me. At first the doctor was trying to tell me I was not going to walk again, [but] I wasn't listening. You will probably be able to do everything you did before [I was thinking]. I still haven't accepted that; well, I've accepted but I still believe there is a chance I might walk. I may or I may not. If I do, I do. If I don't, I don't. It is hard. That was the hardest thing to accept, the fact that I may never be able to walk. . . .

I am lucky to have the wife I've got. It's probably harder on her. I worry more about her than I do my not walking again. Look what she is going through, the worry, having to take care of all the responsibilities and all that. Knowing that her life is half wrecked just like mine is. We will be able to do lots, but there will be a lot of things we did together, we can't do. But then maybe now we will be able to spend more time together. I was always busy doing something. I worked ten, twelve, fourteen hours a day. I ain't going to tractor [his work] no more. That kind of bothers me. I am not going to sit in some old building working. I will do something else. My wife is in the antique business, and I've always helped her before. She always has repairs. There is a big need for brass and copper polishing. I can do a pretty lucrative business doing that. Working with her fits my lifestyle. I don't like to be at work at 6:00 A.M. or punch a time clock. It's more leisurely and I will be more on my own time. . . .

My wife handles the household, the kids, animals, all the problems that arise, and her business. The kids have been very good. The children can help with a lot of heavy work, like carrying out the garbage. There's a certain amount of hunting that I will no longer be able to do. I still can deer hunt and shoot from a van though. My wife can now do pretty much on the rehab ward what the nurses do. She wraps my leg in ace bandages and puts the brace on better than most. Faster. It is easy to get in the habit of having somebody push you [in the wheelchair] when you can do it. Or have somebody go and get something when you can do it. You are here to learn to take care of yourself. When you get home, you are not going to have somebody sitting beside you day in

and day out. Do you think that she is going to want
to dress me every morning? That stuff is going to get
old and tired. Pretty soon I am not going to have any
wife. She is not going to baby me. She is only going
to do what I can't do. The rest that I can do I'll do.
. . . After all, who wants to baby-sit a cripple all of
your life and not be able to go out and do things on
your own? She [too] is going to want to go out and do
things on her own. Certain things she will have to do
for me. If she wants to go someplace for the day, I am
not going to say she can't. I know we will have a good
life. I am not going to worry about her when she is
out.

And again, Mary:

I feel like I am helping my husband. He tells me that
he misses me when I'm gone. . . . Before the accident
he did sanding and repairing and I did varnishing and
refinishing in my shop. He can continue to do that.
He can help in a small way in the loading and
unloading of merchandise. He can help on trips.
Instead of my going back East on trips alone, we will
be able to drive back. Go to flea markets together. I
will load up his wheelchair, and he can take things
back to the car. Also there's a need for brass and
copper stripping and polishing, which he can do now.
. . . I am constantly telling him, "What do you mean
you are not going to be able to do that? I don't want
to hear what you can't do because how do you know
until you have tried it?"
　　　There are going to be some bad times because
he has said to me, "How are people going to treat me
when I get out of here?" [My reply:] "They will look
at you not because they are being cruel but because
they don't understand. You are going to have to be the
one to make them feel comfortable." I let him know
that there is not going to be anything that he is not

going to be able to go and do because he is in a wheelchair. It is ridiculous to think that way. . . .

In the past he was able to run to the store in the middle of the evening to get a candy bar or whatever. Now that will be harder. I will probably ask and he will go, but it will be harder. He will want to paint the house but will not be able to reach the high spots. I will have to do that. Lots of little things he will find it harder to do. We love to go to the beach, but we haven't figured out how to get there in the wheelchair. Before when we were traveling, we stopped at motels; now we will have to make sure there is a room at street level. There will be a lot more things I will have to pay attention to, like handicapped parking, ramps, and things. We will have to do some reconstruction of the house but not a lot. . . .

I know when he gets home he won't be any more demanding than now. I get upset with him once in a while now when he says, "Get me this or that." I say, "Haven't you ever heard of the word *please?*" Then he'll catch himself and ask please. He feels so frustrated at not being able to do things for himself.

Now Peter again:

It's the shits to be paralyzed. You lose your sense of balance. The first time they sat me up on the mat, I couldn't do anything. I couldn't sit up. I was like a little baby. I still have my hands and upper part of my body. It is amazing what you can do, but it takes much longer. Yes, it does bother me that I will be dependent on my wife. I won't want her waiting on me. It has kind of ruined her life too because she has got to take care of me. However, if it was her, I would take care of her, but that is different. I wouldn't mind taking care of her as much as I mind her taking care of me. There will be good times and bad times. You have to readjust. It is hard, hard. It was hard for me to accept that I was going to have to depend on a wheelchair, but after being in bed for so long, that son of a bitch looked pretty good! Let me get in and try it out. . . .

She builds me up. She tells me I will be around more and we can spend more time together. "You will be able to travel with me, go on buying trips." Do you think I would polish brass or do any of these things before? Hell no! I didn't have that kind of patience. Now I guess I am going to have to learn it. The reason I didn't have the patience before was because in the back of my mind I would rather be down working on my tractor. I would throw things down and walk off. Maybe now I will have a little more tolerance. Particularly take more time doing it.

I really don't realize the extent of change in my life because I haven't been home yet. Just having to have someone help me get up those two little bitty steps to get into the house. If someone is going to have to help me that is going to really irritate me. If I want to get through a door and can't and have to go around, that is going to irritate me. If I want to get something out of the cupboard, I am not going to be able to reach it. I can tell you right now that I am going to get mad. If I get mad, then she gets mad. If she is sitting down in the other room and I want something out of the cupboard, she can't always get up every two minutes. I am not going to want her to do it and then I am going to get mad because I can get the milk but can't reach the Wheaties. Or something like that. That irritates the shit out of me. So I am just going to wait around until somebody comes around and say, "Hand me the peanut butter." I am not going to call someone clear from the other room. I am going to go without a lot. Self-sacrifice. If she is sewing or something, she is not going to want to put that aside to get me the peanut butter. I don't want to have to reorganize things. Why the hell should they destroy a house just for me. . . . I still plan to go camping. . . .

They haven't talked to me yet about sex, and I
don't know how that will work. We haven't yet, but
I am willing to try. I believe most of sex is up here in
the head anyway. I still have erections. I have to think
about her. Some way, somehow I am going to please
her. I have to. I don't know if I will feel it. I still think
about it.

Mary, after talking about some possible complications, such
as the seriousness of chest colds now or of bladder infections:

We haven't discussed sex too much. It's a wonderful
part of marriage but not the most important part. It's
not totally out of the question from what I have heard.
I will miss it but no more than him. At least I still
have him. It's not important in proving our feelings
for each other. We'll talk about it later. He asked me
one time, what are we going to do about it? I said, let's
just get you well and then we will talk about that.
Since then I have not brought it up because if it is
going to upset him, I won't want to talk about it, right
yet. He joked with two friends about their doing
plastic surgery on him. It is not something that is
completely out of his mind and feeling bad about. He
is still able to joke about it. I hope I am reading him
right. It is going to be like before; it is not the
important part of the marriage. It was not the nucleus
of our marriage.

In summary, in the early months of this particular comeback
phase we can see many of the phenomena noted earlier in this
chapter as characteristic of the phase. For example, we see the
paraplegic with his wife's help beginning to stretch his physical
limitations and to think ahead about putting his and her life
together on a somewhat new basis. We see Mary's crucial role in
some of that, as well as being a body-substitute resource already,

albeit delicately balancing this against the need to make her husband stretch his physical limitations. We sense Peter's early confrontation of at least one of the basic comeback questions: How far back will I come and with regard to what activities? We can also see the beginnings of some of the biographical processes sketched in Chapters Four and Five. This couple may live for many years with more or less stability of the illness and their lives. These years may be punctuated by occasional or frequent acute phases and emergencies and perhaps eventually some physical deterioration on Peter's part and the added strains of that on their marital relationship. However, right now, in this subphase of comeback Peter and Mary are focused intensely on the knife-edge present and the very near future, which they hope will be better.

Case 2: Recovering from Congestive Heart Failure

Again we shall focus on theoretical points highlighted by the particular illness and by the longer span of comeback covered in the case history. The points in this case pertain mainly to body failure, body performance, self-performance, the conditions for and consequences of specific BBC formulations, and something of the spouse's agentry and biographical phasing during her husband's comeback. (See Chapters Four and Five for the abstract discussion of these phenomena.)

The story begins in 1972 with Professor Einshtein's mild heart attack, which was followed by a gradual return to approximately normal life. Then, in October of 1980, he was rescued from a potentially fatal bout of congenital heart failure. Eventually, he was sent home, restricted to his house, instructed not to move around too much at first, given a complex drug regimen, and advised it would be around six months before anyone could know the extent of his potential comeback. The cardiologist was new to the case and did not know his patient's physical capacities but believed—though saying nothing of this—that the amount of recovery was likely to be slight. However, one of the drugs was fairly experimental, so the cardiologist thought it might work well.

During the next three months, the professor faithfully followed the prescribed regimen and waited and hoped more or less patiently for his energy to return. His wife kept a watchful eye on all of this, occasionally suggesting he rest or sleep, for she became expert at reading cues about the likelihood of his immediate "falling apart" before he himself knew it. She also learned to cook interesting meals without salt since a low-salt diet had been prescribed. Indeed, figuring out how to stay within the daily limits of allowed sodium became a joint enterprise during the first weeks until Mrs. Einshtein—an anxious control agent—felt confident enough to relinquish her part in overseeing this crucial aspect of regimen work. She also made certain that her husband was never alone by ordering groceries by telephone or having friends bring them or cover for her while she was shopping. Hence she was juggling everyday work and the primary aspect of illness work with which she could actually be involved (control agentry, since his regimen entailed work that only he could do: take medications, rest, and adhere to his diet). Meanwhile, for many months, she cut back drastically on her daily volunteer work at an important organization, work that she had been deeply engaged in for three decades. Both spouses communicated very openly about the necessity and problem of the illness work, the handling of everyday work, and their respective biographical concerns. From the beginning of the medical crisis and thereafter, their work together was highly collaborative.

Meanwhile, relieved of his obligations to engage in university work, the professor, while waiting for his body to mend, tried to rest and relax by rereading favorite novels. "That was all I could manage anyhow." Later he progressed to reading Stendahl's *The Red and the Black* in French: "as a sign to myself of progress in concentrating, and as a mild intellectual task." Although he continued to play the piano, his chief hobby, he confined himself to slow pieces and stopped practicing because that either took too much energy or resulted in too much physical stress. In later months he progressed cautiously to playing faster, but for three years he did not allow himself to practice intensively.

There was, however, a discrepancy between his coming to terms with two aspects of his physical limitation. After the professor had, again, become completely mobile, he became reconciled to no longer driving his car and to missing buses because he dared not allow himself to run for them; yet he has never quite come to terms with seeing his wife lift baggage off the airport luggage belt, though she has developed techniques of sharing that division of labor by getting nearby males to do the heavy work that her husband can no longer do. After hospitalization, he was reconciled to temporary bodily limitations that prevented his doing his share of the daily housework, but even four years later he could never quite adjust to being unable to relieve her of heavier tasks such as vacuuming the carpets and taking out the garbage.

In January, as the start of the new teaching quarter approached, Professor Einshtein arranged to teach a small graduate seminar at his house. At first he had sufficient energy to guide the seminar discussion but not enough to talk very much. Gradually, he participated more vigorously. Soon he was also allowed to attempt walking a bit outdoors; however, he was unable to do this because of the almost immediate appearance of agina pain that was otherwise held in check by medications. His own trajectory scheme was to get going as fast as possible with his walking because of his layman ideas about good exercise (although warned by the cardiologist not to do much of that). As another month went by and he still could not walk, the professor was disappointed in his body's performance. He was puzzled too because paradoxically by now "my head was completely clear, and in fact I had already, in mid-January, embarked on writing the monograph that I'd planned actually to begin in October."

He was writing a few hours a day, again under his wife's watchful eye and her occasional reminders: "Don't you think you should rest now?" and "You've worked enough today; knock off now." He wrote by hand rather than using the more energy-consuming typewriter because lowered energy was *the* most disruptive symptom in his life. Energy was a central resource that he could never quite count on despite careful pacing of his activities. Then, as even now, four years later, he had to adapt to unpredictable low-energy periods, mostly in the morning or late afternoon, by not engaging in work until the period passed or he had napped a bit. So he was frustrated all the more that this part of his life was being fulfilled but that walking, again an essential

part of his hoped for—indeed assumed—future, was out of pace
with his thinking and writing activities. As he phrased it:

> My mind was normal, working effectively, as long as
> I was not in a low-energy period, meaning mostly in
> the morning hours, but my body was lagging far
> behind. I could not even walk a block without angina!
> Sudden and unpredictable loss of energy, which
> plagues cardiacs like me, sometimes even now four
> years later, was tolerable, but the prospect of not being
> able to walk for month after month was not.

In short, his "normal" scholarly and teaching work was in
alignment with his visualization of appropriate comeback pacing,
but his mobility was puzzlingly and frustratingly off schedule. His
mental comeback quite literally prevented him from confronting the
possibility that a fair degree of physical comeback would not also be
earned by adhering to the prescribed regimen of drugs, diet, rest, and
sensibly paced activities. After all, the signs of some physical recovery
were progressively encouraging, especially in terms of gradually
increased energy, lessened need for sleep, and so on.

The professor comforted himself with the memory that his
cardiologist had warned him that it would not be until about April
that the degree of his comeback could be known because it would
take that length of time for the physical mending and the effect of
the drugs to permit a fairly accurate assessment. Nevertheless, in
mid-February the patient expressed his frustration and puzzlement
to the physician, who quite forgetting his earlier statement now said
bluntly. "You may never walk again." For the recipient of this
announcement, the statement constituted a comeback crisis—not in
the sense of having suffered a dramatic setback in his physical
condition but in having his trajectory and biographical projections
crushingly contradicted.

Of course, the physician's pessimistic announcement resulted in a great deal of biographical work for the patient as he
began, with dismay, to imagine a life confined forever to his house
and without his university position, a possibility he had not
seriously entertained for two or three months now. However, only

a couple of months later, when indeed he was walking some and finally allowed himself to attend a concert (or rather his wife allowed him to attend!), did he learn from a chance meeting with his internist that the cardiologist had recently expressed astonishment at his current progress since none whatever had been anticipated. "He expected you to be a cardiac cripple." This knowledge plus the recent rapid but still limited progress in mobility fortified the professor's belief that he could get still better and that his determination to do so, in conjunction with continued careful adherence to the regimen, would contribute to that progress. His conception was not so much mind over body as mind working *with* body to improve the latter's condition and performance.

There was still the looming key question, however, of how much farther the mending of his cardiac system, abetted by drugs, would take him along the comeback trail. As is characteristic in many cardiac recoveries, Professor Einshtein was still having unpredictable but not unexpected minutes or hours of light-headedness, occasional days of low energy and general listlessness, and frequent episodes of late afternoon "falling apart" when he had no option but to sleep. Most distressing of all was his inability to sustain dependably the longer conversations he was now having with friends or the work sessions with individual graduate students despite careful scheduling with his visitors. In short, his daily and even hourly physical condition was not yet, and might never be, predictable.

Although he was often impatient at the slowness of his recovery, the professor handled the situation with a fair amount of cheerful resignation—especially since his scholarly thinking and writing were progressing steadily—despite more than occasional impatience with his flawed body. He kept his anxiety about the future in check through his *resolve* to get better and by putting off as best he could any thoughts about a possible homebound future. He and his wife watched for, found, and eagerly discussed all bodily cues and performance markers that suggested or indicated any regression.

Mrs. Einshtein firmly believed that the will to get better was contributing to her husband's progress and concealed some of her own doubts, although unwittingly she signaled her continued anxiety and fear of a setback by focusing on the necessity of his staying well below the sodium limits set by the cardiologist. Indeed, as the need for her control agentry decreased, her own biographical phasing shifted to more overt anxiety about his not breaking that diet. She also carefully monitored his ordering of food at restaurants until later he persuaded her that he was ready to cross that barrier to normal existence too.

The central importance of performance trials and their successes was vital during this period. No longer was it simply enough to be able to walk a couple of blocks. The professor now was able to walk farther, to spend increasingly long hours with visitors, to go to a small and undemanding dinner party, to entertain a small group at home, and to attend a concert. During all these trials he found himself complimenting his body when it worked successfully and being annoyed with it or reconciled to its slow comeback when it failed him. His attitude now was that the body itself (as an acting subject) was on trial during the performance trial. So his body was both object and subject simultaneously.

Eventually, he passed a very difficult and significant performance test. He accepted an invitation to give a guest lecture in one of his colleague's classes. At the conclusion of his talk, he was elated. "felt marvelous both psychologically and physically." That performance represented a turning point for his self-confidence, optimism about further comeback, and faith in an astonishing body—astonishing even to the cardiologist by now. The professor did not deceive himself, however, that his comeback was due solely to a mending body and perhaps his determination to succeed, for "without the drugs I would have been dead in no time."

Finally, ten months after his hospitalization, Professor Einshtein successfully completed a carefully planned trip to a professional convention in a distant city. His wife reluctantly permitted the trip only after he had promised to limit his activities to receiving a professional honor and visiting with a very few friends, "but no running around—you can't do that yet, and anyhow I won't have it." A month later, he was back teaching classes but this time only small graduate seminars. He had decided against ever again teaching the more energy-depleting larger classes.

He also changed his usual teaching schedule from late afternoon, when he was most likely to be very tired, to the more manageable early afternoon hours. His physical recovery continued for perhaps another six months. Then unexpectedly, to himself and his physician, the professor's physical condition abruptly improved; his lowered energy and slight dizziness virtually disappeared. In short, his two-year plateau had risen to another level. Plateau, of course, involves not merely his physical state but all the implicated illness work, everyday work, professional work, and the intensity or amount of social interaction that he could maintain. Understandably, too, the jump in comeback level profoundly affected his views of his body (his BBC) and his expectations about his future years.

As for his wife, once he had returned to work a year after hospitalization, she felt that she could resume her own work life. However, her biographical phasing was different because, understandably, she still was experiencing anxiety about leaving him home alone, albeit happily at work there. She experienced the spouse's not uncommon difficulty in letting go. After all, for an entire year her days had been devoted to aspects of necessary illness work and to housework.

A final analytical remark about this comeback case should be useful. The professor had to face a critical decision about the patterning of his work life. For two decades, he had organized and led small research teams, one after another, and had obtained considerable amounts of funding for that research. His last funding ran out about two years after his hospitalization. Was he to continue with this research pattern, was he up to it, should he settle perhaps for working collaboratively with one or two people, and if so, then write fewer or no monographs but settle rather for writing papers? Implicated in those questions were trajectory and biographical considerations. To be sure, the decision was made neither quickly nor without inner turmoil. Even after his decision to put off any attempts at raising grant money for a time at least, with a further wait-and-see attitude, the actual rearrangement of his work life took many months to iron out. It involved not only coming to terms with his decision but setting up an organizational pattern of partly working alone on his own projects and partly working vigorously with several individual friends on joint projects. This arrangement seems to suit his current physical capacities, his need to monitor and husband his energies, and the general necessity for pacing work so as not to exceed his perceived physical limits.

Although he can now do scholarly work on only a slightly reduced basis, he is reminded of his limits by more than occasional "low" hours, infrequent listless days, and sometimes annoying angina while working. On the other hand, he is happily surprised by those rare days when he awakes and feels

> quite as I used to before I ever became sick. I feel light, springy; there is ease and delight in moving, and unself-consciously so. Anything seems possible, even for my head. I don't necessarily feel like plunging into work, for it seems like the work will be easy to do when once I get to it. I have to remind myself that it can't last and won't. And of course it is all likely to vanish within some hours. It's a reminder, but not a sad one, while it lasts, of what life and you used to be like. What days and activity used to be like. And so it's a reminder of what you have actually come to terms with. No regrets are allowed, or you would have to reopen that Pandora's box. If not the workhorse I was, at least I have pretty much come to terms with my limitations and my life.

But to summarize what he recently confessed to his wife: "Nevertheless, I know there are invisible changes taking place inside that ailing cardiac system of mine. I don't kid myself about that—but I try not to dwell on that."

In closing our discussion of this case, we suggest the usefulness now of reviewing the list of conditions for a successful comeback given on pages 175-176. The professor's case history fits perfectly each of the necessary conditions listed there. Of course, one must not forget that the nature of a cardiac illness, involving its characteristic lowered energy and tendency to angina, is also a central condition affecting both the form and content of this particular variant of a comeback trajectory.

Case 3: Recovering from a Stroke—Four Phases of Comeback

In this case the physical symptoms again greatly affect the specifics of the comeback. The main problem in recovery from stroke is mobility. Therefore, the comeback here primarily involves improvement in stricken limbs, including the return of sensation and the ability to navigate somewhat normally again.

In presenting the analytic features of this case, we shall highlight additional characteristics of the comeback phase after severe physical and psychological trauma. Thus, an understanding both of the variations in comeback contingencies and experiences and of the general patterning of this type of phasing can be deepened. The chief analytical focus will be on the important subphases of comeback. Since various types of work and their relationships take their coloration from and lend character to the different subphases, these features of the phasing will be front and center in our selective account of the long climb upward by a celebrated dancer-choreographer, Agnes de Mille, as described vividly in her eloquent *Reprieve* (1981). The biographical accompaniments of her phasing are also prominent in her narrative and our quotations from it.

De Mille's illness trajectory began, as usual, with an initial awareness that something was wrong with the body. It no longer performed as it should and once did. We shall term this the *discovery* subphase. The discovery in her case was sudden; she had moved into an obviously acute phase of illness. De Mille was rehearsing a group of dancers for a gala opening night at the theater. In the midst of the rehearsal, on the afternoon preceding the performance, she suffered a stroke and was rushed to the hospital. The physician's prognosis was grave. He was not sure that she would survive the body assault. However, she believed that she would live.

Once settled into the hospital, de Mille had a series of trajectory and biographical reviews through which she came to contextualize the illness into her biography. She describes compar-

ing her present body state with her body before the stroke and the
changes in her self-conception that resulted from this comparison.
She refers to the sane, excited woman of the morning as now a
"depersonalized lump that could hardly babble her name and had
begun to drool, an aged, crouched husk of a creature" (p. 29). She
also writes of a symptomatic review in which she gave light to her
present situation by relating it back to her high blood pressure and
unheeded signs of impending trouble, such as having in the past
lost track a couple of times of what she was saying or doing. She
projected forward in time and asked, "Will I recover my speech,
vision, mobility, memory?"

As in all crisis situations, the peripheral aspects of life are
trimmed, and so at first her life revolved around and was caught up
in the basics of survival. "I was taken up with the minutiae of
living. Everything was so extraordinarily difficult and so new to
perform. Every single act became a contest of skill, and games can
be tiring" (p. 46). Eventually, however, the basics became routinized, and she began exploring the extent of her limitations, arriving
at the realization that her body had indeed failed her. There
followed feelings of extreme anger. There was "no exit" from this
situation.

However, she did not give up; she decided that she wanted
a future, although one that would be different from the present. And
so, she writes, "I tackled my strange and maimed existence" (p. 64).
Thus, she moved into a second major subphase: *embarking upon
the comeback trail.*

Four important conditions for embarking wholeheartedly
and successfully now come into play. First, there must be an
initiator, someone such as the physician who initiates the medical
and rehabilitative plan and then sets it in motion. Second, at the
same time, the affected individual must have a hopeful biographical
projection and goals to work toward, while accepting the medical
and rehabilitative scheme as necessary to achieving those goals. All
the rehabilitation in the world will not bring back a person who has
suffered a stroke and who for one reason or another refuses to do
the necessary assigned work. Third, he or she must be mobilized.
Mobilization comes as the result of having accomplished the
prerequisite biographical work in confronting the situation and

coming to terms with it at least provisionally: accepting limitations but believing that they can be stretched and therefore having confidence in a better future. De Mille, explaining why she and those in situations similar to hers are willing to do the work required of them, writes: "The work requires iron discipline, because one hopes to be useful and effective. . . . There was only one single thing that was ours; the determination to do what we wished to do no matter how awkward, how maimed, how slow" (p. 68). Fourth, the total plan must be right, right medically, rehabilitatively, and biographically. If it is found wanting, then one must revise the plan until there is a fit between it and oneself.

All four conditions being met, recollect that comeback requires not only long, tedious, and at times superhuman effort by the affected person but also the coordinated efforts of other workers who share in a division of labor according to their respective specialties and abilities. In short, comeback requires teamwork. Each participant moves in and out of the division of labor according to the trajectory phase and its associated contingencies, including the biographical. In de Mille's case, the team consisted of a variety of members. There were her physicians, who developed and implemented the therapeutic plan and initiated the rehabilitation. They spent long hours watching over her and monitoring her physical status and progress. They ordered diagnostic tests to give clues as to what was going on within her body. They intervened to prevent crises. There were her nurses, who not only carried out the regimen and provided for her basic physical needs and comfort but also urged her to stretch limitations by participating in her own care as much as she was able to. There were the various body retrainers—the occupational therapists, physical therapists, and speech therapists who provided the actual stretching exercises. They also supervised her own attempts at rehabilitation. There were her spouse and son, who let her know that she was loved and needed. They also gave assistance in little ways, praised her efforts, and worked at keeping her spirits up although at times they were down. There was her friend Mary, who took over the work of notifying other friends about the illness, screening calls, and handling the mail. There were her many friends and associates who called, came, and sent flowers to let her know that she was cared about. Each person in his or her own way contributed to de Mille's comeback.

At first, most of de Mille's efforts were directed at body mending and the stretching of physical limitations, tasks that used up most of her time and energy. Eventually, those tasks became routinized and insufficient to meet her growing desire to move beyond where she presently was. At this turning point, the biographical processes came to the fore; that is, reknitting was added to mending and rehabilitation. Reknitting begins when the ill person reaches the point of wanting to get on with normal life. It may become prominent at somewhat different points in the comeback phasing, depending on the degree and type of body assault sustained and the importance of various activities affected by the body's failure. The nature of early reknitting varies according to a person's unique biography. For some, the reknitting may take the form of seeing specific friends, others may begin to call business colleagues, and still others may begin to manage their homes from afar.

De Mille visited with family and friends, using the telephone as soon as she was able. One of her major reknitting acts was to send for the manuscript of the book she was working on before she became ill. She knew that she could not resume her dancing and choreography but could attempt another important and, at least currently, more feasible aspect of her self: writing. Strikingly evident in this period was her frustration yet determination, as she attempted to manipulate her papers and get her thoughts down. Because the papers kept slipping through her fingers, falling to the floor and even out of reach, she kept them on a special table next to her where they would be constantly visible. When she couldn't work on them, she let her eyes rest on them. They represented a means toward the future, a goal she could obtain through work in the right now present. "I thought of them in the night and they were a promise. It is not enough to live in 'now' as we have been told. We have to surmise 'tomorrow'" (p. 76). And she asked the temporal biographical questions: "Will I begin lecturing in six months? In eight? Can I take a theater job in a year? How soon?"

Retraining an uncooperative body is not only hard work, it can also be frightening. Normally the body parts work in unison and can be controlled at will; but the failed body often becomes the frighteningly uncontrollable body. "I began the real exercises, the exercises that were not boring, like hand therapy, but frightening. I stood between the couple bars, one hand on each, which was comfortable and felt safe, except that the right hand was of no use and kept falling off." Also, she was encouraged to stand and then walk. It was terrifying. "Every time I put the right foot out, I trusted the whole of the rest of the mechanism—my head and my breath and my heart and my viscera—to what?" (pp. 83–84).

One's past biography is more than something to look back upon with grief: it can become a crucial resource to enhance development of a better future. In de Mille's case, people were constantly expressing sympathy as to how hard it must be for her, a dancer, to be faced with so many limitations. Her response to this statement was that precisely because she was a dancer and had submitted herself to the physical and mental discipline required to train her body, she was able now to meet the strenuous demands needed for retraining her body.

Often, as noted earlier, a comeback course is marred by setbacks or interruptions that may result in a temporary or permanent standstill or, if severe, a reversal in progress already painfully made. De Mille experienced such a setback when she developed an embolism. The rehabilitation and reknitting, of course, came to a halt temporarily while the focus of everyone's attention was again on her potential crisis.

During the interim between the development of these symptoms and the time that medical action was finally taken, de Mille felt as though she was slowly slipping away from life. She did an accounting review of her past life and through it gained closure, coming to terms with both her past and projected near—future death. However the medical crisis was to be resolved, she had reached a critical juncture on the comeback trail, for the continued assaults on her body weakened her will to live. Again, the physician stepped in, weighing the medical risk of sending her home against the emotional risk of keeping her hospitalized. He opted for sending her home. Again, this emphasizes the importance of the right person's coming up with the right plan at the right time if comeback is to progress further.

The transition from hospital to home often forces the ill to confront their limitations as trajectory and biography considerations again come together in new ways. De Mille now faced a biographical crisis since the future and what to do with it, along with her past, now confronted her. She knew that she could never entirely recapture her past, yet the future loomed ahead. She was standing at a crossroad and had to move on, but what direction should she take?

The biographical decrystallization that took place as she confronted the present and probable future, and the subsequent recrystallization that occurred as she began to work through her problems moved her upward to a third subphase of comeback, *finding new pathways to a meaningful life.* "I was going through this gray area to a new kind of life with entirely new rules and new values. The question was: Could I survive the spiritual shock as I had survived the physical one?" (p. 159). She wanted to get well. She wanted to regain as much functional ability of her body as possible. She wanted to find biographical fulfillment. There was work to be done, but by whom and how? In this illness, as in many others, the regimen work was strenuous and was now largely her own responsibility. She had been sent home with many, many drugs, "together with a printed list of instructions, single-spaced, a full page long, giving me a daily schedule, so complicated that I had to follow my orders line by line" (p. 157).

In addition, de Mille had to visit the hospital daily for rehabilitation therapy. There was also a home to manage and business affairs to attend to but limited energy and mobility at her command. So how did the work get done? Again we see a variety of workers doing a variety of tasks, the articulation of the two lines of work shifting between her husband and her. He, for instance, besides planning carefully for her homecoming, took over the physicians' and nurses' monitoring of her condition. Then he acted as a comeback coach, prodding her to stretch her physical limitations. He teased her "like a football coach towards health, cheering me through the exercises, baiting me to try in all daily matters. Try harder, try better" (p. 192). His vigilance and love, along with that of her son and sister, kept her from despairing during these trying times. Her husband also did body work for her, acting temporarily as a "trained nurse." In turn, she had to learn to live with that.

For stroke victims, comeback also means moving beyond present physical boundaries, often a painful, exhausting, step-by-step process. "I took my pronged tripod and I started out. Shuffle. Close. Shuffle. Close. With pain, with exhaustion and, yes, with fear. As far as the laundry door. . . . As far as the first stairway" (p. 173). This subphase of finding new pathways also involves learning again about bodies. The boundaries of physical or mental limitations must be discovered and rediscovered under varying conditions of living. Sensations and bodily alarm systems, once taken for granted, have to be relearned in new and sometimes very subtle forms. For example: "I would have to learn these different pains . . . learn the tingling that meant I had a wrinkle in my stocking as opposed to the tingling that meant someone was standing on my foot" (p. 180).

After much hard work, people like de Mille begin to see the fruits of their labors. The body has mended to some degree. There is more energy and less mental confusion. The person finds that the boundaries of limitations have moved outward and so is less dependent and can engage in more meaningful activities. A future different from the near past and even the immediate present lies before one. This recrystallization of the self mobilizes the person to move to the next comeback phase: *scaling the peak*. The summit is in sight; one only has to make the final effort to reach it—perhaps not regaining full normal processes of performance but at least a satisfying level of performance. What happens now is that the ill person, inspired by past and current progress, increases efforts to make the final effort needed to ascend to the peak: "Finally—and this is very difficult—you must realize that your situation is changing. As you become increasingly less dependent, you must push yourself to do for yourself as far as you can, no matter how exhausting, no matter how troublesome" (p. 191).

Also very important is the simultaneous accomplishment of coming to terms with physical limitations. For there may often be final residual limitations that must be dealt with on a daily basis. Sometimes these boundaries seem unimportant. At other times they come rushing in before one realizes what is happening. De Mille, along with others who suffer from the aftermath of strokes, was confronted with limitations and the subsequent identity blows. In speaking of her son's wedding, she describes how the bride went into her father's arms to dance, while her son at this point should have reached for his mother. Instead, he danced with the bride's mother. It was then, at another crucial turning point, that de Mille felt the full impact of her physical limitations.

Normally, illness and its limitations are thought of in a negative sense. While very few people would deliberately choose this path, when placed on it they at least sometimes do come to terms with it. They do this by letting go of the past, grieving in the present, and embracing the future. Some not only come to accept the situation but even manage to transcend their limitations by giving new meaning to life and finding in it the means to an even more rewarding future. De Mille's transcendence is expressed in sentences such as this one: "I went deeper and deeper into states of being I had never dreamt of before, states of perceiving and feeling that had nothing to do with achievement or business or duty or morals. I was awake" (p. 205). And looking back on her life, she could view "the entire middle age, as stale, used up, worn out, faded—in short, old—and the new life which had begun since the stroke as a fresh gift (pp. 205-206). Sometimes one has to take a step backward before one can take a giant leap forward. De Mille's step backward came with the crushing news that she would have to wear a leg brace. Before her flashed visions of herself as a cripple, "like a polio victim." Again, the right person moved in at the right time to provide her with the needed push; this time a therapist explained that the brace would help her to feel more confident when she walked and allow her muscles to strengthen. To her astonishment, she found that although the brace is cumbersome, it does provide support and comfort. She even came up with a biographical device to soften the blow—wearing beautiful Chinese style silk pants to cover the brace. Moreover, reaching a later style of comeback also can be signaled by some dramatic event. De Mille threw away the blacks, grays, and browns among her clothes, replacing them with bright colors. "So, another flag went up the mast to signal my recovering and making my new life a happy one" (p. 223).

Ill people reach the final subphase—or perhaps *one* of the

final steps of comeback—*validation,* when they reach a juncture where they feel sufficiently mended, stretched, and biographically reknitted to more or less fully take their place among others in the world at large. Validation occurs through a series of successful performances that prove to oneself and to others that there has indeed been a genuine comeback. The consequence is the feeling that one is contributing, that one is fulfilled. This moving out into the world is usually accomplished gradually, although there may be a crowning validating event. The legitimizing activities may be thought out and deliberately set up or occur as unexpected contingencies. In this proving of oneself, other people are essential as audiences, and sometimes they are fully aware of participating in the validating events.

A year and a quarter after her stroke, de Mille felt ready to add to a considerable return to a normal life by also resuming her professional career in the dance world. While still hospitalized, she had been sent scripts for two Broadway shows, one of them very appealing. She sent word that she was ready to discuss the show, only to find the work had been given to another choreographer. The identity blow was severe. It led to a biographical confrontation in which she made an accounting review of her past and future. She asked herself: "What have I truly accomplished? Have I accomplished the creative work I always intended?" The answer was no. What she wants is to leave behind a legacy, a truly creative work that will leave her mark on the world of dance. There followed another recrystallization in which she realized that her life had changed irrevocably and that she would have to take direction more fitting to the present than to the past. Thus she moved into the validation phase of comeback. But to prove oneself, one must have opportunities. De Mille's first major opportunity came when colleagues offered to present an entire evening of her works at Lincoln Center in New York. She was able to take part in the rehearsals. Of this time she later wrote: "I was not tired. Here was health and rebirth."

Even at this point, setbacks can occur. De Mille suddenly suffered a coronary. She was hospitalized but kept the fact secret since she did not want anyone to know for fear it would invalidate her proclamation of health so that henceforth no one would be willing to take a chance on her. She wanted "to rejoin the living, the doers" (p. 272).

During this second hospitalization, the Joffrey Ballet reconstructed her dance *Rodeo,* which proved again to be a thundering success. With this in mind, after a short period of recovery, she approached the director of the Joffrey with the idea that his company do her *Conversations About the Dance,* the piece that had been abruptly interrupted by her stroke. He agreed. Once the work was in progress, she found herself not only happy to be back at her work but able to move her arm and hand more freely than at any time since the stroke. However, the work was strenuous and, for her, risky. Her husband asked why she felt compelled to take such risk, to which she replied: "I had to live, I felt I had to function the best way I knew how . . . I needed activity. I must *do*" (p. 274).

Final validation came in dramatic fashion. De Mille worked hard to make the ballet performance a success. So did those around her, her collaborating colleagues, the dancers, and the stagehands. The night of the performance, even the audience joined the team, coordinating their actions with hers, making validation a cooperative endeavor. She says of that evening: "Would I remember? Would I hold onto myself? I said the first sentences without notes and there was a cracking laugh. . . . They were with me. They were ahead of me. They intended that I succeed. They would not let me fail" (p. 285).

While her performance was marked by more drama than would occur for most of us, such validations as we saw earlier in the instance of Professor Einshtein's guest teaching are frequent turning points in the lives of people struggling to make successful comebacks. It is worth reemphasizing that validations are more than events; rather, they are constituted by successful performances, a passing of crucial self-tests, in which audiences are likely (whether aware or not) to participate. These validating performances are different from other important tests because they put the recovering person metaphorically as well as physically over the top.

In this long case narrative about Agnes de Mille, we have selected only those features that highlight major subphases of this and other comebacks: (1) discovery, (2) embarking on the comeback trail, (3) finding new pathways to a meaningful life, (4) scaling the peak, and (5) validation. Moving from subphase to subphase, one can readily recognize the shifting specifics of the work types entailed and their subtypes, as well as the various work processes (resource calculating, mutual sustaining, etc.), the sequencing of biographical processes, and the evolution of interaction processes through which actual work gets done. Implicit but not underlined in our selective narrative are the outer rings of the conditional matrix discussed in Chapter Seven that constitute sets of broader conditions bearing on all of this phasing and its associated phenomena.

Summary

Theory. A quick scan of our opening theoretical points about the comeback phenomena will help to bring this chapter full circle, for the experiences of the actors in all three case presentations run true to them. Each story, however, is analyzed and selectively presented to emphasize certain features of comebacks. The cases concern (1) a paraplegic and his wife doing individual and joint biographical work in the face of his physical disaster; (2) a cardiac whose story illustrates body imagery, body-mind distinctions, rehabilitation strategies, plateaus and their psychological meaning, and his spouse's agentry and some of her biographical phasing; (3) Agnes de Mille's partial comeback from a stroke, illustrating especially trajectory and biographical phasing, types of trajectory work, work processes, and crucial relationships with her life's work and its audiences.

Applications. One practical implication of the major theoretical issues brought out in this chapter is that because comeback is really a threefold process made up of medical, rehabilitative, and biographical interactive strands, one must when planning interventions assess and consider each both individually and for combined interactive effects.

A second important implication is that health professionals should help to create the conditions that will foster comeback. These conditions include helping people to establish realistic expectations, to develop schemes that are amenable to their lifestyles and biographical needs, and then to coordinate these schemes to the types of work to be done by the various workers. Most of all, however, health professionals should give the ill the push, the motivation to get started and to keep going, especially when they experience setbacks or when they seemingly get stuck at plateaus.

Finally, practitioners need to be aware of the subphases of comeback and the fact that the types of work and where the emphasis is placed differ with each phase and that the performance of each type of work requires sensitivity and even adaptability on the part of each worker. For example, assistance given in one phase may be detrimental if continued into the next; on the other hand, failure to provide that assistance when needed may kill motivation. Only the ill person involved can make a comeback, but comeback itself requires the supplementary, supportive, and directive efforts of other people in coordination with the needs and efforts of the person coming back.

9

Stable Phases: Maintaining an Equilibrium

Throughout this book we have emphasized that the management of chronic illness and/or disability at home involves work and that this work affects the lives of the ill and their spouses. In comeback, downward, and unstable phases of trajectory the intensity of work and its impact on living is easy to visualize. But how many of us realize what it means to live with a chronic condition that is fairly stable day after day, year after year?

The purpose of this chapter is to depict the giving and taking, the strength and fortitude, the courage and creativity demanded of those who are considered to have a stable chronic condition, and at the same time to portray the tension, frustration, sweat, and sometimes tears that arise from trying to juggle the management of severe chronic illness or disability along with other types of work so that the ill or disabled and those close to them do not have to foreclose on living. Stability is not merely a physiological state but very much a matter of keeping illness work, biographical work, and everyday work in a balanced and mutual relationship.

To convey all of this, we shall present excerpts from interviews that describe in the words of couples in our study what they face and how they manage. But before doing so, let us step back momentarily to reexamine some general properties of the management of stable phases discussed earlier in order to direct them specifically toward the interpretation of the case materials that follow.

Properties of Stable Trajectory Management

Stable phases are those in which all three major lines of work are in relative equilibrium because the illness or disability is in a somewhat steady state (moving neither rapidly upward or downward). This allows for the routinizing of the various types of work. That is, routines are established for articulating the work by obtaining and using resources, providing a division of labor, and sustaining motivation for work performance. One of the major problems, however, is that work performance occurs so much by rote and habit that the amount of time, energy, and effort actually put forth to keep the illness itself stable (and to keep some sense of balance among the major lines of work) is in many instances not recognized either by health professionals or those actually engaged in the work at home. As a consequence, the negative effects of these efforts are often insidious. They develop gradually and become well established before they become apparent. They finally emerge when illness complications bring about conflict between the spouses or even illness in the once healthy partner.

An important feature in keeping an illness or disability stable is the requirement that the illness work be *continuous,* as are everyday and biographical work (Schneider, 1985). Then, too, there are regimens (Conrad, 1985) and body limitations to manage: How can I go out to dinner at seven o'clock with my friends, when I have to eat by six because I am diabetic? Or, how do I get to the corner to catch the bus that I see coming, when running gives me angina but knowing that if I miss the bus I will be late for my scheduled appointment? Such situations present challenges that one must face, complicate the performance of any one or combination of the types of work that one must do, and create the potential for disruption of a delicate balance among the lines of work.

To help keep those lines in balance, the ill and those around them usually establish routines for work performance. Yet routines evolve slowly and over time. Why? First, the ill must learn about their illnesses, their bodily responses, how best to carry out regimens, and how their bodies respond to the regimens where there is disability; moreover, they must learn the limits of their disability and how and when to push their limits outward so as to accomplish important biographical and everyday work. At the same time they must also learn how not to stretch beyond their limits and so bring about temporary or even permanent dips and drops in their illness. Furthermore, they must learn how to perform biographical and everyday tasks under new and possibly difficult conditions. Doing all of this means discovering ways of handling the tasks successfully.

Second, since illness work takes place within the context of daily living, the management routines are often interrupted by contingencies arising out of that living. If not anticipated or handled properly, a trip, dinner out with friends, or working overtime can have a detrimental effect on the ability to keep the illness stable and life stable or even seriously impair later functional ability. Moreover, planning does not necessarily forestall the occurrence of the unexpected. Conversely, the advent of an illness or disability-related complications or an increase in symptoms can disrupt daily routines. In fact, most people who have been ill for some time have developed a set of alternative routines—routines to cover for the usual routines—for dealing with just such situations.

However, one cannot talk about the management of stable phases without talking about the *intrusiveness* of illness upon living itself (Fisher and Galler, 1987). Being out in the world means that the ill and disabled are constantly being confronted by what is going on in that world. In turn, being ill or disabled (although "stable") frames what they are able to do, how they do it, and how others respond to their doing it. Of course, not all ill people feel the effects to the same degree; even those with similar types of illnesses and degrees of physiological impairment will experience their effects differently. Nor is illness always in the foreground. Much depends upon the circumstances in which the ill find themselves, including life-style, the type of household and family composition, their biographical schemes and projections, and the importance that the performance of certain biographical tasks has for them.

Reviewing the examples above one might ask how important it is for the diabetic person to go out to dinner with those friends or how important it is for the person prone to angina to be on time for an appointment. Such confrontations place the ill in situations in which they must either knowingly stretch their limits or come to terms with their limitations. How they respond when faced with these dilemmas has consequences not only for the illness course but for their lives. For instance, a lover of gourmet food may be willing to accept a low-sodium, low-cholesterol diet when eating at home but find the diet very constraining when eating out with friends. In this situation he or she may stay within the limits of the prescribed diet or simply ignore them, possibly to the consternation of the onlooking spouse. Also, while a dependent person may have come to terms with having to rely on a spouse for certain activities of daily living, he or she may later find an increase in dependence (brought about by an acute illness) unbearable. Even the best-adjusted stable person can feel the renewed intrusiveness of illness or disability under new or differing life conditions that force him or her to face the meaning of that illness or disability once more. This leads, of course, to more rounds of biographical work (a coming to terms again and again).

Usually, to get around just such situations, the stable ill develop personal routines to manage their illness, their biographical performances, and everyday occurrences. For a diabetic, this may mean eating a snack at six o'clock before going out to dinner and then taking extra insulin to compensate for the additional intake, or it may mean informing friends of a need to eat at an earlier time. For a cardiac, it may mean quickly taking an extra nitroglycerin tablet before engaging in any physical activity known to bring on angina or alerting others ahead of time that he might be late for an appointment. Health professionals can provide guidelines for management, but the ill are left very much on their own in discovering how to implement such guidelines! Sometimes the ill make errors in judgment or find that social situations do not allow for an alternative course of action. When this happens, they are left to deal with the consequences. These may be minimal—a couple of bad hours—but at other times the error may result in a lengthy illness complication that puts the ill farther behind in their biographical performances or daily chores.

Thus, much of the "invisible work" and many of the insidious consequences accompanying the maintenance of a stable phase are actually derived from *constant* adjustments and shifts in *routines,* shifts made in response to management obstacles presented by illness, biography, or everyday contingencies. These shifts are vitally necessary to keep the three lines of work in balance. With this in mind let us turn to the case illustrations.

The following cases are meant to illustrate how people

manage to keep their illnesses or disabilities in a stable state and at the same time actively engage in living. The cases differ in terms of the type and degree of illness or disability, the period in the life cycle they represent, the biographical schemes and projections involved, and the management styles that evolve. They illustrate different salient features of stable phase management, some people's situations being more complex than others. What they share in common is that all of the people in them are engaged in an active life, despite their own or their spouse's illness or disability. Therefore, they are faced with the challenge of meeting the obstacles that living places in their paths.

Case 1: Maintaining Stability Through Close Collaboration

Our first case presentation is that of the Jorgensens, a middle-aged couple whose children are grown and have left home. Mrs. Jorgensen has suffered from rheumatoid arthritis for many years. Notice how her pain and functional disability act as conditions that frame her performance of daily chores and affect her marital relationship and work outside the home yet how it is the latter rather than the former that is the focus of her life. While Mrs. J. is now in what might be called a stable phase—meaning there has been no visible change in her condition for some time except for minor dips—there were times when she was far more disabled than she is now. Both partners pursue their respective careers; and both have their own as well as mutual interests.

The words of each spouse will be interspersed throughout the case in order to present a more complete and vivid picture. The salient feature of stable phase management that will be illustrated is how routines function to keep the major lines of work in balance. Not only have this couple developed routines to handle these lines, but they have also come up with an alternative set of routines to draw upon in contingency situations such as traveling. When illness or life conditions change, thus bringing about different circumstances, or the partners see the same situation from different perspectives, then they work out routines for these too. Our presentation is organized in terms of the various categories that have evolved from the analysis of such cases.

Routines for Getting Up and Getting Out. How do a couple manage to arrive at work on time, when one partner awakens in the morning with stiff joints that make it difficult to carry out even the simplest of life's daily activities? Here the Jorgensens tell how they have articulated these activities. Notice how they have worked out a division of labor in which Mrs. J.—using "limitation stretching devices" and a lot of grit—does her part of the work, and how Mr. J. acts as a body resource in certain activities.

According to Mr. J.:

She gets herself out of bed, then she sits on the edge while I make the coffee. [There is also] the routine of the elastic stockings. Sometimes she has episodes where the skin on her legs gets very sore, and I try to stretch the stockings in such a way that they don't rub the skin too much while going on. Then she gets herself into the bathroom—where we have a high toilet—and in some magical way does most of her dressing, while sitting on that high stool. She has a routine that she goes through; and sitting there makes it easier to get into her pantsuits. I usually stay here until she is dressed because she may need help with some parts of dressing, depending upon how she is feeling.

And now Mrs. J.:

We have a routine for morning. Every morning when I wake up, I have all the little bottles on the bedside table and I play pharmacist. I put them in a little container. I get my coffee sitting on the edge of the bed, while I take my pills and begin to move all of my muscles. He listens to the moans and the griping. Mornings are hard. Right now I am going through a nice period, so it is not too bad. But there has been many a morning where he has had to point me to the front door and literally pour me into the car to go to work. He plays it very cool and does anything he can

to help: he hooks my bra and puts on my shoes. To
make it easier to get dressed I have adjusted my
clothing, and he puts on the elastic hose.

Routines for Handling Public Places. The Jorgensens often
eat out or attend theatrical performances. This too can pose
problems. How do you get out of a chair, negotiate stairs, walk long
distances, or wait standing up? But just as important are the
questions faced by Mr. J.: When does he step in, hold back, and
why? These questions pivot around dependence and independence.
The former represents the need for bodily or emotional resources;
the latter pertains to preserving the integrity of one's own or the
other's identity while providing this assistance. Managing this
situation calls for asking oneself, "What in this situation is most at
stake?" Mr. J. has this reply:

> For someone like her you need to know when to come
> or not come running or how to help. Part of it is things
> like moving around the chairs in a restaurant. If she is
> sitting in a chair where she can scoot it against the wall,
> I don't do anything. I just stand there and watch her
> struggle. She doesn't want me to grab her and pull her
> out of the chair. It hurts her anyway. There were times
> when I have had to lift her, and for her these times were
> embarrassing. I guess everybody in a restaurant must
> wonder why I stand there and watch her. But we have
> a system. What I do is hang onto the chair so it doesn't
> slide and she gets herself up.

How Interactional Routines Evolve. Articulating a division
of labor so that two people act in unison, each moving in or moving
out at the right time, takes a great deal of sensitivity and problem
solving. The more experienced the couple, the more likely they will
have worked out a repertoire of routines for handling situations.
Again, Mr. J. explains:

> When you are together all of the time, you work out
> a protocol. I can guess when or when not to come in

on almost all of the activities. After several years you have been through almost everything—that is, you have been through or come across it somewhere.

Routines for Handling Interactions with Others. How do the Jorgensens perceive that other people respond to Mrs. J.'s disabilities? How do the Jorgensens respond in turn? Here are Mrs. J.'s words on the matter:

People so often treat you like you are deaf, dumb, blind, and retarded. People's attitudes . . . as a company we belong to a trade association and some of those people! I was asked to be on a committee and when a man found out I had a walker, he was very concerned because I was to be one of the hostesses. What difference does it make when all I have to do is stand there and talk to people? Other people at a later date felt that I was perfectly competent and that I could even handle a seminar. In fact, they moved my seminar from the ladies' program to the general program and from the second day to the first. They made the adjustments and never thought about it. They put the podium in the wrong place and I had to crawl up the stair. It truly didn't enter their minds. That attitude was almost too much the other way, but I would rather that they don't see you as needing special accommodation than to have them think you are retarded or something.

Routines for Doing "Dirty" Work. Certain tasks in life must be done even though they are unpleasant. But even dirty work doesn't seem quite so dirty if you develop tricks for its performance. Mr. J. describes one routine:

About the only thing that bothers me is getting up in the middle of the night and going through the ritual of putting her on the bedpan. I am sleepy but other-

wise it doesn't bother me particularly. Interestingly
enough, over the years I have worked out ways of
moving with the bedpan so that I hardly ever smell a
thing.

Routines for the Performance of Personal Activities. We take
many aspects of bodily performance for granted. We bend, stretch,
and turn without much thought. Not until we lose this ability—
temporarily or permanently—do we realize what it means to be
disabled. Being disabled means one has to depend on devices and
other people to act as body resources even for the performance of
the most personal daily activities. When these resources are not
available, the ill person just has to make do. Mr. J. states:

Usually she sits in her walker in the shower. She has
a brush and if she is a little stiff on a given day, she
will ask me to come wash her back. The main thing
I do is take care of her feet. There is no way she can
trim her toenails. So we have a routine we go through.
While she watches TV she soaks her feet for a while.
Then I bring my cutter in and do her toenails.

The interesting thing is that I do work some
evenings and she does manage to do things by herself.
Like the bedspread, if I am not here, she manages to
pull it to one side and she can at least get into bed.
Most of the time she can get her bra unhooked but she
can't get it on. I am not sure how she does it. I don't
think I've ever seen her do it. She can't get the elastic
stockings off though. She has to sleep with them on.

Routines for the Performance of Household Tasks. Here
again we see a division of labor based on ability, and the use of the
other partner as a bodily resource. We also see how the division of
labor is rearticulated under differing circumstances. Again, Mr. J.
explains:

She can cook dinner in the wheelchair. But I worry
about her spilling something on her legs because she

moves a lot of hot things. When I hear something
drop in the kitchen now, I go in there because there
is no way she can pick things up off the floor anymore. She does a good part of the cooking. I do things
like cooking the rice partly because I like the rice
better. If she does a big dinner, then it is pretty much
her role to supervise the kids.

According to Mrs. J.:

When I want to do the family shopping, he goes with
me. I used to do all the gardening; now he has to do
it. I used to do a lot of the painting or little things like
that, which now are his responsibility. We cooperate
a lot. Like at meal times, I prepare the dinner and he
clears the table and puts the dishes in the sink. There
is a lot of sharing of the work. Of course, there were
times when I was so ill and down, I didn't know if I
would ever come back. I had to spend a lot of time in
bed. [Then] he just took over totally. He would see to
it that the kids got their dinner and the dishes were
done, the whole bit.

Planning Ahead: Establishing Routines to Handle the
Expected and Unexpected. It is fun to do things spontaneously. But
having a chronic illness can limit spontaneity. For example, before
embarking on a journey or an outing the couple must articulate
certain situations and then come up with appropriate strategies. A
determination to live life to the fullest (within the limits of one's
disability) and the ability to anticipate problems and establish
routines for handling them both seem to be conditions that make
undertaking a voyage or other biographical schemes possible and
successful. Mrs. J. notes:

We work around a lot of situations. For example, I
have run into places that have impossible facilities, so
now I have a portable toilet seat that fits into an
athletic-like bag. It goes with me whenever I travel,

just in case. We also have a motor home that my
husband has remodeled to make it easier for me. Over
the past four years, it has enabled us to travel 25,000
miles.

Additional Conditions that Sustain Work Performance. One
characteristic of stable trajectory management is that the work is
constant. Having routines helps to ease the strain of its constancy
by enabling people to respond habitually. Keeping up with the
work also requires having and sustaining motivation, as Mr. J.'s
words make clear:

> What the illness has done is make the marriage much
> closer knit because there are things that really need to
> be done. I can't just kiss her goodbye and leave in the
> morning. There are things I have to do. That could be
> a nuisance for some personality types, but it doesn't
> bother me. I've never really gotten tired, angry, or
> resentful, partly as a matter of an act of the will and
> partly because I am a very religious fellow and I
> consider it improper to do that. I am the kind that
> takes it as it comes; whatever is necessary, I do it. I
> don't think in the meantime either one of us ever
> spends time dwelling on her impossibilities. . . . My
> wife is the kind that doesn't give up. That is very
> important to me. It means that the things I do for her
> work.

Mrs. J. comments:

> I think we are probably closer now than we ever were.
> I was talking with this friend of mine: "If I had to put
> it on a scale to pay him back, I never could." I try not
> to whine or do the hypochondria bit.

Trajectory Projection: The "Looming Potential." Stability is
only one phase; with arthritis there is always the potential for
progressive body failure and increased disability. Progressive

deterioration stands out as a looming potential—a fateful contingency that can have great biographical consequences. Important here are not only the Jorgensens' respective trajectory projections but their schemes for managing both illness and biography. Here is Mr. J.'s trajectory projection:

> I think the odds are good that she will get worse. There is some evidence that she is going to have real problems with her feet sooner or later. . . . I do worry about her. However, I am fundamentally an optimist and figure that somehow we will figure out a way to get along with it. We will do whatever is necessary. . . . What scares me the most is losing her, and this illness, while it is debilitating, it doesn't threaten life.

And here is Mrs. J.'s trajectory projection and biographical scheme:

> As to the future . . . I am at the point that I want to do everything I can do now before I can't do it, although there is the possibility with rheumatoid arthritis that it may go into remission with the end of menopause. I want to keep going as long as I can. That is one of the things about this motor home. We just get in it and go to see our children or go out to the lake and do things. Of course, I can drive.

Personal Modes of Intervention for Handling Symptoms and Disability Contingencies. Developing personal modes of intervention is an important aspect of stable trajectory management. Such modes not only help to keep symptoms under control but can also serve to prevent a small dip from becoming a deep drop! They are also designed to minimize interactional friction. Mr. J. provides an example:

> When she has pain, there is nothing I can do about it. You just have to try and keep your wits about you and also to try to avoid making it worse. For instance

when I hand her something or take something from her, if I am behind her I try to take it in a way that does not pull her shoulder back. Her movement is pretty limited in some directions, and it is pretty painful if she goes against the "stops." So I try to remember when I hand her something to hand it way around in front. Sometimes she wakes up in the night with something hurting. If it is leg cramps, sometimes she will want me to rub her legs. There isn't much you can do. You get the sense sometimes she wants to be left alone. If she gets into one of those spells where she is having a lot of pain. Sometimes she gets depressed. When that happens I try to cheer her up and in a few days she seems to feel better. If there is something like a massage that she thinks will help, then she usually asks me.

Mr. J. goes on to explain some of what he, too, has had to come to terms with.

Her changed appearance [from steroids] and the illness have not made that much difference in terms of our relations. From the standpoint of affection it hasn't made all that big a difference. The sex life is not a big deal. It has slowed down a lot. I don't find that a big problem. The arthritis, unless it is very acute, doesn't have a severe effect on the sex life.

It is painful in a way to see what has happened to her. On the other hand there are a lot of things that have happened in the world that are worse than this, like our friends who are going through a divorce. My feeling subconsciously is that we can get along with it somehow.

Identity Work. One of the important types of biographical work pertains to making people feel good about themselves and not like a burden despite their disability. This is an interactional process, with each person responding sensitively to the other. As Mr. J. puts it:

> I see her as handicapped but not really ill . . . partly because in my mind she isn't really. When she becomes depressed, I try to cheer her up, and also I think it is very important never to portray a sense of being troubled by helping her. That would depress her if she thought she was bringing trouble to the world around her. It would anybody.

Summary. Because of the nature of Mrs. J.'s disability, her husband can be very involved in her care. These excerpts show how the partners have achieved an articulation of the major lines of work and kept them in balance through an effective routinized division of labor. This consists mostly of her pushing herself to do what she can within her body limits, while he acts as a body resource in those situations where her body fails her, and of his acting as an innovator of devices, resources that she uses to extend her physical abilities. Mr. J.'s motivation to continue the work is sustained not only by their occasional camping trips (that renew him) but through her continued efforts to stretch her limits and through his seeing that his coordinated actions enable her to do so. Mrs. J. keeps pushing, and Mr. J. gives her the necessary resources. This couple has been able to work out and maintain a collaborative type of working relationship. It takes two committed and sensitive people working closely together and an adequate pool of resources to maintain this type of relationship over the long term.

Case 2: Maintaining Stability Through Complementarity

Mrs. Moore is a diabetic whose illness is stable and relatively easy to manage. Therefore, it is relatively unintrusive. Nevertheless, considerable work is necessary to prevent complications, and a sensitivity to cues and resources (money, information, devices) is necessary to keep the illness and life stable.

Mr. and Mrs. Moore are an interesting couple from the standpoint of management because of the specific features of their articulation. Basically, the day-to-day management of the diabetes rests with Mrs. Moore, as indeed it has since she was an adolescent. Yet even with Mrs. Moore's relatively stable illness, Mr. Moore plays very important complementary roles. Without his efforts, her physical condition would be far less stable.

The Motivational Agent. Mr. Moore is a motivational agent: he gives his wife the inputs necessary for her to do her work. What motivates him to motivate her is his fear of consequences. These mainly include the long-term complications, which he learned about in the diabetic classes, and the couple's previous anxiety-provoking experience with retinopathy. As Mrs. Moore recalls:

> The classes for couples on diabetes interested him in giving my evening insulin. Before that, it was "She is a very healthy person and has very good control. She can handle it by herself." [Now] he has become more involved.

Critical Management Periods. Pregnancy and retinopathy drew Mr. Moore into becoming an illness management resource for important tasks: providing backstopping interventions, assisting with decision making, providing support, and gathering information. According to him:

> The pregnancy and eye problems were critical periods in my opinion, and that is why I was so involved. I wanted the best thing for her. I wasn't sure she would get the best care so I went with her to make sure she got the best. I went with her for her examination to the eye clinic, looked at the results, and discussed it with the doctor. All three of us discussed it. What we were interested in was understanding what was going on, what the treatment would be, and what the percentages of success are. Then we went and talked to the doctors.

Control Agentry. A breach in regimen management is usually the stimulus that prompts a spouse to take over. This role is crucial but can be difficult for the spouse. Motivating him or her is an ability to foresee (usually from experience) the implications of failed control—not only in terms of illness but also in terms of potential interruption of important biographical performances. Thus, the spouse, too, has much at stake in keeping the ill partner stable and usually does not hesitate to move in when that partner fails at control. The timing and manner of the intervention are very important in determining how the ill partner will respond. Such responses range widely, from gratitude to antagonism. Mrs. Moore explains her own circumstances:

> Even before the pregnancy, if we were out to eat he would say, "I really don't think you should eat that." Or "I don't think you should go back for seconds." He would say it quietly so no one else could hear, but I would get the message, and usually I agreed with him.
>
> Since the eye problem he has been much more involved in my control and maintaining my physical health. But he knows better than to come on too strong saying "I think you need some help." If he had, I would have replied, "If I need your help, I will ask for it." He knew better than that, but when I ask for help or need to talk something out, he is always ready to do so.

Symptom Management Responsibility for the assessment, monitoring, prevention, and treatment of symptoms lies with Mrs. Moore. According to her, the conditions for this are the following:

> He doesn't watch for symptoms of hypoglycemia or hyperglycemia because that would take a lot of time together, and time together is something we don't have. He gets home late and we spend time with the child. Then maybe we watch television for a while and go to bed.

And according to Mr. Moore:

My wife can pretty much handle her reactions by
herself, because of her training and the fact that she is
normally in good control. . . . And unless I am paying
real close attention, I can't tell that her blood sugar is
low. She has to tell me.

Articulating the Division of Labor. Effective work performance entails the coordination of the spouses' respective actions.
However, before that can occur, preliminary types of work must
take place: learning about the illness and the tasks necessary for its
management, finding out which person is best equipped to handle
given tasks, and deciding who should move in to do what and when.
Mr. Moore notes:

It has been a matter of learning how best to help her.
She has had reactions, and I have helped her through
that. Mostly I give moral support because I guess it is
kind of scary. My wife can usually tell when her blood
sugar is low, even before she gets a reaction. When she
does, it is either in the middle of the night or because
she wasn't paying close enough attention to herself,
and then it is too late to prevent. Usually she can
handle them by herself. If she can't I get her some
orange juice or a sugar cube.

However, Mr. Moore has not learned one basic thing about
Mrs. Moore's illness. This affects his responses and, thereby, the
smooth functioning of their division of labor. Mrs. Moore says:

I often get bratty when my blood sugar gets low,
especially before meals. I wish he would recognize
that. We should sit down and talk about the reason I
get that way. Perhaps he knows, but he hasn't told me.
To my knowledge he doesn't know when I have a
reaction, except when I have a severe one in the middle
of the night. . . . Sometimes I think that it has been
a hard adjustment for him, but it has also been one for
me. I have expectations for myself that I couldn't

realize because I would be out of control one way or
another. . . . I don't think of the diabetes as a big part
of our life, only when it needs to be.

Coming to Terms. Both partners have to come to terms with
the illness and its implications. Many conditions enter into the
situation to ease, hinder, or complicate this evolving process, as
Mrs. Moore explains:

Actually I don't think he has had that much to adjust
to because he sees me as basically a healthy person. I
think that his adjustment has come over time, from
living with it and doing lots and lots of reading. The
more he knows the less afraid he is. Being a diabetic
is like being a natural person only more intense.
Sometimes your physical needs are more intense and
you need help fast. I am glad I am married for that
reason, though I am alone most of the day. But I know
I have neighbors nearby if I need help.

Mr. Moore adds.

Once in a while I think about what the future has in
store, but it doesn't matter to any great degree. I feel
that is totally out of my hands. As far as I am concerned, it is in God's hands. I leave that up to him.

Planning Ahead for Potential Instability. Planning for
potential illness instability is important. For instance, Mrs. Moore
explains:

We bought a dextrose machine to measure blood
glucose. We have had to struggle with whether or not
I should get pregnant again. We have talked with a lot
of doctors. We are willing because the other child had
no complications and because the picture is brighter
for women with complications in pregnancy. The fact
that I have had retinopathy and we were looking

forward to another pregnancy was the impetus for
buying [the machine]. We wanted to have the most
optimum conditions we could. No more guess work!

Routine for Managing Emergency and Potential Crisis. In
emergency situations, Mrs. Moore explains, she does the preventive
work and her husband does the comfort work:

> When I have convulsions from the hypoglycemic
> reaction, I need him to hold my hand and be there. He
> is very good about that. I usually have them in the
> middle of the night and become frightened, and he is
> reassuring. I am able to get something and pop it into
> my mouth before I start twitching. Once I start, the
> fear comes. I know I have covered the sugar aspect of
> it, but the uncontrollable twitching scares me. Until
> about a year ago he was frightened as well. Then when
> he realized all I need is reassurance, that somehow I
> have taken the sugar, then he was okay.

A Critical Set of Events in the Trajectory. The consequences
of Mrs. Moore's retinopathy included a forced coming to terms,
changed trajectory and biographical projections, and a closer
marital relationship. Mrs. Moore concludes:

> The retinopathy was an experience of total fear. [Also]
> it was the closest to true depression that I have ever
> gotten. I was concentrating so much on the fact that
> I might lose my vision. But it also made me realize
> that I might be losing my other vital organs soon. I
> have known other people with eye disease, and five
> years later, they were dead. I was trying to deal with
> my own demise I guess. My husband and I did a lot
> of talking. It helped very much to work things out.
>   Our faith increased and our relationship in
> God increased together. We felt that he would not
> bring something into our lives that we couldn't
> handle without his help. And R. told me he would

still love me and take care of me even if I was a blind
person. What I had to work through was that I
thought he might not love me and that I wouldn't
appreciate myself and all that.

Summary. In this family, where the illness is relatively easy
to control and there is no related disability, the illness impacts very
little on daily or interpersonal life. However, there could be
considerable impact if the illness were to worsen. Therefore,
keeping major lines of work in balance consists mainly of keeping
the *illness* stable. The couples' work is articulated by means of a
division of labor in which the day-to-day illness management rests
on the wife, whereas the husband plays a supportive role that
consists of gathering information, providing assistance with
decisions, doing comfort work, and so forth. His actions comple-
ment hers by enabling her to do her work more efficiently and
completely. Also sustaining the couple's motivation to continue the
work is their mutual desire to prevent any complications that would
have consequences for their respective and mutual biographies. We
call the type of working relationship that this couple has developed
a complementary one. This is because the husband's work is such
that it need not be highly coordinated with the wife's but is
supplementary to hers. By complementing each other's actions they
keep her illness, as well as the other aspects of their lives, stable.

Case 3: Precarious Stability and a "Limited Functional" Marital Relationship

Mr. Smitt was in an automobile accident about three years
after he was married and as a result is a paraplegic. At the time of
the accident, the Smitts had two toddlers and his wife was pregnant
with a third child. The children are now in school. Both Mr. and
Mrs. Smitt work outside the home.

The severity of Mr. S.'s disability allows us to examine the
issue of dependence: having to rely upon others for the performance
of tasks that are necessary to maintain the disabled person, the
household, and satisfying biographical performances. What
becomes especially noteworthy in Mr. S.'s situation—a stable phase,

but one often interrupted by contingencies—is how the work is still articulated through the usual work processes and the implementing interactions of the spouses.

In the case presentation you will see how Mr. S. relies on his wife as a resource, the conditions for this, and some consequent problems. Articulation for him means maintaining his wife as a resource (and finding substitutes when she is not there), negotiating an acceptable division of labor and timing for work performance, and providing her with sufficient "payback" to keep her motivated. Complicating his ability to articulate is, first, his need to perform other types of work and then the occurrence of disability and life-related contingencies that compete for his time and energy. For Mrs. S., articulation involves coordinating her husband's body work with her everyday chores and biographical performances; this articulation is further complicated by having three children and two part-time outside jobs. Considering the total amount of work to be performed and the complexity of their situation, the couple's ability to fit their mutual tasks together places considerable responsibility, effort, and stress on each partner. As a result, their ability to maintain a balance among the major lines of work is precarious.

A failure to articulate any of the work processes properly or to further articulate when they are disrupted—in light of this precarious balance—can result in feeling burdened and feeling like a burden. These are not continuous states but tend to fluctuate in degree and duration. Several conditions seem to affect their degree and duration: the total amount of work to be performed, the degree to which both partners have come to terms with the disability, the verbal and nonverbal messages that are given during the work performance, the relief time away from the work, the availability and use of backstopping resources, the ability to work out routines to facilitate work performance, the perception of how hard oneself or the other person is working, and the amount and type of compensation received. In this particular family the precipitating factor that triggers feeling burdened and feeling like a burden is the disability-derived or biographically derived contingencies that unexpectedly disrupted their work routines.

Such disruption appears to give rise to management obsta-cles that call for further articulation if all three lines of work are to continue. For Mr. S., this means finding alternate resources to do the work, or renegotiating the division of labor or timing of the tasks, or providing his wife with additional compensation. For Mrs. S., it means redefining her work priorities (including the biographical) in terms of salience, while letting go of tasks that she has no desire, time, or energy to carry out.

Feeling burdened is a self-interactional process (I'm tired, overworked, not appreciated) that turns into another interactional process when verbal or nonverbal messages indicate these feelings to others. Such messages (depending on the dependent person's perception of them, the degree to which he or she has come to terms with the disability, and so on) in turn trigger the ill mate's response of feeling *like* a burden. The latter feeling may also stem from the belief that he or she is causing the spouse so much work regardless of how the spouse perceives the situation. This, too, is related to the degree to which the disabled partner has come to terms with the disability, perceives the actual extent of the work load, can offer compensation for the work, and so forth.

Considering the Smitts' situation and the number of contingencies they are encountering, the couple do a remarkable job in articulating the three lines of work and in keeping their lives and the disability stable. However, one cannot help but notice how their demanding situation generates considerable stress and strain and prompts one to wonder what looming potential lies ahead.

"Feeling Like a Burden": A Flip-Flop Process. Note the conditions that make Mr. S. feel like a burden and how he has come to terms with this feeling and himself. Also note the other conflicts generated in this dynamic interplay between the spouses and his interaction with himself. Finlly, note the effects of disturbed routines and physical contingencies on the situation.

> I still do flip-flops about whether or not she is being burdened. Of late I've been feeling like I am burdening her. The reason is that I've been having trouble with my bowels and bladder that complicates and adds to all she has to do. Let's face it—the daily routine is a drag for her. But still she gets frustrated, particularly when I am not feeling well. . . . If our routine is upset,

she gets frustrated and angry and takes it out on me. I start feeling sure she is going to feel that way, but still it makes me angry that she responds in that manner. Then I start feeling like a burden. I say, "It is not my fault; there isn't much I can do about it." And she replies, "Well it is not my fault either. . . ."

When I have a complication, I become very focused on it. The thing about it is that when she reacts and brings things out in the open, most of what she says is right. When I refocus and begin to get outside of myself a little bit more, things get better. But then I get to feeling that she wants me to be superquad. And she retorts that I want her to be superwife.

Another part of the problem is that . . . she accuses me of bitching and complaining. I say, "I can't even talk to you without your getting frustrated." On the other hand, I say to myself, "She is right. Why lay out all that stuff." As I say, it is a flip-flop process.

Social contingencies affect the routines and so, again, Mr. S. feels like a burden. Notice how he views this as a no-exit situation.

It is hard to keep the work she has to do for me out of the focus in our relationship. Like tonight, though there is the school meeting to go to, it is bowel care night. The more I think about it in those terms, the more I feel that she has taken on a monumental task. Then where do I go from there because I start to feel sorry for her again? That puts me in the same boat as when I was first hurt. Maybe that is why I don't like to think about how hard it is on her. So even if I think about how hard it is on her, what am I going to do about it anyway? It is a dead end.

Reciprocating. As mentioned earlier, being able to reciprocate in some form or another is an important condition that mitigates feeling like a burden. Here we see how Mr. S. does this. However, he must juggle his time and energy because of disability-related complications. Meanwhile his work with family finances, his need for body work, and life contingencies, all become constraining variables that hinder his willingness and ability to reciprocate.

> I help her running around with the kids. I also make stops at the grocery store. She hates grocery shopping. I also make phone calls that relate to financial things. Sometimes my doing these things correlates with seeing her overworked. Sometimes I do it because I am in a good mood, relaxed, and happy. When I feel tired or have personal problems, like the bladder problem, then I don't go out of my way. I work eight hours a day and drive one hour each way, and there is only so much energy.
>
> I like to take my wife out to dinner. I feel good that she is served. Tonight there is a school meeting for her and tonight is also bowel care night. I would like to take her out to dinner before the meeting, but the activities of daily living take priority.

By minimizing the work load Mr. S. places less of a burden on his wife. "We seldom go on long trips because for my wife it is more of a hassle than it is worth. It is clear to me that this is extra work for her and so I don't take this for granted."

Falling Short For this couple, articulating is a particularly delicate process since it involves a difficult joining of two crucial matters: what the other perceives as important to sustain himself or herself and doing those things that the dependent person (at least) feels are necessary. Both spouses estimate that Mr. S. sometimes falls short on this account, mainly because of increased competition for his limited energy and time. Yet he is not always certain about falling short, so Mrs. S. is faced with a dilemma and perhaps increasing frustration. She, too, is caught in a double bind.

> I am probably more demanding of his time and attention now. Because he is now so much out in the

world, I don't feel I get the attention I need from him
and that is important. It was the glue before, kind of
like the reward. . . . You do come to expect it. You
want it regardless of what their outside interests are.

Mrs. S. has tried to articulate the wife-nurse relationship:

I've always been up front about all of the physical
work that has to be done. I dislike doing it, and
sometimes I mind doing it. But I am the only one that
can do it. So I guess there has always been the
underlying thing that in return I expect him not to
treat me as a nurse. I want him to say, "You are my
wife and I care for you and not for your nursing
abilities." That is something I established from the
beginning.

   Now that we are both working, we have trouble
setting aside time to be together, but I think that is
really important. I can see it immediately slipping
into a nurse-patient relationship, and I have to really
fight because I know the consequences of that happening. It just would not last.

   There were times, are times, and will be times
when he does become the patient to me. Most of the
time I am working with him, I have an impersonal
approach to it. It is like I was washing the walls or
something. I think it has to be that way to some
extent. . . . A lot of humor has brought us through
much of this.

   Being in a One-Down Position. Being dependent on another
person places one in a position of trying to minimize the burden
of work placed on the other. It can also place the dependent person
in a position where he or she cannot express anger or push the other
too far. The other person can make the dependent person feel in a
one-down position—not able to make extra demands or even
negotiate a change in behavior in the other. This constraining of

demand—sometimes desire—has its untoward consequences for oneself and ultimately for the marital relationship.

> Sex is a problem, but it has been since we were first married. Because of the injury I kind of put it on the back burner [as] just one more hassle. The last time we talked about it, she saw it as another pressure put upon her. She is just not that interested, and the few occasions are sufficient for her. But I think I am on hold in terms of rocking the boat. The few times we have it, she initiates it. I find that easier than putting pressure on her. Before I could get angry and walk out of the house. I could get into the van and leave, but now it is such a hassle. If I did not have the disability and was not already putting so much pressure on her, I would feel that I could put more pressure on her in regard to the sex. The disability has changed things in that respect. It affects how I handle situations. I am not as forceful.

Articulating Body Work with Outside Work. Mrs. S. acts as her husband's body resource. The quotations below (the first from Mrs. S., the second from Mr. S.) also reveal what a strain the constancy of the body work can impose on both spouses.

> I get up at 5 A.M. to do his care so that he can get to work on time. I also have a job four mornings a week, but I leave after everyone else has gone. He leaves by seven. I get him out of bed, then he washes what he can and shaves. I dress him. We have it planned that he gets his bowel suppository on weekends and once during the week. He probably should have it more often than that, but it is hard to fit it in any more often. Sometimes the suppository is given at night, sometimes in the morning.

> I do not have an attendant not only because of the cost—the state fund only pays part of it—but

mostly because of the intrusion. We did try it for a while. I still remember the way she (the attendant) would come in the morning and say, "Good morning, Mr. S., rise and shine!" I felt like strangling her. When my wife gets frustrated, I say, "Well, what are our options? We can get an attendant. I could move out. Things can stay the same." Once in a while, when things get rough, I think about moving out. Not really being separated or divorcing her, but of relieving her of the work. But monetarily that would defeat the purpose. . . . My wife seldom gets away alone. She will go away on retreat next weekend and the kids will take over. My wife has very little help. It is totally on her.

Here Mr. S. explains how both partners seek to handle Mrs. S.'s peak periods of feeling frustrated and overburdened:

The stress of all she has to do builds up to a point of frustration at times, but then it blows over and everything is okay until the next emotional crisis. Lately, there have been more and more crises because of my physical problems and the extra hassles they mean. When my wife reaches one of these points of frustration, she might scream, then retreats, and doesn't talk to anybody. Sometimes she just sleeps. I just let her be. She has told me a number of times, "Don't try to talk or reason with me during this time. Just let me be." Usually that works. Usually what provokes her is my saying I am going to do something and then not doing it, if I am capable of doing it or if she feels that I am capable of doing it. It is a very complex situation.

I am able to pick up a small object. It takes a long time, though. When I am alone, I do push when I want to accomplish something. . . . My kids by not always reacting to my request keep me from using the disability as a crutch. My wife also keeps me honest in that way.

According to Mrs. S.:

When I think he can do something I just say, "I don't want to do this anymore. I know you can do it." That is not hard for me to do as long as I know it is something he can do. Now, if we are in a hurry or something, I will do it.

Trajectory Projection. Mr. S. describes the biographical impact of trajectory projection:

It scares me to think of what lies ahead down the road and that illness may creep in. That would be a double whammy. I guess I just have to take it one step at a time.

Summary. Articulation of necessary work through the work processes is particularly difficult and complex in this family's situation because of the heavy work load, minimal resources, and the drastically unequal division of labor. These conditions create a precarious balance among the three major lines of work. The balance is easily shattered by the many contingencies that further strain the couple's already stretched resources. The management of contingencies requires a reevaluation of how resources are used, a redistribution of the work load, and increased motivation to sustain performance. However, this couple's ability to do those things is limited. At night Mr. S. is tired from work and the long drive home, has little reserve energy, feels unsustained in some ways (mainly sexually), and thus finds work more difficult at home. Mrs. S. often feels overworked and undercompensated, which leaves her unable to find the reserves that such situations demand. The couple does handle the contingencies, but in a patchwork manner generally unsatisfactory to both. Each functions, but in a limited manner that often destabilizes the balance among the three lines of work. As a consequence, marital strain surfaces. When the contingencies pass, routines again set in and the lines of work return to precarious balance, with the marital strain becoming submerged for a time. In light of all this, we have termed their working relationship a limited functional one. Usually, the couple function in a manner that allows for work performance, but when contingencies arise, the Smitts' decreased functioning limits the quantity and quality of the work put forth.

Summary

Theory. These cases contradict the usual assumption that once "stability" is attained—usually with medical means and often after an acute period of illness—then all that is needed is the proper treatment and regimen to maintain this state. If the equilibrium is delicate, then of course great care must be taken, while treatments may have to be changed or supplemented occasionally and the regimen adhered to even more rigorously at home. Overtones of compliance and noncompliance attend this view of the matter, one that has been criticized as too medically oriented in perspective and that underestimates the active role played by the ill in their own illness management (Conrad, 1985; Zola, 1982).

This chapter reinforces that criticism by demonstrating and illustrating the tremendous amount and many types of work that must be engaged in to keep the major lines of work effective in controlling illness. Regimens or aspects of regimens may be abandoned, altered, or supplemented not only because patients are careless or irresponsible—or for that matter disagree with author-ities or prudently experiment with regimens—but also because various conditions and contingencies affect the way those regimens are carried out as items of work.

Each case in this chapter underlines those points while at the same time illustrating and clarifying the varying experiences that the ill (and their spouses) undergo despite their common problems. The cases also illustrate the different measures of success and failure experienced in dealing with their respective lives. Of course, some illnesses are so mild that maintaining stability is not particularly burdensome; yet some work must always be done and some cautious handling of body limits must be observed when someone is confronted by potentially destabilizing conditions.

As the cases also demonstrate, if we think further about the more successful instances of stability even in the most durable of those calm phases, we can sense that there is always a potential for destabilization. If some of the stabilizing conditions change—death or disabling illness of a spouse, the loss of a job, a sufficiently radical symptomatic change—the hidden seed of the "looming potential" may begin to flower. Then the marital partners need to (if indeed they can) shift or supplement their resources and divisions of labor and perhaps draw on sources of commitment not yet tapped, at least until stability is again regained and thought to be secure.

Applications. When chronic illnesses are stable practitioners are least likely to be involved in the care of the chronically ill and their families. Yet as our cases indicate, a great deal of work still goes on at this time. What can practitioners do for the ill when they are in stable phases? One of the most important contributions to management is an awareness of what these people are going through to keep the illness, their biographies, and their everyday lives in balance. Rather than being accused of noncompliance, couples need to be helped to find creative solutions for resolving conflicts among the three lines of work by effectively handling the contingencies that come along to upset daily routines.

It is also important to make couples aware of the physical and emotional wear and tear that the long-term management of illness can bring. Then they must be informed that the more assistance they can get along the way (in the form of routines worked out together, helpful devices, outside help, breaks from the work, good times together and alone, and so forth), the better they will be able to continue the work over the long haul. Attention to the work processes is especially important during stable periods, perhaps more so than during any other, in order to prevent complications that might destabilize illnesses or lives.

10

Unstable Phases:
Facing Disequilibrium

Difficult and wearying as maintaining stability may be for some ill people, they experience something else if and when their illness takes a turn for the worse. Short of developing a permanently deteriorating condition (to be discussed in the next chapter), the ill may move into an unstable phase. Of course, they need not necessarily lose hope of making a comeback, even when the instability is of considerable duration. Furthermore, an unstable phase may turn out to be of short duration, representing only a temporary, though nevertheless distressing, period of physiological stress and personal duress.

Unstable phases have other properties such as variable frequency of occurrence, number of body systems involved, physical severity, controllability, and degree of comeback attained thereafter, as well as an impact on social relations, everyday life, and biographical concerns. In addition, of course, an unstable phase may precede, succeed, or even alternate with comeback and stable phases or, more unhappily, move into or accompany a permanently deteriorating condition.

The hallmark of an unstable phase, especially when it is severe physiologically and in terms of personal impact, is working hard to keep one's personal life in some sort of order—and, potentially, to avoid death. One's life may be in disarray, not merely physiologically but socially and biographically as well. Until this phase has either been conquered or has physiologically run its course, one has to endure. Under such circumstances, there is plenty of experiential—and existential—drama.

236

Unstable phases are analytically different from what are commonly called medically acute phases, which may, for example, be brought on by an asthma attack. In such instances, skilled medical care is usually necessary, a physician and often a hospital staff serving as agents who try to get the ill person back on his or her feet relatively quickly and at least somewhat improved. During acute phases the ill person's life slows down at the very least and may well come to an abrupt halt until the person is "himself or herself again." Of course, acute medical phases can be of considerable duration, one's life actually hanging in the balance for some time. However, under that condition the living per se is likely to be carried on in a hospital, a nursing home, or if at home then certainly in much reduced form. By contrast, unstable phases, as we have noted, may make a shambles of ordinary existence, but still one struggles to continue as a citizen in the real world.

The cases presented in this chapter illustrate three main patterns of instability. We shall illustrate the first two patterns briefly, devoting most of the chapter to a more detailed account and commentary on the third pattern. We do this because the period of instability in the case illustrating this third pattern was so severe and prolonged. This third case is not only very revealing of the consequences of a severe, prolonged unstable phase, it also provides additional information about the experiential characteristics of the other two patterns of instability.

The first pattern of instability arises when a long period of stability turns unstable—sometimes to an extreme—because of a pivotal contingency or set of contingencies. After a time, the pattern may be controlled or vanish, and the ill person may return to stability. Our example will be that of a woman whose pregnancy occasionally contributed to the destabilization of her relatively stable diabetic trajectory. The second pattern constitutes a kind of permanent instability: for example, a cardiac patient who is on a downward course is constantly in danger of having unexpected bouts of severe angina, which are not associated with immediate physical exertion or any other discernable event and, yet, not necessarily so severe that the patient requires hospitalization. The third pattern of instability is illustrated by what happens when someone with no apparent chronic illness—or only a mild one—

suddenly develops one or more illnesses that throw him or her into physiological and personal disarray. As with the first pattern, the duration of this third pattern of instability varies. In our case illustration, stability is regained after a little more than two and a half years, during which the ill person experienced infrequent among otherwise constant instability.

Case 1: A Period of Potential Instability

In the preceding chapter, we discussed the case of Mrs. Moore who had a fairly stable diabetic condition, which she managed well with minimal assistance until her pregnancy. She had followed her regimens carefully since childhood. Moreover, she understood her body signs very well, monitored them, and adjusted both her regimen and behavior in accordance with any warning signals. By this method she could usually prevent unstabilizing physiological events, and, thus, stop any potential downward cycle from proceeding out of control. However, occasionally she had insulin reactions severe enough to require short periods of hospitalization. Her generally stable physical condition depended, of course, on scheduling regimens, managing diet, and so on. And in order for Mrs. Moore to attend social events special arrangements for travel and food had to be made in advance.

Diabetes sufferers are vulnerable, in varying degrees, to disturbances in physiological functioning. Daily or weekly contingencies—both physical and environmental—can cause a very rapid shift from a relatively stable status to a critical one. With severe diabetes, this delicate balance can be upset by any alteration of life-style—even as slight as when a young diabetic child eats too much candy—or changes in physiology brought about by physical development—as when a child moves into adolescence.

When Mrs. Moore became pregnant, at first neither she nor her husband—nor even her obstetrician—was particularly concerned about her seemingly stable diabetic condition. She and her husband thought themselves well prepared for the pregnancy. They read pertinent literature assiduously. They talked together a lot about the potential hazards of a diabetic's pregnancy. They felt confident they could manage the potentially upsetting contingencies. Mrs. Moore watched her diet carefully, primarily out of concern about birthing a normal child, not out of her concern for herself. Yet she had several life-threatening insulin reactions, apparently because she could not always read her body signs when she was pregnant as accurately as before. About the time of Mrs. Moore's pregnancy, her husband said: "Though usually she can feel [the insulin reactions] coming . . . when she [is] pregnant she [can't]." So, he occasionally monitored her physical condition while she was sleeping, waking her for sugar intake if her signs indicated a probable insulin reaction. Once when her signs were very severe, Mrs. Moore was hospitalized in an intensive care unit for two or three days. The doctors continually asked Mr. Moore what drugs she was on, but she was not taking any. At the time, she was "spaced out . . . scary," and her speech was unintelligible. The doctors talked of brain damage, perhaps permanent brain damage. Finally Mr. and Mrs. Moore, together, convinced the physicians that she was having a particularly severe insulin reaction.

Because of these experiences during Mrs. Moore's pregnancy, the Moores now monitor her body signs even more carefully than before—especially Mr. Moore, because when his wife is having an insulin reaction she is not necessarily aware of exactly what is going on. The couple believe they have "learned a lot from the pregnancy. We learned what to watch for. . . . During the pregnancy, it was difficult. She couldn't tell if she was going out. It was a new experience for both of us, and we had to learn . . . by going through it. We know a lot more now." Since this major contingency in her life, Mrs. Moore's physiological condition has been relatively stable.

It is notable that the pregnancies of women with certain severe illnesses other than diabetes—for instance, cardiac diseases or asthma—are also marked by close monitoring for signs of developing physiological instability. Sometimes this instability cannot be easily prevented; sometimes control of the illness is highly successful (Corbin, 1987). One final note on this first pattern of instability, the destabilization does not always develop into a clinical crisis or emergency necessitating hospitalization, as in Mrs. Moore's case. The destabilization may be mild or very transitory. Also, the general phase of instability usually passes with the contingency that causes it, whether it is the gradual settling back into a prepregnancy physiological status or, as in the case of a teenage diabetic, learning how to control the disease after the onset of a new developmental stage. So there is a clear distinction to be made between an unstable phase and an acute phase, even though the former can pass quickly into the latter.

Case 2: Permanent Instability

Mr. Smigel is elderly, and has a progressively worsening cardiac disease. In recent years his condition has been very unstable, sometimes moving very quickly into an acute phase and a medical emergency. In fact, he has been hospitalized ten times in the last two years. He is now subject to sudden anginal attacks that appear without warning, sometimes even at night while he is sleeping. Neither he nor his wife are able to pinpoint the immediate causes of these attacks. They do not result from overexertion, fatigue, failure to follow his regimen carefully, or any other contingency of which the couple can be certain. None of their experiments—such as "preventive resting," sitting in different positions, or cutting back on social engagements—seem to make the slightest difference in the frequency or intensity of Mr. Smigel's angina or any of his other symptoms, such as occasional sudden drops in blood pressure. The same inconclusiveness marks the cardiologist's experimentation with the type and dosage of Mr. Smigel's medication; sometimes these experiments seem to have an effect, and sometimes not.

Nevertheless, Mrs. Smigel constantly monitors her husband to be certain that he is taking his medications on schedule. She does this out of fear that if she does not check he might quickly slip into a crisis again. As well, she does this despite her reservations about the medication: "I think in his heart he doesn't think that the nitroglycerin does him that much good. I don't know that it does either."

Consequently, we can characterize Mr. Smigel's condition as one of constantly living with instability and the possibility of death. So, while his destabilization derives from his very deficient physiological functioning, it has psychological and social concomitants. The Smigel family lives with a very high level of anxiety and fear, which escalates to panic during Mr. Smigel's recurrent medical crises. The Smigels are fortunate in only one sense: Mr. Smigel's symptoms can usually be controlled by taking simple medications and careful adherence to his medication schedule. Yet his wife is constantly alert: "If he isn't around [in the house], right away I go into his room to see if he is all right. He may just be listening to [talking books on tape]. And I don't say anything, but if I just see him sitting in a chair, I have a pretty good idea that he is not feeling well." Then she goes into action, giving medications. "The doctor said I can give him three nitroglycerins five minutes apart. . . . Then, within an hour, do it again." To that statement, she added what is probably a great understatement: "So you are never completely free from worry." As for the Smigel's social life, they can never plan far ahead. "You go from day to day. In fact, you go from hour to hour." They still socialize, but they never serve dinner to friends at home anymore because of his unpredictable condition.

Most often, however, Mr. Smigel is neither so acutely ill nor so debilitated by angina attacks that there is any real life threatening danger. On the other hand, he is not lucky enough to be able to hope for many weeks or even days of freedom from these attacks. Like a nation permanently at war, he is permanently unstable.

Case 3: Severe and Prolonged Destabilization

Our next case presentation illustrates additional aspects of the struggle and drama marking unstable phases. Anxiety, bafflement, frustration, anguish, desperation, and other extreme emotions can be—and were for the ill woman portrayed here—part of living with and through a prolonged and severely unstable phase. We have deliberately selected an extreme case to illustrate major analytic points that are more muted in less severe cases of destabilization. We have also selected a case of a single woman to highlight the additional stress of having no spouse to aid in the necessary work of managing illness.

What one can readily see in the sequential account of events in the life of Debby Jones is the following:

1. A two-and-a-half-year phase of instability, alternating with some brief periods of only relative stability.

2. The many contingencies that throw her into dips, drops, or crises. These contingencies derive from external events, internal physiological events, and reactions to prescribed drugs.

3. The ill person's discovering and experimenting with strategies for minimizing the possibilities of these contingencies or handling their consequences after they appear, as well as her strategies for waiting out the contingencies.

4. Attempts to locate appropriately astute physicians who will make accurate diagnoses and come up with effective medical interventions for her various illnesses. Both treatments and treating agents are on trial.

5. These ad hoc medical interventions are attempts to gain and retain some measure of stability in the face of current instability, and it is hoped, to make a genuine comeback to more or less permanent stability.

6. The respective parts played by the ill person and her physicians in discovering, trying out, monitoring, assessing, evaluating, and deciding on successive medical interventions.

7. The exacerbation of the management problems by multiple diseases—and thus multiple bodily systems involved, multiple symptoms, multiple diagnoses, multiple physicians, multiple interventions, side effects, monitorings, assessments, decisions—and the cumulative impact of all this on daily life and biographical concerns.

8. The great difficulty in making accurate self-diagnoses. Things get out of control, her assessments tell her they are getting worse, but what has happened? What to do? Which physician's services to request or use?

9. Crises are potential if not frequent, and their management consists largely in waiting out the episode. (Once her body was so out of control and life generally so desperate that she prepared to commit suicide.)

10. Strategies must be devised anew for staying on top of everyday-life requirements; that is, she must make do by cutting back

and cutting out activities, by adjusting their pacing, by delaying, and so on.

This particular ill woman, Debby Jones, happens to be single, living alone, doing advanced studies at a university far from her family, with minimal financial resources, as well as being extremely physiologically unstable. So, all of the phenomena listed above take place within a context of lessened resources (especially womanpower), the necessity for a rearranged division of labor, relatively minimal psychological support from others, and a heightened—and almost impossible—set of articulation problems. She has to do almost all of the work of keeping herself afloat in the face of her combined physiological-personal fate.

She sees her body, first of all, as undependable, often out of control; second, as immensely puzzling and distressing; and third, as temporarily (perhaps) so affected in appearance as to be personally distressing. Her major set of biographical questions is "Will I ever come back, and how far, and if not how can I survive as 'me'?" Until she could answer those questions, she essentially had to delay for over eighteen months in facing up to the central biographical issues of her life. Rather, she focused on (and is still primarily focusing on) (a) persisting through one dip, drop, and crisis after another; (b) persisting with *some* version of her immediate biographical plans (university work); and (c) meeting her immediate personal obligations. After the many months of extended instability, which always reappears even after some stable phases, she is beginning to grapple with her permanent limitations and the issue of adapting to them.

In this case presentation we shall give a partially chronological listing of events with some accompanying comments by Debby Jones. The quotations from her (précised) account capture more explicitly fragments of her accompanying activity, reaction, and experience. The interview was conducted in the spring of 1985.

In early autumn of 1982 Debby got the flu, which persisted until she was diagnosed at the student health clinic as having developed an allergy. She had trouble breathing and "ran downhill." Then she had an acute asthma attack. "Before then I thought of myself as a healthy person."

The attack was probably triggered by an allergy. According to Debby, after the diagnosis, "I couldn't get stabilized" even with the medication. She was diagnosed by a private physician, since the clinic staff could not diagnose.

Then Debby went back to the clinic because the private physician was expensive. By July, however, she was dissatisfied and returned to the same physician, who did a workup for allergy.

She told herself that she should be able to go back to her classes. Some days she did very well; other days she felt "in outer space." By Christmas, she was "feeling out of control." She increased her prednisone dose but got no response; she was having trouble breathing. At about the same time, she and the physician talked about further increasing the prednisone.

She then developed pain, sometimes so constant that she was afraid to drive. This came from osteoporosis, but she thought at the time that it was lung pain.

By the spring of 1983 Debby's breathing was "not bad" and things "turned around." She took three courses that spring. As she puts it, some days she was "pushing," proving that "I could do it." She finished two courses and felt good about that. But then her parents had their fiftieth wedding anniversary, so she went home, which was 3,000 miles away. She arrived, exhausted. After returning to school with three weeks of spring quarter yet to finish, she had to take one incomplete because "there was no way I could function."

In June she was overwhelmed by pain from not being able to breath: "I saw myself as ill; I didn't know what was going to happen." She found her body unpredictable. For instance, she would get half way to the grocery store and then realize she should not have left home. Or she would do one thing and think maybe she could do another. If she wanted to do two things outside the apartment, she would do one, return home, wait three or four hours, and then do the second chore.

She kept on living alone: "I didn't think to have anyone stay. My eating was peculiar—whatever was in the house. . . . Independence was the big thing, and I kept thinking [the illness] would go away—or would get less bad." She and the private physician juggled her medications, and life became "more sane."

Debby was still thinking this was an acute phase of something, "but when I didn't come back, I was questioning. But I didn't think in terms of dying." Most questioning about that came a year and a half later.

All that summer, Debby says, "things were out of control . . . some days I couldn't get things together. [In August] my menopause manifested itself. I missed my period. There were a lot of problems, hormone-related in retrospect now; it took time to put the story together."

As she got further into menopause, her allergies, asthma, and premenstrual symptoms worsened. That summer her physician had decreased the prednisone, and she had continued taking the lower dosage in the autumn. She was depressed and anxious, wondering what was going on. Her face was "particularly bad" because of her allergies, although no one knew the cause at the time. She had "multiple problems which tend to interact. The hardest time was in terms of asthma, for I didn't know what was going to happen."

In October of 1983 she thought of suicide "things were so out of control." For three nights she thought she would die, her breathing was so bad. She made preparations: "The first night I got rid of my letters." The second night, she mended her underwear. "The third night—I didn't give a damn." She had seen the physician but decided "if this is the quality of life I can expect, it's not worth it."

A couple of months later her physician was no longer available to her. She "had terrible times," was ready to give up. She was in debt to the extent of borrowing money from other people and taking money from her retirement fund. "If this is to be, let it be."

She did register for classes. But during that week, she again began to feel out of control and cut back on the number of courses she would take.

Then she almost ran over a bicyclist while she was driving and feeling out of control. She knew she had to do something, so she and her allergist talked it over and decided her allergies were related to her environment. She made up her mind to move.

But I knew I couldn't move alone. In spite of my independence, I had to call my sister, ask for help. It

was difficult. [She did not use friends because] you
cannot ask them to help for ten days. You use them
to take you to the physician or to get groceries. . . . I
thought that with the move, it would be fine: of course
it wasn't [what] with more dust, the parking worse.

By February of 1984, Debby's asthma was acting up, and the
spring allergy season was coming. "It's crazy: one handles some
problems, then another shows up." By March she was exhausted.
She had some "crazy bleeding" and went to a gynecologist. It was
"something menstrual-cycle related," although with medical
treatments, her cycle was now more predictable.

In July she again thought she was going to die. The
gynecologist decreased her estrogen. By August Debby once more
had severe asthma. She was sleeping sitting up and awakened every
hour or two; she was panicked because she was getting no air.

Then "eighty things fell into place: estrogen was the
culprit." She asked the gynecologist for a diuretic to get rid of some
fluid. The gynecologist told Debby that she was not taking that
much estrogen and directed her back to the allergist for more
prednisone. However, Debby decided against that, knowing it
wouldn't help. She went to the emergency room for a diuretic. The
next afternoon she lost fluids and was thus able to breathe more
easily.

The allergist thought someone should check Debby out.
According to Debby, "Once you get a feeling what the problem is,
you can get the physician to listen and say that makes sense. He
said, 'Figure out when your period comes and make an appointment in advance, so the gynecologist sees it at its worst.'" Then the
gynecologist gave up her practice, so the allergist referred Debby to
an endocrinologist, who changed her estrogen. But in October, after
undergoing a series of hormone studies ordered by the endocrinologist, Debby stopped the estrogen and started on natural progesterone. By November she was having her menstrual period and felt
good.

However, during the preceding summer she had picked up
an infection, which probably intensified her breathing problem. An
antibiotic then killed the infection; but because of it, she went off

progesterone. Then she felt wonderful, but "figured it would end," as it always had.

In December Debby had the old windows of her bedroom replaced with new ones. This stirred up lots of dust, so her allergies became bad again. The situation was complicated by the painting of her apartment that same month.

Then she missed a menstrual period, but her physician showed "good patient handling." He told her not to panic and figured out that her problem was related to when in the cycle she was taking the medication. Together they worked out a new medication schedule, and in January of 1985 they added an estrogen suppressant.

> Now I am coping with drug side effects rather than the primary illness. I don't know who I am anymore. My body is giving me different messages. A lot has to do with the endocrines. The cycle itself is different. But I can cope; I don't have to stay home for a week at a time.
>
> *Now:*
> I am stabilized.
> I am focused on side effects.
> I have learned you can't really count on remaining stable, that my allergies are seasonal.
> If I have learned anything, it's that you can't count on anything, can't plan anything.
> I'm hoping to get through school. If I remain OK, in six months I will have a paper done for my qualifying exam.
> I do social things on the telephone when [I am] not up to social obligations. When I feel well, I take myself to dinner because I don't know when I'll have to cancel a date. I hate to break commitments.

How does Debby assess her symptoms? "Sometimes it's almost like record keeping you do for a patient: like charting, graphing your symptoms. I had to learn for myself. Deciding what to do for what set of symptoms has taken a long time to discrim-

inate.'' Recall that her pain was not a lung problem but turned out
to be osteoporosis.

During rough periods and crises Debby first used the
emergency room and later her primary physician.

> During bad periods, it's usually more than one
> problem occurring, and I'm sick, immobilized, and
> fall to pieces. One problem you can differentiate, can
> better decide on proper treatment.
>
> The crises fortunately are somewhat self-
> limiting. I always know the longest period will be
> about three hours; I get myself through it. Eventually
> I pass out and go to sleep and the pain gets less.

Debby keeps a three-day supply of drugs. She changes the air
filter of her respiratory machine periodically and takes it with her
everywhere. Taking a shower or bath is exhausting, so she plans
that in terms of other activities. She has some backup people, other
students, to take her grocery shopping, but she keeps that flexible
because sometimes people are unavailable.

She says her body image is bad. (Her face is puffy from the
estrogen and prednisone.) "I know I don't look so great. . . . I don't
like the way I look these days." (She has been taking a diuretic and
looks better at the moment.) She also has a "terrible time" wearing
her bra because of a back problem and pain and because menopause
treatment—estrogen—has led to breast development, putting
pressure on her back. "I have a real fear of my body falling apart.
Mind falling apart. What will come back, will anything come
back?"

Her body is "unpredictable" so she is thinking about taking
a written qualifying exam since she does not know how she will
perform orally on any particular day. She is currently more
optimistic, and the treatments seem to be working. "But I must
accept that I will never be completely well." She is gradually
making adaptations and restructuring activities: for example,
making arrangements to meet friends at the stadium for football
games rather than walking with them there, because she can no
longer keep up with their pace. "When I begin a job again, will they

have handicap parking? All of a sudden you realize that is where you are at." She started thinking about such things in the spring of 1985.

In October of 1985 Debby reported that she had had a bad summer. The prednisone and estrogen had led to fibroids, so she was thinking of having a hysterectomy. She had switched to another gynecologist. Also her asthma had been bad. She had discovered that when her estrogen count was high, her writing was confused, so she had learned not to write papers when in that condition.

We shall not follow Debby's trajectory further except to add that some months later her physiological condition stabilized sufficiently so that she could squarely face the issue of what do do about her career. She took a supervisory position in a good hospital and many months later told the authors of this book that she planned to keep this position until she had built up enough savings to resume her graduate studies at the university.

Summary

Theory. In this chapter three major patterns of instability are illustrated by case examples. The first pattern is presented through the case of a woman whose pregnancy disturbs her otherwise stable diabetic trajectory. The second pattern is demonstrated in the case of a man suffering from severe cardiac disease who is in a state of permanent instability as his condition progressively deteriorates. However, his instability does not always culminate in acute phases that necessitate hospital care. The third pattern of instability is illustrated by the case of a single woman who has previously thought of herself as healthy, but suddenly develops asthma and other complications. This destabilizes her for more than two and a half years. We describe her experiences in considerable and sequential detail because her illness trajectory clearly presents features of destabilization that are more muted in less drastic instances of instability.

Descent into a severely unstable phase presents a major problem for the ill person: how to come back to normal physical and social functioning. Analytically, we might conceivably think of efforts to return to normal as a "project," which quite like any other project must entail a goal, a generalized plan for attaining it, some specific means for operationalizing it, an approximate schedule for its pursuit, and some means for evaluating progress along the scheduled path. For relatively mild instances of instability, and especially when the ill person has had considerable experiences with instability, that project model would nicely fit the sequences of imagery and action. However, with very severe instability (as in the case of Debby Jones), while the project goal is clear enough, everything else is exceedingly problematic. The generalized plan evaporates in the face of evolving events, and each new, more specific plan and its implicated operational means must be reformulated, experimented with, modified, or discarded. Envisioned schedules of progress are shattered. Progress is nonlinear and difficult to evaluate anyhow. Experientially, the victim of her or his own body—and perhaps of less than competent or astute physicians too—lives through, as best as possible, at worst a true nightmare (or at least depression, if the instability is not so shattering) in which the goal of genuine stability may recede at times into the far distance. The more specific aims then become just staying in place and not getting worse. Severely unstable phases often pass and are succeeded by comebacks to long-lasting stability. In the instance of more or less permanent instability, the only operational means of handling oneself is with routines, such as resting, taking it easy, or just waiting out the worst moments, days, or weeks with as much patience as one can muster.

Two final remarks will help link this chapter with some of the preceding ones. First of all, note how the severely debilitated have to juggle the three main lines of work (illness, everyday, biographical). Illness work becomes dominant; during the worst dips and drops it floods the other two lines of work. Everyday activities are curtailed, delayed, cut to a minimum, and even dropped. Biographical work, as suggested earlier, is almost restricted to present concerns, the future being held in abeyance in a kind of biographical limbo (which for Debby Jones lasted for a great many months). Biographical work, then, is linked tightly with staying afloat in matters of personal concern: for example, how to manage sufficient work at the university to remain a legitimate student or how to travel and live through a family celebration that is taking place 3,000 miles away.

Second, in Chapter Seven we discussed four central work processes that enable work to be carried out: resource flow, division of labor, mutual support, and articulation. Debby's nightmare of effort and experience was due in some part to the relative failure of the four essential work processes (although the fault is certainly not hers). Her successes were due—aside from native physiological processes, perhaps—entirely to her ingenuity or luck in finding and maintaining proper resources, in establishing workable divisions of labor, in gaining sufficient psychological support, and above all in developing great skill at articulating all of the types of work and work processes involved in managing her illness and her associated life. When the unstable ill person is fortunate enough to have a cooperative partner, the successful functioning of these work processes (and their articulation) is greatly furthered.

Thus, the unstable phases, especially when severe or with unanticipated developments are more devastatingly problematic, are more pervasively dominated by illness work per se, and are perhaps more acutely pressing upon the necessary work processes than the stable phases discussed previously. The burden of maintaining at least some semblance of normal life is more obvious, even if life itself is not in question (as in the acute phases of trajectory that usually take people to the hospital). When a period of instability is prolonged and more than a trifling intrusion in the ill person's life, then the essential work processes are interfered with. The destabilized person must either be very resourceful, as was Debby Jones, or very fortunate in having a cooperative and highly supportive marital partner, as were Mrs. Moore and Mr. Smigel. With ill people whose physical instability is more or less permanent or frequent, even if their physical condition is not deteriorating, stability is represented by only infrequent moments of calm in a relatively choppy sea of existence. Those are the moments for which they hope and live.

Applications. The role of health practitioners in unstable trajectory phases is one of supportive assistance. No other trajectory phase is characterized by such frequent physical and emotional ups and downs. Lives can be completely disrupted while the afflicted seek to find means of controlling their symptoms if not the course of an illness itself. Most important is that the ill person be assisted to find his or her way through the medical maze and obtain appropriate medical care. Important also is the giving of assistance in finding temporary services to help with daily work (the grocery shopping, cooking, picking up medications, housekeeping) when symptoms are out of control. When unstable, the ill need someone who can look in on them periodically. Finally, they need, especially when they are depressed, emotional support from health practitioners as well as from relatives and friends.

11

Downward Phases:
Encountering Deterioration
and the Approach of Death

We turn now to trajectory phases whose direction is downward. Downward phases are, alas, all too familiar. Virtually everyone knows some friend, acquaintance, or family member who is experiencing, or has experienced, an increased measure of disability, and many of us have known people who died from fatal illnesses. There is a considerable technical and lay literature about the psychological and social accompaniments of physical deterioration and a comparable literature on dying experiences. Moreover, some discussions in our previous chapters bear on those situations. So what have we to add to all of that?

First, we provide some additional conceptualizations that may aid in an understanding of the experiences of people who are deteriorating. Second, we link those conceptualizations to our earlier analyses. Third, we offer a few cases and case vignettes to highlight the new analytical points. We present those cases in detail, for the quotations graphically illustrate certain features that attend deterioration and dying.

It is useful to make an analytical distinction between two types of downward trajectory phases: deteriorating and dying. Some chronic illnesses do not lead directly to death. On the other hand, some lead sooner or later to death, or are apt to. When that happens, as with some cancers or heart conditions, then the actual dying (as defined by those most involved with it) is preceded by a period, often lengthy, of gradual bodily deterioration and accompanying so-

253

cial and personal disabilities. Such deterioration can also lead indirectly to death. Thus cancer victims can die from pneumonia because of systemic weakness. In an analytical sense, it is also useful to note that some people may suffer from a nonfatal debilitating disease, for example, bronchitis, while simultaneously dying from a "terminal" illness.

Running now somewhat ahead of our story, we need to add that when physiological-physical deterioration is translated into symptomatic debilities, these in turn are translated into bodily limitations, and these in their turn are then translated into performance limitations and failures. But, of course, each of these factors is affected over the entire course of the trajectory (whether it moves downward quickly or slowly) by available resources and by two other work processes: division of labor and motivational commitment. In short, social and psychological conditions may affect the pace and degree even of symptoms and the disease course itself, not to mention social and psychological performance.

With both the deteriorating and dying phases, a time line is involved. In the instance of deterioration, the temporal issue is How fast, when, and how much deterioration? For dying, it is How soon? One way to visualize the time line is to imagine someone who is thinking about his or her disabilities and/or about dying locating himself or herself on a continuum: immediately, soon, later, not for a long time, never (from this illness at least). This continuum allows us to reason analytically about phenomena such as the following: Someone who is not medically defined or self-defined as dying but is deteriorating markedly from an unknown cause or a wrongly diagnosed cause is finally correctly diagnosed as having an inoperable brain tumor big enough to cause death within a few months. Or again, diabetics expect a great many years of stability but realistically do anticipate a possibly radical deterioration late in life and know they may or may not die from their diabetes. Self-location on the time line is enormously relevant to how the ill organize their lives and how others' lives are organized with respect to them. (We shall see this locational and parallel organizational relevance in the case illustrations that follow.)

But is there a major issue that spans the distinction between deteriorating and dying phases? Yes, there is, and it can be summed up as a question: What keeps people going despite increasingly severe disability *or* knowledge that they (or their spouses) are dying or will die in the relatively near future? Most ill people struggle to maintain as much of their desired styles of life as possible in the face of increasing limitations and perhaps despite expectations of their dying rather soon. The work of managing an illness and getting around with disabilities is vital in allowing as high a level of attainment of this desired living as possible.

But the effort and the greater struggle attendant on the increasingly severe disabilities or decline before death should alert us to the centrality of biographical processes (and for both spouses). These include contextualizing, coming to terms, reconstituting identity, and reconstructing biography (see especially Chapters Four and Five). Since by definition the downward phases involve successive drops in physical and social performances, biographical work is likely to be called for at critical points along the time line. This is done under different conditions at each point. Just as the juggling of the three major lines of work will require review and rearrangement, so the biographical work itself will entail reviews, revisions, and reconstructions of inner life and self-conceptions, and so of the resulting overt behavior. In all of this, progressive changes of biographical body conceptions (BBC) are crucial. One especially prominent feature of the BBC in the materials of this chapter will be the conceptions of mind-body relationships held by the ill and their spouses and linked with their biographical time conceptions and self-conceptions.

Deteriorating Phases

By definition, bodily deterioration is the chief physical feature of a deteriorating phase. Translated into bodily limitations and then into behavioral and interactional limitations in performance, this deterioration leads the ill and their spouses to adapt in various well-known ways. They modify or cut back on or cut out certain activities. They devise clever ways of getting around actions they formerly took for granted, such as opening faucets or managing flights of stairs. The ill conserve their energy by resting before visits with friends. (An increasing number of publications about the chronically ill vividly portray the many varieties of managing despite disabilities.) In the lives of the ill there is a delicate balance between adapting to limitations and stretching them by innovative uses of resources and by a fighting "with will" against the limitations (Forsyth, Delaney, and Gresham, 1984). The danger of overstretching is not merely that one may fail in some public performance but that the overexertion may contribute to a worsening of the disease or lead to further disability. Hence the paradoxical requirement that the ill must come to terms with disabling limitations while at the same time fighting them.

If now we focus on deteriora*ting* rather than deterioration, still another picture emerges. A key to a deeper understanding of the experiences of the increasingly disabled is that their organization of mind, body, work, and behavior can only be temporary. While their diseases may stabilize for long periods of time and even afford occasional comebacks at higher performance levels than previously, nevertheless, overall decline is the name of the game. Each more or less permanent drop in ability requires yet *another* round of redevising, revising, rearranging, reviewing, reconstituting. It requires also a "reprioritizing" of activities and social relationships in light of increased limitations. The more severe the drop—not simply in bodily terms but in its impact on performance and identity—the more sharply confronting are the changes in life.

Understandably, some ambiguity attends this necessity, indeed this inevitability to redo one's life because the ill are not always certain that a new symptom or the worsening of an old one is permanent. In addition, they have memories of preceding comebacks and therefore may have problems in assessing what is really going on. When the symptomology is stable for a period and personal reorganization is stable too, then images of future deterioration are easier to push to the back of one's mind than when one experiences the threat or actuality of yet another decline in capability. During these latter periods or immediately after an acute phase, which often takes the ill to a hospital (the hospital functioning as a backstop for the illness and sometimes for a weary or thoroughly exhausted spouse), the ill are more likely to plan realistically for future deterioration. Then they envision probable scripts for unfolding events and figure out how best to make the plots turn out more favorably. Of course, people do not often imagine worst-script possibilities, either in amount or speed of decline of their own or their spouse's resources. For this reason they are sometimes caught dreadfully short when the worst does occur. They have, in effect, put out of mind the ultimate looming potential of their illness. How the ill and their partners handle these ambiguities in imagining, reasoning, and behavior is very much linked, then, with respective past experiences along the trajectory time line and how they currently locate themselves along that line.

A metaphor or set of images for this type of trajectory phase experience may be useful here. Think first of a scale for weighing objects, a pan on either side. Equal weights on each represent a stable phase in which life is on one side and illness impact is on the other, however delicately balanced this impermanent stability is. When a decline occurs, the illness weighs more heavily and the life side less so. When both illness and life are restabilized, then again there is a more equal balance of weights—even if life is really less satisfactory than before. The more that deterioration sets in, the more difficult it is to reestablish a satisfying balance. So although life and illness may continue to seesaw in this manner, with life being reconstituted on *some* basis that is more or less satisfying, the ill when struggling to maintain some semblance of a satisfying existence may find that getting the scale into proper balance is now existentially more difficult. Yet remarkably few opt out of life, and this of course is the poignant drama. Indeed, the ill may try very hard to live as fully as possible while dying, however little the windows of opportunity (see the case of Henry Lawson that follows) may still remain open to familiar and beloved scenery.

The four cases presented in this chapter illustrate some of these general features of deteriorating phases. Other more specific points will also appear, along with some variations in experiences that derive from differences in both life circumstances and the particular disabilities. We begin with the story of a friend of one of the authors who has since died from progressively disabling Parkinson's disease.

Case 1: Extreme Deterioration and Disability

This case illustrates a late phase of deterioration in which the husband can perform virtually no self-care, except to take pills as given, and no daily work. He lives in a microspace and within virtually a minute-to-minute or hour-to-hour time frame. Nevertheless, he is still very much alive, not merely existing. At the moment, his life reflects a kind of stasis in which the struggle just to stay alive with a minimum of discomfort and a maximum of quality of life (however now constricted) takes precedence. Yet near the very end of this interview, you can see the next phase moving in as he begins to think about a self-induced death.

The couple in our case have been married for fifty years and are now in their early seventies. Illness forced Mr. Lawson's retirement from university teaching about ten years ago, and with the increasing burden of his care, Mrs. Lawson gave up her modest craft business. Parkinson's disease has had him in and out of the hospital frequently, and his ability to move about has gradually become severely limited. During much of the day, his muscles are so locked that he is not able to move. If he needs moving, his wife must exert great strength to hoist him to his feet and maneuver him over to the toilet or bed. He is often confused or so completely exhausted that he falls asleep for many hours at a time. During the day, he is really in the world for only a very few hours—hours that we have termed *windows of opportunity*—when he actually thinks, interacts, and is like his old self.

At the time of our interview, Mr. and Mrs. Lawson were thinking of moving from Minneapolis to Los Angeles, where their married son lives. They had been considering such a move for seven or eight years, but because Mrs. Lawson could not come to terms with such an uprooting and despite much encouragement from their son and daughter-in-law and friends in Los Angeles, they were still not certain about such a drastic move.

The interview excerpts below bring out particularly the microspace and microtime within which Mr. Lawson lives. For him, major issues include his lack of control over his movement in space and his management of the environment and people in it so as to allow him minimal discomfort or terror. He faces additional terror in contemplating the relationship of his mind to his body and what this relationship means for his current and future existence. Since life is enormously constricted (he can no longer even read, scarcely concentrate long enough to listen to taped versions of written books) and his wife is carrying an increasingly exhausting burden, even empathetic friends wonder why he does not choose to die. At the end of this account, we shall see him finally getting to that question. Meanwhile, he struggles against his almost total limitations, the struggle being carried out on a microscopic but paradoxically heroic human scale.

We begin with excerpts in which Mr. Lawson comments on the immobility of his body and consequences of that:

Last night I couldn't move, in effect, and I had to find a chair and sit in it in the bedroom. James [his son] was very tired and fell asleep. My wife also had fallen asleep, and this left Lucille and myself, and I could see she was anxious to get home. James suddenly woke up and they began talking about going home, and I said, "You are going to leave me in this house sitting. I may be sitting in this chair all night." So I began making a list in my head of things that I had to have done if I could get to the bed or they could help me to the bed before they left. It made the night appear very desolate. In fact I felt abandoned and this feeling . . . the fact that you are extremely alone is hard to take. But finally when Joanie woke up just before they left, Lucille said, "We weren't going to leave you alone anyway." It was very thoughtful. She is very sensitive. . . .

What do I do when I freeze and my wife is asleep? Well, you have to be aware that you sometime will unfreeze, but you don't know how long it will be. [He had described earlier going to the toilet at night and finding himself "frozen" on the way back to bed and having to remain there terrified for a couple of hours.] If I'm standing, I sit on the floor. I've become aware of how tall I am. I'm frozen. I'm standing and the floor seems a tremendous distance. . . .

[What goes through your head when you are frozen?] How do I get out of this? is the first thing I say to myself. How do I get out of this? How can I get

into a safer situation? Then also I consider two
possibilities. One is how to secure myself and become
safe, but then as soon as I get safe I want to get safer.
[The only really safer place I guess is in bed when
you're like that. Or in a soft chair.] That's right. You
find your body is twisted, and one of the things I
learned in relation to being in bed is that you do not
evaluate your discomfort points too clearly. You can
stay relatively quiet and do not need to be concerned
about your discomfort if it isn't too great. The longer
you can stay in the first position the better off you are,
because if you move, then you've got two positions to
think about. And you say, "I was better off before than
I am now." So you move again, and you don't know
if you can get back to it right.

Also with Parkinson's, if you get into the
position where your drug has worn off pretty much,
then you are quite stiff. Also, the blankets on your bed,
you see, become quite stiff. So you can't turn them.
Then the blankets get heavier, and you are more of a
prisoner of the position, and you can't rightly . . . I
was always a restless kind of sleeper. I can't afford to
be restless now because I can't turn that much. I can't
change my position. The body will be so strange to
you. The body lies around and plays pranks on you,
too. That's what I don't like. On the other hand, it can
torture you.

Next Mr. Lawson describes how he lives in microspace. Note
another of his dominant body images and also the additional
problems he has with people and his body limitations:

I find that people don't respect my things. When I get
into bed, I get my things when I'm able to walk and
put them in relationship to each other where I can get
them in my place in the bed. Like drugs, books, and
TV. I'm relatively self-sufficient, but nobody respects

my things; so they come in and they move my table just a couple of inches, and they don't see anything wrong with it. But by moving it a couple of inches they change [things]. I have to be careful. I can't readjust them, if I can, while they're here because they'll move them again. . . . One of the terrors of life is my urinal. If somebody moves my objects too much and without the possibility of my relieving myself, it makes me anxious, and it usually then starts signaling my body to urinate. Your body becomes a principal torturer in that way. . . .

If you sit down on a toilet and if you turn around in order to position yourself, you need a handrail. So you see in a sense what we are talking about is all sorts of intimate actions that are no longer easy. And also another thing: . . . several people would want to help me . . . the thing is that I have to be aware of what they want me to do. If somebody helped me to come and sit down, if they explain, "I'm going to turn you around now"—but usually they start you out and you're off balance, or you don't know what they want as you are coming around, and then you suddenly discover if you follow their directions, you're going to fall down.

Next Mr. Lawson comments on his body in relation to his lack of control over it. He is talking now explicitly about mind-body relationships as he conceives of them. This leads him to comment on what his bodily limitations mean for not being able to reciprocate people's favors, a failure in his life that hits hard at his sense of what makes the world deeply human and what he cannot now share. Then this brings him to relationships with his wife.

[How does it feel being frozen?] The sense of being a captive. You know you're going to get over it, but you don't know when. I have never been able to relate [beforehand] how I feel with how long I'm going to be frozen. I have not been able to discover [this], although I've thought about it and wonder at the relationship between my condition at one time and the possibility of how I'm going to get out of that condition. It works in unexpected ways. You respond many times through your own will, what you'd like to do, how much you can get your mind off yourself, and things of this sort.

I know there are two aspects of this disease and that social situations trigger it in some ways. If someone comes and visits, there are a lot of people I don't . . . well, I find myself alerted to the social situations in unfortunate ways. I'm not sure, but I think sometimes I use the physical problem I have to escape. Well, it's like a self-fulfilling prophecy. I say, "Don't get excited, don't get upset," but I do get upset. . . . When I first had Parkinson's, one of the things I was trying to do was to find out whether I was being motivated by the social situation or myself.

[The psychiatrist and neurologist] said it was not a separate problem. But your new relationship with people is the thing that's troublesome because you cannot pay back for your assistance. I mean when somebody does you a favor, you can't rush down and pick up your groceries and go up those stairs. You're constantly taking on a "taking" sort of situation. As a matter of fact, in so many ways you're demanding of the other person, who for instance gives of himself. You are demanding. But again you have to evaluate the assistance that they will give to you. They may make it more difficult. . . . When somebody does you a favor, you have got to exchange. It's not paying back, it's because you're saying you've done a friendly thing for me and I would like to let you know that I am willing to do something for you. That seems to me one of the most generous aspects of human experience, interaction that has meaning to each other. It's hard, if they have a lot of groceries and they want . . .

you can't help them. As with my wife, Joanie, I am constantly taking from her. And she's never complaining. But sometimes she gets terribly angry with me, which she has never done before in her life. She just gets so god damned fed up with it. . . .

I've had to think over my relationship with her very much, and sometimes I say she might be better off without me. On the other hand, then I begin to redefine situations, thinking about this, and I find that I'm trapped in a situation. For instance, I'm retired, have a certain income, and she may have difficulty living off half my income. I don't think she could live off half my income. I don't know. So I can't say, "why don't we separate? You'd be happier . . . you'd be free." . . . But she wouldn't. I can't say it even.

Fifteen months later, Mrs. Lawson has carried out a monumental set of tasks, first coming to terms with moving to Los Angeles and then carrying out the move itself. She has survived it well, seems no worse off than previously but, of course, has been under enormous strain and is still showing it. She is falling asleep in the evenings and so soundly that Mr. Lawson is now terrified about what will happen if he is stricken while she is fast asleep, with no way to reach her, to reach anyone, especially if he is frozen. Then he speaks to his friend approximately as follows:

Is it worth it? All my socializing with her is between ten and twelve in the morning. She's exhausted at night. She's been getting angry, as she never has before. Last night we yelled at each other. So when she passes out on the bed and says before she does, "I don't want you to disturb me" . . . it's so lonely. So lonely. . . . Is it worth it? [How long have you been thinking this way?] Two months.

Three months later, Mr. Lawson asks his friend whether killing oneself with drugs is legal in California? In noncomplain-

ing words that have surely been going around and around in his
head for months, he explains: "My life is unproductive." He can do
nothing all day long so why continue on and on? His friend advises
him to think it over totally before taking that option and that he
cannot possibly act without talking it over thoroughly with his
wife. They have talked a bit about his dying, he says, but he agrees
to the friend's advice. In the next days, it is clear that he is wrestling
with this potential escape from his otherwise no-exit situation.

Obviously, both he and his wife are trapped in an almost
impossible situation despite a lifetime of very close affection. Yet
their circumstances are perhaps not entirely a matter of cruel fate.
It is possible that the obverse of Mrs. Lawson's great strength as the
care-giver resource is her inability to discover and utilize relatively
inexpensive or public resources that would relieve her work. Under
current American conditions, the burden is entirely on spouses to
find these resources, and clearly this particular couple has not done
that, nor have their physicians apparently guided them to and
through what has been called the agency maze. As a result, the
continued deterioration of the ill leads to a pervasive sense of no exit
and continued desperation or at least relatively unrelieved depression for such couples.

Dying Phases

Recollect the time line along which people who define
themselves as dying locate themselves. From this, we can extrapo-
late various subphases of expected dying: immediate, proximate,
farther in the future, far away but still inevitable (or gradually
happening). At any subphase the primary question for the organization of the self and life is "When will it happen?" (Stoner and
Kranfer, 1985).

Other questions the dying pose: How will I physically die
(painlessly, with full faculties)? How will I know I am actually
dying, the manner of facing dying (courageously, sustained by
religion), the quality of life while dying, the issue of living with the
idea of final death itself (life after death, reincarnation, or nothing),
and what will happen after my death to others significant in my
life? All of these questions are addressed in one or another of the

three cases presented next. The questions imply the usual biographical processes, variable though they may be in terms of content, life circumstances, and individual response.

As noted earlier, a growing literature describes and to some extent analyzes dying experiences. Our data parallels much of this discourse. There is no point in repeating what has been written elsewhere. Rather, we shall present, in their own words, two courageous and thoughtful women who are facing death in the ambiguously proximate or later future—or miraculously perhaps not at all. Then we shall discuss briefly some biographical subprocesses that occurred during one man's dying.

Case 1: Dying Complicated by Other Phases

This case presentation clearly shows how the trajectory phases are not necessarily neatly distinguishable from one another. They can appear in combination or in rapid alternation; in this instance they appear in relation to what is basically a dying phase.

Mei Yuan was a close friend of one of the authors. Several excerpts from her letters to him and his wife during the first six months after her diagnosis of thoracic cancer give a graphic and evolving picture of those months, December 1982 through May 1983. She lived for another two years, suffering gradual physical decline but living through alternating phases of stability and partial comeback that allowed her to live as much life as she was able to, including the fulfillment of academic obligations, until her death. In her last months, she was still able to focus on planning research for which she had written a proposal although it was quite clear in her own mind that she might not live even to begin the research.

In these early letters, written when she was on a downward path to death but before the later physical decline, we shall be reading mostly about comeback. It is comeback that is very slow, very small, and under the shadow of Mei's fear that she will die. The fear shows through her lines only intermittently as she describes her symptoms, her progress or lack of it, what her body appears like to her and what its altered state means, what it is like to live at such low ebb, what it is like to squeeze in bits of real living here and there, what it takes to maintain continuity in one's radically altered life. Letters like these to close friends, we can surmise, represent one way of enhancing that continuity, of keeping in touch not only with them but with herself.

In the first letter, we see how Mei handles the announcement of her illness to her close friends. We see also, of course, how she is handling this immediate postdiagnosis period in her life, or the first steps in the contextualizing drama.

> December 20, 1983
> Dear Fran and Ans,
>
> This *is* meant to be a Holiday Greeting, but there is no getting away from the necessity of also having to convey bad news—very bad news so far as I'm concerned. I should have called you, but events overtook me, and now it will be some months before I can talk to you. The above address may be familiar to you. It is one of Mayo's hospitals, where I am convalescing from a "near total" laryngectomy. My Chicago MDs sent me up here as the only alternative they knew to total laryngectomy. Major difference between the procedures is what kind of voice one can get back with "rehab." A surgical team up here has developed a procedure which should eventuate in my gaining something like a normal voice. But that is some months off. [Then in a few lines, she describes the surgery.] I had somewhat over two weeks to contemplate the probable diagnosis and type of surgery. Cancer of the larynx it was, and no way to save my voice. Curiously, I was not so horrified about the potential threat to my life as I was focused upon the mutilative character of the surgery. That gave me the horrors, waves of horrors—until, after sufficient looking at it, the horror level went down, and it began to appear as something a person could live with.
>
> So that's where I am. Morale pretty good. Prognosis is very good. After a few months I will start using what kind of voice I'm going to have, although

it will entail months before its potential is reached.
Not having speech is dreadful, just dreadful, but it's
only temporary. I should be going home in a few days
after Christmas, and then I can write you letters on the
typewriter so you can read them. . . . I don't mind
spending Christmas in the hospital. Having got over
the horrors, I've landed on the other side of the stream,
where I'm grateful to be—to be as such as possible.

In the next letter, dated January 21, 1983, we see the
beginning struggle with her drastically altered ability to speak—at
first with an electronic device and later without it albeit hoarsely
and with effort. Moreover, since speaking is at the very heart of
communicating, Mei is beginning to discover what her new life
entails.

I had thought that when I got home to my beloved
typewriter I would really set to expressing myself, and
I had visions of thick letters winging to the far seas
and shores. Somehow, it didn't work out that way,
which is still puzzling, because I am so endlessly,
wordlessly frustrated by unexpressed words in my
daily life. In my previous life, I probably went along
quite content to be silent a good deal of the time. What
is so galling, I think, is the interruption of the
spontaneity of speech. This is a particularly apropos
punishment for me, because I really was the strong,
silent waspy type in my youth, brought up to believe
that one did not speak unless one had something
worthwhile to say . . . over time I learned to enjoy
talk, talk for the sake of relishing talk, as well as for
playing with ideas. . . . Now I am rendered relatively
inarticulate—or at least I have to be spare in my
language. Not *all* bad, in forcing me to search for the
most telling words, accompanied by the extra challenge of finding phrases that come over better through
an artificial larynx. I'm pretty good at it now. . . . Still
not very good over the phone, though, and that has

been the occasion of some of the most uncomfortable
moments. God, are people freaked out by this device!
Don't blame them—it is quite grotesque.

Her words shortly afterward move from the disability to the
looming possibility of death and then away to the quality of life.

Until the last week or so I hadn't given much thought
to the life-threatening aspects of my situation. I was
all bound up in the emotion of the mutilation—of
which there is a good deal in this damned surgery,
over and above the obvious voice problem. Now I
realize I was also all bound up in simply surviving the
huge surgery. . . . The real horror of modern medicine; they may save your life—no guarantees, remember—but leave you wondering what is left.

Mei is also discovering what else a comeback entails
physically:

No sign of a shunt voice developing. Healing in the
right areas has been delayed because of a stupid
fistula. That kept me in the hospital almost a month
. . . still isn't completely healed. . . . Anyway the
beginning of radiation therapy is being held up also
because of the fistula . . . so there is a grim little
balancing act being contemplated now: I go up to
Rochester next week to be seen by my hotshot surgeon,
who intended to pronounce me fit for radiation. Now
what will he do?

She is discovering, too, some of the social and personal
consequences of her voice change. None of her friends had

put a finger on what was going to loom as most
salient: namely, the change in my status from whole
person to handicapped—a kind of nonperson, or
limited, at best. I should have known better myself, so

it has been quite shocking. And I have had some
emotionally bad encounters, in which I allowed
myself to feel diminished; but I'm learning to avoid
that, or counter it. . . . In a year or so this will
presumably be all past, but this transition period is
rugged. . . . It is not particularly profitable to engage
in theorizing about what conditions some people to
do better with me and other people to really louse up
what relationship we had. I'm just grateful for the
people who handle it well.

Next Mei touches on what satisfactions life is still offering
in and around, and against, the ever-present background of her
current disablement:

I am just beginning to make some serious moves
toward getting back to work. To be sure, it has only
been within the last week that I have had any time left
over from the demands of taking care of myself. . . . I
found myself pooping out very quickly when I tried
playing the piano [and a problem managing one of
her arms now]. However, it will and is coming back.
. . . I am enjoying having my students and younger
colleagues come to see me. And now we are getting
down to their and our work, this week. . . . I'm going
to a concert later this week. Have been to a couple of
movies . . . So it goes. I find it becomes difficult to
write; my mood is so mercurial, ranging from glee, to
sardonic, to black . . . that I worry about the tone of
what I put down on paper.

In her March 2 letter Mei begins with thanks for some
exciting piano music sent to her. Then she writes of lassitude
"which seems to be a major side effect of the damnable radiation
'therapy.'" She is looking forward to the time when the effects of
her last radiations will vanish. "Another few weeks before the
crappy feelings go away: a series of usually minor pains and
discomforts, from fantastically burned and painful throat, itchy

skin, to weird headaches, strange and sudden weakness, etc. And constantly the lassitude."

About the radiation itself and its relation to her body and body conceptions she says:

> It is just dreadful, all the more so, perhaps, for being a silent assault. It doesn't feel so silent as creepy, dragging away at your life. . . . I sometimes fall asleep under the machine, even though I am trying very hard to help things along, magically, by visualizing a war between the good beings and the bad beings, the good ones being bronzed maiden warriors; the bad ones Joe McCarthy type male slugs.

Then she writes of squeezing in a small slice of life and accomplishment: "Oh well, I am capable of making some larger moves. Last night, for the first time, I took over a three-hour seminar that a colleague has been handling for me all quarter. I'll finish the rest of the quarter. It went all right, which was a great boost to my morale." Then a last sentence that underlines the communication issue that has so beset her: "The students had no trouble hearing me."

When giving specific answers to a query, made by her friend in his previous letter, about whether the lymph nodes had been involved in her operation, she makes the following comment:

> Doesn't sound all that encouraging on the surface. Doctors and loved ones have hastened to be hopeful. The five-year survival rates with lymph involvement are about 50-50, but my surgeon hastened to tell me that most of the bodies in those figures were much worse off than I, so my chances are really much greater.

Mei ends this comment by laconically remarking, "But your physician consultant will have already told you this." Death is on her mind, but not so prominently as to take precedence over the daily struggle to cope with treatment side effects and the immedi-

acies of day-to-day living or her preoccupation with the central
comeback questions of how much and how far.

Her April 26 letter opens with lines that reflect her difficulties with an unpredictable body and the beginnings of coming to
terms with its irrevocability; then again, however, her words reflect
how the unpredictability and ambiguity of comeback complicate
the process of coming to terms.

> On the other hand, one inevitably has to accept the
> irreducibility of body limitations. One's body not only
> goes awry, it goes unpredictable. No, that's not quite
> what I want to get at. There is another dimension
> here. It has something to do with the notion of "trust"
> in one's body: when your body "lets you down." . . .
> For sure, my notion that one month past radiation I
> would be getting on the path to "normality" did *not*
> turn out. Such a spooky business, as if those rads are
> still beating into my tissue and turning me into milk
> toast. Except, I think maybe there are some signs of
> bottoming out and turning upward in the last few
> days.

Then follow a couple of lines that suggest either her
puzzlement or just plain frustration about her rate of comeback.
Months later this will turn into much greater anger about horren-
dous side effects, which the physicians either could not or would not
predict to her.

> It is striking to me that you [with your heart problem]
> can recite a precise degree of limitation communicated
> by cardiologists, as compared to the vague, noninfor-
> mation which seems to be the style of radiologists. I
> think much about clinical and functional uncertainty
> these days, and wonder to the point of paranoia who
> is putting me on about what.

Mei estimates that she is about where she was three months
ago, or maybe worse "since my muscle tone has deteriorated so

much more." At Mayo's, where she is going for a checkup next
week, maybe she can get "some more concrete help and timetables
about developing a voice." She then describes a setback in speaking
brought about by radiation side effects and relates this again to the
physicians' inability to either predict or control treatment side
effects—but with overtones of dying in the background of her
writing:

> But going back to the feeling of being misled by my
> medical authority, this is my primary area of guts and
> fury right now. Damn their eyes. They made it sound
> like once the shunt opened up acquiring speech was
> a breeze—only a couple of sessions with the speech
> pathologist were necessary. It would all come. Shit. I
> can't tell whether my air shunt still needs to open
> properly or whether the whole scenario is myth.

Then she turns and writes in a lively vein about New York
City politics, civil liberties, sociology, and her seminar. This
represents some of the continuity in her life and of herself. But a
month later, on May 26, she writes about "the difficulty of keeping
up a regimen when it doesn't seem to be going forward, and instead
keeps slipping back. Taking a longer perspective I can see that there
has been forward movement, but it really requires a multi-month
perspective, much, much longer than I had anticipated." In short,
a revision of her temporal ideas about the comeback is taking place.
At least partly in consequence of that, she notes: "I have also
dropped into such a depression that it foreshortens my energy level
. . . it has gotten to the point where I am pretty sure that much of
the time when I don't feel like playing the piano, it is depression."

But there is also the matter of her voice—besides energy,
understandably, her principal concern. She is asking herself
whether she is *ever* going to get a workable voice again. If not, then
this is *the* identity blow, with totally radical implications for a
changed life. To prevent that she is even willing (although very
reluctant) to submit to another minor surgery on her now incredibly
painful and swollen throat.

No doubt the thing that has most disheartened me has
been the voice. My surgeon and speech pathologist are
disheartened too. No doubt about it, I was supposed
to be speaking by now. Actually, all the surgeon
offered me when I was up at Mayo's was a species of
hope: it was not so utterly peculiar, not to be speaking, because I still have a lot of edema, and it is not
so long since radiation; and if there is no improvement by next time, there is something he can do. go
in and prod the air shunt open. Sounds terrible, but
he has done it before, and it worked. So I came back
with higher spirits about it, and practicing making
sounds with more zest—*and* more effectively. For a
week or so. Slipped back again, probably because in
the last week my neck has swollen up again and that
may have happened because—would you *believe:* I
have another disease! A gall stone, yet. . . . Actually I
am taking it rather well, and that is probably because,
deep underneath, there was the fear that it could be an
errant cancer cell gone amok.

She continues to expand on that last sentence, and for the
first time really refers openly in this correspondence to dying.

There are comeback trajectories which can suddenly
shift to terminal. Do you regard that as a regular
combination? Presumably everyone is organized
around the comeback, but maybe in the back of some
minds is the potential shift. What about those occasions in which the patient is on a comeback, but
others are secretly on a terminal trajectory with the
patient?

In the preceding quotation does *others* mean the physicians,
her friends, possibly her correspondent? (If the last, yes; he was
thinking what she was thinking.)
Then a final—and to her two readers, poignant—reference to
what helps to sustain her:

intellectualization [is very helpful]. . . . Being an
intellectual is one of life's greatest pleasures, isn't it?
In psychological pain, I find it easier to get in touch
with my intellect than with my sensitivity to art. It
isn't always possible to listen to music, even when I
want to. On the other hand [when walking the
neighborhood], one can be overcome, unexpectedly,
by the beauty around one: suddenly hear a birdsong,
see a flower.

At the end of this letter there was a reminder that significant
others who are not spouses can serve the same function: "All my
love to Fran. (And don't I know how lucky to have someone with
me through this!)"

Some months later it must have become apparent to Mei—
since she was developing a number of debilitating symptoms and
a fantastically swollen neck and face (which she was told would be
with her for life)—either that her comeback would be infinitesimal,
more or less arrested right at that point, or that her death was just
a matter of time. The ambiguity of this earlier phase—part
comeback, part acute, part low-level stabilization, part deterioration—had now been cleared away. What had not been settled yet
was whether she would live with her disabilities and disfigurement
or whether she would die from her illness.

A month later Mei writes to a second intimate friend that she
has just been to the local hospital for another checkup on a
suspected tumor, which has not been found. There she rejected an
oncologist's proposal to do a biopsy on her throat region because
of a very great danger that the wound would never heal. She did
have a CAT scan, which showed nothing, though "it doesn't
distinguish between various kinds of inflammation—like between
a tumor and an inflammation." She continues:

I learned in this period how bad a cancer I had. I
knew—I was told after surgery—that the chances were
worse than 50-50; indeed, worse than that. However,
in my surgeon's opinion, considering my overall
health and the affected nodes, I was probably better off

than that worse figure. I didn't question the statistics any further. I don't know how much it matters to one to be told that the chances are 60-40 or 80-20 or 90-10. Now I gather I have been way on the 80-20, 90-10 end. If you did a little research—which you may have done—you probably already know this. I have been gathering this information over the last few months, and it all came to a horrifying focus during these days of hospitalization. There were all these experts convinced that I had to have a tumor. . . . Then there was the growing notion that they might not be able to make a diagnosis: I would have to try to live with those symptoms, not knowing whether they were killing me or not. Well . . . I lived with the great likelihood of more cancer for a couple of weeks. It was almost certainly *inoperable,* and I couldn't have any more radiation to the neck. . . . Thus I was in for a rather awful death, and within a period of months. *And,* if we could not tell from diagnostic tests, how would I know what was going on in the months to come? When and how would I know whether I was dying? . . . I looked down through those columns of horror for days and days, but only part of the time. I couldn't concentrate on these ideas for more than an hour or so. And then it was necessary to draw on my various defensive mechanisms—of which I am richly endowed . . . the Gammion scan was negative! There isn't a lot of faith in that test but if negative—well, that was the only thing that could penetrate the black box, and it says *I do not have a tumor.*

Next Mei's facial edema went down a bit, then worsened. So a month later she reports: "For all I know, this latest could still turn out to be tumor induced, but I proceed on the infection assumption. It seems as if all this has to be lived with. I think that can be done; it is a matter of trying to get a reading about whether I can expect things to get better, or not. And of course the MDs don't know either."

A month after this she takes heart from having survived two years and the fact that the chances of having a recurrence of the tumor are "statistically nil." After celebrating this watershed anniversary and "settling down to try to arrange a prospective life—with all the iatrogenic mess—I still have a nugget of doubt." Meanwhile, she is doing exactly as she said: living with the illness, with her doubts, and planning a sabbatical and her next research project.

Three months later, Mei died of a hitherto undiscovered tumor.

Case 2: Death or Not, and When?

The young woman in this case, Frances Verdi, is in a combined trajectory-biographical limbo, for she was recently diagnosed as having advanced breast cancer and is now waiting to see the results of presurgical treatment. If it is successful, she has a chance of living; this is because of the possibility of a mastectomy plus further treatments. If the current treatment is unsuccessful, then Frances faces death soon. Even if she is saved by those further treatments, she may not live. However, she is not concentrating on that possible fate right now. Rather, her thoughts and energies are completely and understandably absorbed by the immediate future. She is doing massive biographical work while waiting for the results of current medical treatment. Her eloquent account reflects her struggle to contextualize, to come to terms with current body limitations and possible worst scenarios and the beginnings of reevaluation of what her life has been all about and possibly should be in the future. We can sense, in her words, the backward and forward reviews that have been part of all of this. In the months to come there will be something of the same ambiguity about comeback stabilization and dying that attended Mei's postoperative life, except that for Frances, the physicians have clearly laid out all the odds. Psychologically speaking, in reality she is fated for death either immediately or in the near future. Biographically speaking, she is imagining comeback and stability as well as immediate, proximate, and far off dying.

In response to a request to tell about what she's been experiencing since her diagnosis, Frances's interview begins on an intensely biographical and complex note:

Since I've been ill, I've been captured by the feeling of being struck down in the prime times. There are a lot of feelings I have. . . . I finally after the last few years have been extremely happy with everything that I'm doing. [After a difficult career period] it took about two or three years to get on my feet again and then . . . I was really rolling. I was feeling extremely confident about my ideas and my work. . . . Things were real good. And when I got the diagnosis of cancer, I felt very struck down. [For two months since, she's been unable to read anything but] pieces which speak to the heart and speak to the issues about finitude, death, time, you know. I've only listened to chamber music [by romantic composers, which have a] tragic quality. I'm feeling very tragic about myself, as I said, this image of being struck down at a prime time. . . . So that's the kind of imagery I am working with for myself. How to deal with all of this.

Then, looking forward in combined trajectory and biographical projection, Frances continues:

Because of the gravity of diagnosis, to be followed by anticipated "remission for a while" and chemotherapy and radiation, it's [nevertheless] likely that maybe in three years it could come back. . . . I see myself as having a life of struggle . . . they can't guarantee a cure. Not at this stage. And so I feel kind of . . . I think of a sense of hopelessness, of why begin something . . . why begin writing a book if I only have a year and a half or two years? How can I sustain myself through these periods?

This invasion of present time by future dire time leads Frances to biographical reviews of her life, reviews concerning her past, future, present, and other intense biographical work:

> This is a tremendous question for me and I am
> wondering about the value of my activities . . . I'm
> having a crisis of meaning right now. I don't know
> what is really a hundred percent important to me. I
> feel the sense of time and that I want to cram every-
> thing into life because I don't know how long that
> will be.

This leads Frances to talk about a conflict over choosing
between work and pleasure this very weekend, which is between
chemotherapy sessions. Concerning pleasure: "I'm on a very strict
diet, so there are limited kinds of pleasure that I have. I really used
to love food." This particular pleasure links up with a main theme
that she will develop throughout the interview: her social mobility
and its meaning to her. But, again, with reference to food:

> It's so ironic to me. I came from a working class,
> actually a very poor family, and one of the ways in
> which I went up in the world . . . [The interviewer
> comments here: "You went up on your tummy."]
> Exactly. What do my parents know for food? I learned
> about . . . all kinds of exotic cooking. I turned into a
> great cook. Even in graduate school I would buy a
> bottle of wine just to try and educate my palate. I
> learned how to like all these things. So now I have this
> tremendously sensitive, educated palate and now I
> have cancer, and this particular diet . . . eliminates a
> lot of things I have grown to love. It is so ironic that
> the markers of class mobility have involved food for
> me. . . . People would say, well I have X amount of
> time to live; shit, I am going to have a great time . . .
> but I feel that the length, longevity and lengthening
> of your life is very important. [But the food is] very
> meaningful about concepts of the self that I have.

Then Frances touches on her biographical wrestling with the
place of intellectual work in her life. "So, I'm not sure where the

place right now of intellectual work and creativity and wanting to write and solving intellectual problems is in my life."

She then gives a long account of how her case was completely misdiagnosed by physicians at the medical cooperative where she had been going—in fact she won a malpractice suit later against them—and how she simply was ignorant about incompetent medicine, not challenging the physicians despite an increasingly enlarged breast because her background led her to assume physicians just knew what they were doing.

> I worked so hard at being a competent human being.
> I mean, I come from a family that's not so competent.
> My father is a laborer and my mother is a housewife.
> And they are not sophisticated in the ways of the world, and I worked very hard at being a competent human being, at being good at things . . . to really learn the ways of the world. . . . And the irony again is that I'm betrayed by all those things I worked so hard at. I surround myself with competent people. But the blind spot I have was what was a competent doctor. . . . They [her physicians] missed everything . . . it's one of the grim realities that I have to face, this theme of being done in by incompetence, when I worked so hard at being a competent person, competent in my work, competent in my life. It is extremely painful to me.

So even the conditions of her misdiagnosis precipitate intense biographical review.

She is also intensely debating the direction in which to turn her intellectual efforts; and she is doing so with evident turmoil. Until now, she has written about matters of interest and pleasure to herself rather than what "is useful for other people." Perhaps she should do that now. Perhaps she should write a book for women about cancer *before* they have it, explaining disease processes, procedures, experiences.

I think I have an incredible store here of medical
knowledge. I'm wondering how to make that knowledge useful to other women. And then sometimes I
just get very depressed and I think the hell with
writing. The hell with writing anything. I've been
writing my whole life and trying to make money from
my brains. Why don't I just have these . . . weekends
. . . where I go away and have a good time and not
think about making my writing of use to other people
or solving any problems? Let me have a little peace
and quiet and just not think of these things.

Or, she reasons, perhaps she should put off such decisions
until after her surgery and radiation. (That is, until she is free from
her trajectory limbo, she is also biographically still in limbo.)

I'm still paralyzed by a lot of anxiety that sort of slows
me up in terms of wanting . . . I'm not clear . . . I'm
just not clear on what it is that I want to do with what
I think is the rest of my life. . . . It's a trial of the self
that has been myself for all these years that is very
much . . . is questioned . . . and I feel like in some
ways that I'm still holding my breath from the
diagnosis. And I won't let my breath out until after
surgery.

Then Frances talks about mind-body issues. The main issue
includes an untrustworthy and potentially betraying body, a
disappointment in strength of mental control (or will), and so a
certain distrust of her capacities to pursue a purposeful goal as long
as the body is unreliably out of her control. (Thus she is caught in
a vicious closed circle, at least for the time being.)

I'm waiting to trust my body, that I can depend on my
body to last a particular period of time so that I could
count on my body not to give out . . . let's say if I'm
working on something I'm enthusiastic and happy to
be . . . working on and then boom it's time for chemo

or I get tired, and I lose interest and all of that . . . but also at the same time I feel like, and this may be puritan or whatever, I don't know, but that if I had a strong mind I could whip my body into shape, that if I really decided to write like crazy, if I decided that this piece [of writing] that I'm going to do is important, I can make my body last longer in this period of time that I have, that if I had this purpose, if I had a goal, if there was a productivity goal, that I could push my body into shape. It's like the psycho side of somatics. And in fact, I haven't risked it because I don't want to be disappointed. I don't know if my body . . . even though I tell myself that I could try to do it, I don't know. . . . As it is I can put in four hours a day on my regular job and then I have to come home and take a nap. You know [on chemotherapy] . . . it's unpredictable from day to day.

Here Frances discusses one of the last topics touched on in response to the interviewer's comment about body conceptions and relationships of mind to them:

I always saw myself until very recently as a very plain, ordinary looking person, and only recently have I begun to see myself as somebody who is better than average looking, even pretty in some ways. I saw myself as . . . an academic schlump and never saw myself as looking good in clothes. My body was always a necessary appendage. If I were to draw a stick figure of my mind and my body, I'm sure it would be like a three-year-old child's, with a very big head and a very small body . . . my mind has always been extraordinarily central to my vanity and to my life. I think of my mind as the place where I make my money. And the mind is the place . . . I'm sort of . . . I work with my mind. I labor with my mind. And it's brought me a lot of pleasure, and it's the sort of the central way that I see myself. I mean, I see myself as

a thinker. I see myself totally as having this very live
mind all the time . . . that's why this period of time
right now is so strange for me, and so painful, because
that relationship is altered profoundly. I view my
mind as a way of upward mobility. I got out of being
. . . I got out of many lives by having a good mind.
I got out of many fates. What was fated for me by
transcending that and being smarter than average,
better than average, talented and whatever, fighting to
get out. . . . So my body has just been a source of a lot
of pleasure, sexual pleasure, food pleasure, a source of
pleasure for me. Never a problem and just something
you don't think about. I never thought very much
about my body. . . . The thing now, if this . . . like [a
set of] scales . . . if it was mind-body, it's now body-
mind. My mind was very important to me, but it's just
that it is not a source of great pleasure right now. It's
just keeping me intact.

That is, her mind now is almost totally at the service of her body
and of maintaining her continued identity in the face of the bodily
disasters.

Finishing that thought and further underlining the limbo
character of this period in her life, Frances eloquently elaborates:
"And I have to just do whatever I do to stay alive and use my mind
to just go from day to day. It's like my mind is so engaged with day
to day that I can hardly think about anything else. It's not soaring.
It's not free. It's hinged to my body. It's attached to my body. It's
like my mind has feet of clay because it's stuck in my body."

Immediately after that comment from Frances the interviewer asked a pointed question about self-betrayal through the
mind. "Did your mind fail you because of the mobility business
when you misjudged the cause of your enlarged breast? Do you
think in those terms?"

Yes, I do. I have thought about this a great deal . . .
that was why I said earlier that the one blind spot I
had was that I couldn't see it and you know I think

a lot, since I got sick, about seeing things. How do we
see in the world? How does the sociologist see? How
do the doctors see? We use machines to see better. Why
couldn't I see? My vision failed me. My mind, my
sociological vision failed, something failed me.

In sum, Frances's articulate account portrays vividly and
accurately something of what it is like to live in a trajectory-
biographical limbo, as well as the issues that the biographical work
addresses during this period, the issues that it puts on hold until one
can face the ambiguity of maybe yes (life) or maybe no (death). If
Frances lives, this is *not* a predying phase but the beginning of a
comeback phase. For us as bystanders, this phase is ambiguous and
should also plunge us, empathetically, into the reality of her limbo.

Case 3: Living While Dying

Journalist Cornelius Ryan, given a totally unexpected
diagnosis of cancer, probably fatal in two years, returned immediately to his office and began dictating his thoughts and activities.
After his death, Mrs. Ryan published these notes, with additional
ones of her own (Ryan and Ryan, 1979). Ryan's great concern
besides his wife and children was to write—and finish—a last book,
A Bridge Too Far, for which he had collected a mass of notes. He
felt an obligation not only to himself but to all who had heroically
fought in the battle described in that book. In Ryan's autobiographical notes, one can easily discern a number of biographically related
activities and biographical processes characteristic of phases of
dying when death is expected, although not immediately or even in
the proximate future. We shall simply list these, for they are easily
understood. Of course, not every person facing death would
encounter or experience all of these biographical phenomena but
certainly some of them.

- Assessing and reassessing trajectory location concerning
  potential dying and death
- Rearranging life in terms of the prioritizing of goals and
  activities

- Living intensely: savoring moments and experiences, having flings, cutting loose
- Keeping thoughts about dying from spouse, children, friends
- Fighting the looming potential: activity, resolutions, ignoring the future
- Employing prolonging strategies: following regimens, praying, using the hospital to ensure longer life
- Asking the question How long?
- Swinging between hope and despair; fighting panic
- Fighting to stay normal and alive; fighting one's way out of depression
- Pacing when work is possible and when it is impossible because of pain, energy, loss, etc.; juggling so as to conserve energy for work rather than other activities
- Deciding whether each new type of treatment suggested by the physicians, as one goes increasingly downhill, is worth it
- Talking oneself into believing there is hope despite all signs of failing
- Staying on top of one's work, using every minute, albeit intermittently because of intruding symptoms
- Experiencing increasing identity blows (body and performance failure) and their cumulation
- Self-validating performance to show oneself one is still the same person despite deterioration
- Reviewing death as one moves closer to it; being unable to keep the looming potential out of mind
- Looking past death and planning for the family more concretely
- Occasionally assessing how much longer one has to live
- Preparing oneself for the actual dying and also preparing one's spouse and children
- Finishing one's work properly, gaining closure on that aspect of life
- Counting one's blessings for having lived long enough to finish one's work
- Making last public performances and "willing" oneself to carry them off properly
- Giving up the fight; drawing the final curtain and withdrawing into oneself

- Coming to final terms with death, while recognizing that one is dying right now
- Achieving final closure with one's spouse and family—and granting them closure

Even closure acts, which generally are thought of as occurring only near the end of life, represent a complex set of activities. Ryan's running account includes the following activities more or less in chronological order.

- He begins closure with his initial session of tape-recording immediately after the diagnostic announcement despite the fact that his future is still open if problematic.
- Before a crucial surgery, he puts his will and papers in order.
- Just before the operation, he achieves a muted closure complicated by a pretense of optimism shared by his wife; he invites a priest in to visit; and he tape-records a message for his wife, just in case he dies.
- He goes on outings with the family so that after his death his children will remember him as a good and interested father.
- He carries out a Christmas party for all his friends and instructs his wife to send out, the first Christmas after his death, cards with his photo on them.
- He carefully makes an outline of his book for his wife and secretary, just in case. . . .

We skip an equal number of closure acts to end with two actions Ryan performs as he is about to die:

- "My poor little girl, my Katie." She is looking down at him in the bed, and he is looking up at her.
- And with his teenage son, looking at a picture of a fisherman casting, which happens to be on the hospital wall: "The wrist. . . . Remember to use the wrist." The son says he will, and Ryan smiles.

Once again we can see the biographical ideational processes outlined in our earlier chapters very much at play as this coura-

geous man, during his last months and days, contextualizes the
illness into his life, comes to terms with his dying and forthcoming
death, reconstitutes his identity, and undergoes biographical
recasting of his life, though recasting not so much in direction as
in detail.

Summary

Theory. With this chapter on deteriorating and dying we
conclude our discussion of types of trajectory phases. Here, we place
biographical work and biographical processes in the foreground,
while keeping illness and everyday work much more in the
background. The major concepts brought out here are those
developed in Chapters Four and Five and include the BBC chain
and its disruption, contextualizing, coming to terms, reconstituting, identity, and reconstructing biography. These concepts are not
only reflected concretely but are seen in their various forms in the
different case situations.

In progressively deteriorating but not life-threatening
illnesses, while many everyday-life and biographical adjustments
are made with each downward step, the thought of death is
nevertheless more distant. It is the daily effort at coping that is
salient. However, with potentially life-threatening diseases, the
adjustment problems are even more complex. Because every
downward step may mean that death is that much closer, there is
a struggle to stave off death, finish one's life work, handle identity
blows, and make closure acts, while also dealing with a failing body
and its daily ups and downs of performance that impede or interfere
with important biographical and everyday work.

Applications. Both types of deteriorating trajectories are
dealt with in this chapter because of similarities in the biographical
processes that each person undergoes. Yet the practical issues are
not the same for each trajectory. The looming potential of death is
not always hanging over the person who does not have a life-
threatening illness but does have a progressively deteriorating
illness. In some ways this may make the thought of living with
one's failing body even more distressing, for then there is no escape
through death. Rather, one has to learn to live with increasing

performance failures, and then with each step downward to contextualize, come to terms, reconstitute identity, and recast biography all over again. In these situations, practitioners can be helpful in several ways. They can help the ill find the resources they need, such as home health aides and helpful devices (for example, handrails and body lifts), as well as assist in working out new ways of doing old things, and discovering useful things that the ill can do to fill their otherwise empty time. Practitioners can also assist the ill and their spouses to do the biographical work that should accompany each downward turn by putting them in touch with support groups, listening to their problems and frustrations, suggesting professional counseling when necessary, and allowing them to verbally and otherwise explore alternative paths.

As for those who suffer from life-threatening illnesses that are in deteriorating phases, practitioners should strive to achieve a balance between helping the couples deal realistically with their situation while at the same time maintaining some hope. This calls for a great deal of sensitivity and good timing in providing help with biographical and illness work. The important kinds of biographical work here are coming to terms with illness, with life, and with death and performing the necessary closure acts. This work can be especially difficult for those who find the identity blows suffered—as a result of performance failures and thoughts of death—too painful to talk about.

The handling of physical pain is another important issue faced in this trajectory phase and something that professionals must deal with individually since each person's level of pain and pain tolerance is different. Also, dying people inevitably have questions about death: When? How? Where? For many ill people and their spouses, dying at home can be a frightening experience even though they may consider it preferable to dying in the impersonal atmosphere of a hospital. For these people, the support of an appropriately trained nurse or professional can bring physical and emotional comfort. Yet even with illnesses such as cancer, deterioration may be slow at first, sometimes with long periods of stability after the initial diagnosis and treatment. During this time the chronically ill may need encouragement and support for reengaging in life after the initial shock of announcement and treatment;

they may also need help with finding new ways of doing things should there be any residual body limitations. For these people, support groups can also be very important. The very last subphases of this type of trajectory phase have, of course, been extensively written about by and for health practitioners. It is the earlier subphases that are less well charted. Yet combined as they are with brief comebacks and weeks or months of stability, these subphases call for great psychological sensitivity, empathy, and interventional ingenuity on the part of health practitioners.

12

How the Spouse Is Affected

The stress and strain of living with and caring for chronically ill people are well documented in the literature (Klein, Dean, and Bogdonoff, 1967; Stuifbergen, 1987; Eckberg, Griffith, and Foxall, 1986; Brody, 1985; Goldstein, 1981; Archbold, 1980). Yet the problems associated with prolonged caretaking still exist. Why does the strain build up even to a crisis state? Why aren't resources available for spouses (and other caretakers) to call upon to ease their physical and emotional burdens? Or if such resources are available in a community, why aren't they discovered and better utilized (Chester and Barbarin, 1984)?

There are several reasons. First, the caretakers live in communities surrounded by healthy families; and since they often do not have the opportunity to talk with others with similar problems, many caretakers believe they are alone in their feelings of fatigue, depression, anger, and frustration, and they are ashamed of these feelings. They believe that if they were to tell others, somehow they would be perceived as inadequate—or even worse, as "bad" spouses. As a consequence, the healthy people around them (sometimes even their own children) are not aware that such feelings or problems exist. It is probably true that the healthy don't really want to be bothered by the details of what caring for an ill person is like; for the most part, they find these situations too depressing to dwell on, however sorry they might feel for the caretaker.

Second, in the United States people are expected to take care of their own—this is not the responsibility of the state. Rather, it is the *duty* of the spouse, parent, or adult child to care for his or her debilitated or disabled partner, children, or parent.

Third, caretakers are often reluctant to burden others by asking for help. They see their children, kin, and friends as having lives of their own. Not until they reach a crisis state do they call upon others to provide physical or emotional assistance.

Fourth, the impact of stress and strain is cumulative. It builds up over time, and even the caretaker may not be aware of it until he or she reaches a crisis state or is simply too worn down to take counteracting steps.

Fifth, even though resources (discussion groups, respite services, and home health aides) may exist, many caretakers are unaware of them or believe they don't have the extra money to pay for them; and some caretakers have no one to come in and care for the ill partner while they attend a potentially helpful group.

Sixth, many caretakers feel trapped, that there is no way out for them so why bother.

The purpose of this chapter is to describe what trajectory management means from the perspective of the spouse. We wish not only to portray their plight but also to emphasize *how* it comes about. Though our picture is certainly not complete, it will draw attention to the depth and scope of spouses' problems and add to what is certainly reflected in the technical literature. In the next section the discussion revolves around both general and specific aspects of the impact of trajectory management on the well spouse. The remaining sections focus more on the development of those consequences.

The Impact of Trajectory Management

In general, we found the spouses in our study eager to talk. Sometimes they seemed ready to burst: they had so much to tell and had held it in for so long. Often they would cry as they described their experiences. Sometimes, too, their vivid and often poignant life stories left us feeling drained and somewhat helpless. Usually all we could do was listen, offer words of comfort, and assure them that they were not alone.

Sets of Conditions. Before discussing what these spouses of the ill said, we should note that some well spouses feel the strain of living with an ill partner more than others do. In addition, the problems they must contend with and the manifestations of the underlying stress and strain do vary. In other words, (A) chronic illness or disability does not necessarily lead to (B) high stress and strain, which is then manifested by (C) certain behavior. Some of the conditions for the variation have been spelled out in previous chapters (especially in the interactional model presented in Chapter Eight); however, for emphasis, we will note a few here.

1. The type and severity of the illness or disability
2. The trajectory phase or subphase
3. The degree of related body failure
4. The degree to which the ill person has contextualized and come to terms with the illness and reconstructed life around it
5. The degree to which the ill person is able or willing to control symptoms, participate in the regimen management, prevent and handle crises
6. The work style that the couple have developed around the illness management and how well they have been able to articulate (singly and together) the resources, division of tasks, and sustained motivation to continue the work
7. How well the ill mate balances limitation stretching against overstretching

Additionally we might note some of the biographical conditions that affect well partners.

1. The degree to which well partners also have contextualized the illness into their lives, come to terms with it, and constructed their lives around it is extremely important. They too ask questions: What does this illness mean in terms of my life? How far will my mate come back, when, and for how long? What changes does this change mean for me? Will I have to go on alone? What will it be like? Well partners also often live with uncertainty and fear; but they don't want to add to the illness burdens borne by their spouse. They want to spare the spouse's already drained energies so they hide their feelings.

2. The salience of those aspects of the self that are lost because of a partner's illness—for example, those pertaining to sex, a job, or traveling—have a tremendous impact on well spouses.

3. The degree and type of deterioration of an ill partner and the relevance of this to a well spouse in terms of his or her partner's failed performances can be significant. For a wife to see her once handsome or strapping husband physically deteriorate and become disabled by illness or accident can be difficult and depressing. It can be even more disheartening to see him struggling with a simple task and to be unable to prevent that struggle, or to see him in excruciating pain and to be powerless to ease it. (It is not unknown for a spouse to help with a mate's suicide when his or her situation becomes hopeless or the pain too severe [Wertenbaker, 1957].)

4. The length of time the illness endures, the consequent interrupted biographical processes for the well spouse, and the sheer amount of cumulative work to be done can be exhausting.

5. The ingenuity of the well spouse to utilize resources and to develop management strategies to ease the burden (Holaday, 1978) is significant.

Moreover, additional macro and micro conditions bear on the situation. These range all the way from government regulations and disbursement of Medicare funds and the present rate of economic inflation to the age and health status of a spouse and the composition of a household. All of these *conditions* together result in the *impact of an illness trajectory* on the well spouse. This impact includes the numbers and types of *problems* that spouses must contend with, the total amount of *work* to be done, the *contingencies* that arise to upset daily management routines, the *resources and support* available for work performance, how and to what degree the *work load* can be *divided,* the amount of motivation and emotional *sustaining* that is needed and the degree to which it can be provided, and, ultimately, what the *consequences* of the trajectory management will be for the well spouse.

Consequences for the Well Spouse. Just what are the range and extent of the impact of a chronic illness trajectory on the well spouse? We had no difficulty in finding specific answers to this question in our interviews. Rather, our difficulty was in limiting the types and numbers we could present. The examples given below use the respondents' own words since these speak to the problems effectively and often dramatically. Each excerpt represents a different problem or constellation of problems. Some of these are as follows: (1) conflict over control of illness management, (2) constancy of the work and the resource drain that it brings about, (3) feeling the burden of three lines of work, (4) spouse overload (see Corbin and Strauss, 1985) and the resulting downward spiral of consequences from fatigue to hidden drinking—or what might be called the caretaking syndrome, (5) juggling of the needs of the ill person with the spouse's biographical needs, (6) sexual frustration, (7) anxiety over dwindling financial resources, (8) fear of the dying, (9) feelings of isolation and loneliness, (10) biographical disruption and biographical limbo, and (11) change in the nature of the marital relationship (including a spouse's resentment) and lack of a mutually sustaining relationship. This partial list gives some conception of the range of problems that spouses face.

The husband of a diabetic admits his resentment:

> I am under a lot of pressure at work and there are times when I come home and I feel that I am being attacked for no reason at all, or I come home and she is sick. I try not to let it affect me, but I know it shows. I come home and she has a headache, and I think, Jesus Christ; here we go again. I have to sit back and grit my teeth. I don't like to see her ill. Nobody likes to see somebody suffer. I may have had a bad day and I get to the point that I become resentful. Okay, I am resentful. I am not making apologies for myself.

This woman describes the physical work required in caring for her ill spouse:

> All night long he would say, "Get me water, put me on the commode." I would tell K., "Let me sleep; let me rest. I don't mind waiting on you hand and foot during the day, but at night let me sleep." . . . He got out of bed one night and urinated all over the floor. I had to get up and clean him up and put him back to bed. I didn't realize he was taking up so much of my energy. That twenty-four-hour stuff was getting to me. . . . After he died, I was so exhausted. . . . I am

still. . . . God was good to me in a way. Had [my
husband] been sick for any longer, it would have
broken me physically and financially.

A woman describes how she felt about having to place her
husband in a nursing home because of her own exhaustion, after
having cared for him at home for twenty-four years:

I feel so guilty. I know that I have no reason to feel
guilty. He has never been alone before and now he has
to be. I admit I wish he had just died. I worked so darn
hard all those years to take care of him, to have to go
through seeing what is happening to him now. I pray,
"Please, take him quickly."

The wife of a diabetic admits to feeling like a victim:

I feel like, "Oh, my word. This dear man, he is pulling
me down, I am pulling him down." I get down. What
do older people do? You can talk to your kids, but they
don't understand. He is tearing me down because I am
always on the lookout. How is he? Does he need
something? The main things that bother me are the
insulin shock and now the congestive heart thing. He
doesn't listen to me and so it is a constant vigilance
with this man. Yet as a wife you have an obligation.
There are times when I think gosh, if only I could
wash my hands of him. But of course, I can't.

Next we hear from a woman whose husband has heart
disease:

I don't allow myself to think about what it will be like
after he goes. I just hope he goes quickly. I try not to
think about it, but I can't help but think about it
because I am concerned. I don't make any plans for
myself for the future because you can't predict what
will happen. Maybe I will go first. You can't let them

know that it is upsetting you because then they get
upset.

The wife of an Alzheimer's sufferer describes her frustrations:

I've been able to get him into the respite care program.
I might add that up until that time I was getting
desperate, just desperate, because it is a twenty-four-
hour thing and you can never get away. They follow
you like children. And then their hygiene habits
become appalling. . . . You can't imagine the pressure. We not only need hospices, we need places for
people who are going to live. Before I sent him to
respite (one week every six weeks), I would speak to
him very sharply. Sometimes he would speak back,
but most of the time he would go to bed. He was
spending a lot of time in bed as a reaction to that
situation. We had always been very close, but I was
getting to dislike him, really getting to dislike him. I
would get up first and I dreaded hearing that voice in
the morning. . . . Another thing is I started to drink.
. . . It is a vicious cycle because the problem is there
the next morning and you don't feel as well able to
cope. Then, of course, it was taking more and more
wine to make me feel good. I gradually graduated to
a gallon. One day my daughter said, "You have got to
stop drinking that wine. You will become an alco-
holic." I was probably well on the way. Then and
there I made up my mind to quit, but it was a struggle.

Another wife describes her own precarious mental state:

For a while I was awfully nervous and I thought
maybe I should see a psychiatrist. I thought well there
is no point in that because it is just the stress of this
situation. And the financial problems are getting
awfully bad. . . . The rent keeps going up. Medicare
doesn't pay the extra doctors they bring in or all the

other extras. I've had to turn in two savings bonds and lose money. . . . I feel sorry for myself because I haven't been able to go to church for two years. I can't leave him. . . . I get lonely. I don't have many visitors. Sometimes when I go out to do the laundry or go to the drugstore, I sit in the lobby for a few minutes just to chat or watch the people go by. . . . I don't know what I would do if he died here [at home]. I think I would go nuts. I don't think I could take it.

We hear next from a man who explains some of the pleasures he has had to give up since his wife's illness.

I am a bundle of nerves because I can't get out and play handball anymore. I have had to give up my sex life. I am a healthy physical man. It is a toughie. You can't masturbate at seventy-three; it isn't going to do you any good. I'll be honest with you, there isn't a dame that I miss when I go out shopping or anywhere. . . . Sometimes I get impatient. She pushes me pretty hard in the morning: "I want my cereal. You didn't do this." I say, "Give me a chance. If you were in the hospital, you would have three or four attendants." I lift her out of the bed onto the commode. I have to make sure of the catheter. I say, "Honey, I only have two legs, two arms, and one mind." I can't afford to have someone living here full time. I would have to mortgage my house. Some of the bills I have received from the doctors are unbelievable. It has been a year now and I am still paying on some. . . . She gets depressed and so do I. . . . Some of my friends are going to Reno on a bus. I wish I could climb on the bus and go with them.

One woman describes the effects of the stress in her life:

When he becomes depressed I get depressed too. There are times in between when I get depressed. I think it

is just the worry, the stress. I break down rather easily.
I didn't do that in the beginning. It's just that it has
been so prolonged. . . . It has been one stress after
another. You can't imagine what it means to have to
hospitalize someone ten times in two years. The days
that he is in the hospital I can't describe the exhaustion that I feel. I know that it is the stress thing. . . .
I've changed. Inside I have had to be stronger. I have
had to cover up an awful lot of my feelings so that he
doesn't see them. . . . I think one of the saddest things
for me is when he said to me in the hospital, "I know
that I am never going to be well."

Finally, a woman whose husband has Parkinson's disease
tells of her own devastation.

I need some help. I am burned out. I am locked in this
house. I am used to going out to work and had to
retire. I didn't plan to retire so soon. We had planned
our retirement. We never did anything before because
we didn't have the same vacation time. So you do all
this and then bingo! . . . Two weeks ago I had a
terrible pain in my ribs. But I can't run to the doctor
for every little thing. How can I leave the house? I
worry, what is going to happen to him, if I have to go
to the hospital. . . . Medicare pays for only part of the
things we need and doesn't pay for medications. That
bottle of medication cost $130. . . . Sometimes he has
to go to the bathroom just when I've finished eating.
It is hard to get up at that instant to do it. You feel
like everything is going to come up. You have all these
things to contend with. People don't realize that
unless they are in those situations themselves. My
sisters definitely don't understand what I am going
through. You have to really see it for yourself, be in
it, to know what it is like.

Note the wide range and combinations of problems that the spouses of ill people face. One can see why they feel frustrated, angry, baffled, isolated, guilty, biographically blocked, worn out, exhausted, financially strained. It is not hard to imagine how they begin to feel trapped, desperate, and pushed to their limits of tolerance, so that the stress begins to manifest itself in overeating, drinking, illness, allergies and skin rashes such as hives, verbal and other emotional abuse of the ill person, and undoubtedly, if rarely, even attempted murder.

Calling attention to the problems and how people react to them is not enough. If we want to ease the plight of spouses, indeed of any caretaker, caught up in the problems of living with and/or caring for a chronically ill person, we need a much deeper, more explicit, and systematic understanding of what happens in such situations.

We turn next to cases designed to illustrate more directly how the consequences for healthy partners develop. The cases show especially (1) how the stresses that well partners experience arise not only out of physical caretaking but also from the emotional drain of living with the chronically ill even when there is little or no physical caretaking involved; (2) how the work of spouses, as well as the impact of living with and caring for the ill, varies according to the trajectory phase; (3) how the well spouses must also do a great deal of biographical work; (4) how the impact of chronic illness or disability is not necessarily all negative but sometimes brings out strengths in the well mates that they did not know existed and thus can affect the lives of both partners; (5) how there is in every situation a looming potential for the physical or emotional breakdown of either spouse or the marital relationship because of constant and sometimes insidious strain brought about by having to cope day after day with managing severe illness.

Well spouses are in a sense a mirror image of their ill mates. We do not mean that the former are exact physical and emotional replicas of the latter. Rather, we mean that the work that *well* spouses are called upon to perform for their partners, themselves, and others is to some degree a reflection of where the *ill* mates are in terms of their own illness, biographical, and everyday experiences (Bray, 1977). As Mary Willis says, "His infirmity reflected on me in ways so subtle that I was unaware of their effect" (Willis and Willis, 1974, p. 167). However, these reflections, like any mirrored image, can become distorted and illusional, depending upon whose eyes see them. Put another way, we cannot examine the impact of illness upon well partners without looking at that in relation to their mates. Both the illnesses and the ill people's responses to them—along with the well spouses' responses to both—set crucial conditions under which the well act.

Case 1: Living Through Trajectory Phases

Several years ago, Mr. Marston suffered severe damage to his spinal cord. From the diaphragm down he has no feeling. He uses his pectoral muscles to breath. With therapy, he has been able to learn to perform his own daily activities.

We shall first take you through the case in a shorthand fashion from the beginning of the disability trajectory to the time of the interview, when Mr. Marston was in a stable phase. The format of presentation is arranged in terms of the conditions present in each trajectory phase, including the action context in which the wife is acting, the work that she is called on to do, and the consequences for her.

Acute Trajectory Phase and Other Micro and Macro Conditions. In the immediate postaccident, acute phase of trajectory the family didn't know the extent of injuries or how badly Mr. Marston's neck or back was broken. In addition, his ribs were crushed and his lungs perforated. He was comatose for a short time and was on a respirator and IVs and had chest tubes. His wife was called on to make decisions about moving him to have CAT scans and possible surgery. Before he was moved, she was warned that moving him might further increase the extent of his injuries or even cause his death. During this acute phase, Mrs. Marston spent most of her time by her husband's side except for evenings with her children. Because her husband was in the military, she had no immediate financial concerns about hospital payment. Both partners' extended families lived nearby. It was this couple's first contact with severe illness or injury.

In this phase the action context was rich in manpower

resources. Immediate resource mobilization took place as neighbor and family stepped in to provide support and child care. "They were very supportive. With living so close to the hospital and having our families, I felt very fortunate."

Mrs. Marston had to suspend all but necessary everyday work and biographical performances. Of the unknown future (for him, her, and them), Mrs. Marston notes: "I wasn't concerned about paralysis at this point; I was more concerned about whether or not he was going to live."

In terms of sentimental and "filtered" information work with the children, Mrs. Marston explains: "I went home every night so I could see the boys and talk with them a little about what was going on. I didn't tell them too much because I was afraid they couldn't handle it. But I had to tell them some because they were afraid their dad was dead."

At this point, biographical types of work for Mrs. Marston mainly involved some coming to terms with the possible death of her husband. Disability-related work was primarily limited to decision making in regard to treatment. Her internal resources were drained by fatigue, fear, and stress:

> I didn't trust myself to make any decisions. I was too emotionally involved. I had to call his brother, his parents, and my parents before I could do anything. . . . At the time of the CAT scan they told me he might die. I became hysterical because I always had it in the back of my mind that no matter what happens he is going to make it. He may not be the same, but he will go on living. When they took that away from me, I didn't have anything to hold onto. I felt that I'd lost control.

Mrs. Marston acted as a body resource for her husband. Although he was fairly independent by the time he came home, she did have to do some things for him, such as those mentioned below, and she had to drive him to the hospital for checkups and rehab. Mrs. Marston also said:

It was hard when he first came home because I didn't
know how to take care of him. I couldn't please him
no matter how I did it. I didn't have to do his physical
care; rather, it was more of setting things up for him
so he could do it. I didn't know how to fix the pillows,
arrange things around him. He wouldn't compromise. It had to be his way. I said, "Fine, fine." After
a while, we finally worked it out. He just told me what
to do and how to do it. Now he can do all of that
himself.

*Beginning Comeback Phase and Other Micro and Macro
Conditions.* Mr. Marston's rehabilitation began in the hospital;
soon, however, he was transferred to a regional rehabilitation center
in another city. This phase of treatment would be quite long, so his
wife decided to move to a city closer to the rehab center. It took her
two weeks to find housing that the family could now afford, that
would be near schools for the children, and that would be wheelchair accessible for her husband.

All decision making in regard to details of the move and the
work of maintaining the household fell to Mrs. Marston. She
received little assistance or sustenance in return: "He just saw what
was there around him. He didn't see what was going on at home.
He really didn't want to know. He didn't want to know about the
pressures at home. He stayed out of it and let me handle it all."

In addition, there was the following biographical
construction:

I had to drop [going to school] plus my job as an
instructional aide at the children's school. I had to
drop all other activities. . . . The only time I went out
of the house during this time was to go grocery
shopping, drive the kids to and from school, and go
to the rehab center. . . . He didn't know about the
move up here, my getting the kids in school, finding
doctors, then traveling back and forth. He couldn't
understand why I couldn't be with him more. Then
some older boys took my second grade son into the

woods—he had no idea at the time about sex—
exposed themselves and said how is your dad going to
do this now? I had to deal with that. I didn't tell my
husband.

Mrs. Marston also had to deal with closed awareness in the
following sense: "Even if I saw him angry and upset or didn't like
the way he talked to me or something, I didn't get upset in front
of him. If I got upset every time he got upset or pitied him, he
couldn't have handled it. He had enough problems just trying to
get better."

At this point Mrs. Marston began to ask: Will he come back
physically, how far, in how long? And if he doesn't, what will this
mean? Of the shift in the division of labor, she says:

> One of the major problems since the accident has been
> having to cope and make decisions by myself. We used
> to make decisions together. I took care of the imme-
> diate things, and he took care of all the future things.
> Since then, I've had to make all the financial deci-
> sions, all the decisions about how to handle the kids,
> where to go, what paperwork to do and so forth. I
> didn't have the experience to handle that by myself.
> . . . He always took care of the car. . . . [Now] I feel
> very inadequate about that.

Mrs. Marston also had financial concerns at this time.

> We didn't have the money to move into off-base
> housing. I had to borrow money from my dad, and [he
> and my mother] helped subsidize us until I could get
> some benefits from the service. . . . I kept getting
> panicky because I kept getting notices about him
> being in the service and what they were going to do
> or not do for us. I wondered who was going to take
> care of us. Were we going to lose our ID cards? They
> were trying to retire him. I thought that meant we
> would lose everything. Finally, I got a lawyer. I found

out if they retired him my benefits would be greater
than if he died.

Sentimental work, for Mrs. Marston, consisted not only of
encouraging, comforting, and supporting her husband but also
bearing the brunt of his frustrations and convincing him that he
was making progress. In terms of sustaining herself: "Most of what
I ever did for myself during this time is whenever I was driving I
would take a break and stop somewhere to eat, even if it was only
McDonald's. I would just sit there for maybe fifteen minutes and
watch the people go by."

Then, too, there was the matter of reciprocating: "Everyone
helped me so much. Therefore, when my sister asked me to watch
her two- and three-year-old kids so she could work, I did. I did that
for six months until my husband came out of the rehab center, plus
running back and forth to the hospital."

The consequences of all these factors weighed heavily on
Mrs. Marston, as we can see from the following quotations.

Robot functioning: "During this time I was completely
numb. I just did what I had to do and was with him as much as
I could. I tried to explain to the kids what was going on without
letting them see how flat I was. I held in a lot. If I had not had my
mother to talk to, I would not have made it."

Self-questioning: "I questioned everything I was doing. I
didn't feel very confident in my opinions, especially concerning the
kids. I would say, 'We are going to do this,' then I would change
my mind and say, 'We are going to do that.' The kids didn't know
where they stood."

Self-neglect: "I didn't take very good care of myself. I gained
a lot of weight. The first three months I gained fifty pounds."

Overprotectiveness: "I wouldn't let the children go anywhere
for a long time. It was very difficult for me to let them go. After what
happened to him, I was extremely frightened. I couldn't handle it,
if something happened to the kids."

Later Comeback Phase and Other Micro and Macro Conditions. After Mr. Marston returned home, he was able to perform
many activities of daily living, such as dressing and brushing his
teeth. For him, coming home meant having to push his limitations

outward in order to gain greater independence. It also meant trying to fit back into the household, only from a changed position physically (from the wheelchair) and emotionally and socially (from the wheelchair). The conditions that motivated Mr. Marston were, first of all, his desire to attain greater independence and not be a burden and, second, the degenerative arthritis in his wife's back that prevented her from doing any heavy lifting or bending.

In speaking of the transition and adjustment that were taking place for the family, Mrs. Marston says:

> One problem we had was who was going to be the boss? When my husband was in the service, he was home mainly on weekends and he pretty much let me handle disciplining the children. When he got home, he wanted (and took) control of it. He felt he wanted respect from the kids and this was the way to do it. The kids didn't like it. They would come to me and say "Dad bawled me out. . . ."

Attempting to redefine her own identity in relationship to his attempts to redefine his identity, she says, "I felt very threatened by his attempts to take over the disciplining because I thought I was doing fine and then all of a sudden he decides he is going to do it all. I felt very left out, and we had a big argument about that."

In terms of diffusing the tension, Mrs. Marston asks, "What do you do when your husband starts screaming and cussing at you and the kids? He never used to be that way. He wasn't just using *shit* or something like that. I told him either to stop it or do it by himself because "the kids and I don't like to be around you when you are like that." He did stop.

The consequences of this later comeback phase were upheaval, confusion, and frustration in the children as well as in their mother. "[They] didn't understand the frustration my husband has gone through and how he [then] put it on them. He wanted to be the father but was superstrict and shouldn't have been. They didn't know where they stood. It was very frustrating. . . .The children fear that since he has been home, he is going to leave us because we fight and we didn't used to fight. Usually when we fight, it is about disciplining the children."

The cumulative impact of these consequences began to take their toll on Mrs. Marston.

> I didn't have much time to myself at all. . . . I developed hives on my hands. They were driving me crazy so I had to go to the doctor to get something for that. . . . Stress also throws my back out. The doctor gave me pills, but I don't like to take them because they make me sleepy. . . . No matter what I wanted to do I couldn't do it. Finally, I reached a point that if I didn't have to do anything, I did nothing. I did the things that were expected of me, like taking care of the kids, but I didn't want to do them. I didn't want to do anything for anybody. I was tired all the time because I didn't sleep. He didn't do a lot to make it easier on me, but I don't think he realized what he could do.

Her emotions erupted into feelings of hatred and resentment, guilt and self-pity.

> A lot of the time, I felt a lot of hatred toward him because I felt that he was treating me like a servant, a housekeeper, rather than a wife. I didn't realize he didn't know how to treat me. He didn't know where he was. It could have broken up the marriage if I had let it get to me. At the time it wasn't that important to me. The most important thing was that he continued to get strong and more independent. . . . I felt that I wasn't getting enough attention and I didn't want to do anything for anybody because nobody was doing anything for me. I felt sorry for myself. At the same time, I didn't like that feeling because I felt it was very selfish. I felt very guilty about it, which compounded the self-pity. It was like a vicious circle.

Stable Trajectory Phase and Other Micro and Macro Conditions. It is now two years later, and Mr. Marston is quite independent. He drives and attends classes at a local college. Mrs. Marston has also started back to school. Because one of their children ran away, the family attended family counseling for six months. "It worked out well because it got the kids to talk."

Although Mr. M. has come back to independent functioning, he still has not fully come to terms with his disability or found new directions for himself. This is a time of searching for him. "Before he knew where he was, what he was going to do when he retired, and where we were going to retire. Now he is going through all of this again. . . . I don't think he has come to the point of acceptance of you can't function one way but you can do other things, feel other things."

Through all of this, Mrs. Marston's mother has been very supportive. "The first thing my mother does when she comes through the door is put her arms around me." The children have also. "I tell the kids when things are really bad—depressed. I tell them, 'You better behave yourselves or you will have a screaming mother on your hands.' When I tell them this, they leave me alone." Mr. Marston does try to help. When his wife is out late, he fixes dinner; occasionally, he does the laundry and takes the boys bowling to give her a break.

Mrs. Marston talks about this time as being a waiting period for her:

> At this point in his life, he is not ready to have me in
> it too. I am there as the mother, his housekeeper, and
> so forth. Now that he has some freedom and mobility,
> he wants to see where he is going to go. Once he has
> decided, I know I will be in it but it is a matter of
> finding out where he is and what he wants to do. I told
> him we needed to talk to someone who can get us to
> talk. He says we can handle it ourselves. I am waiting.
> . . . I don't know, I do a lot of waiting.

Speaking of a physical and emotional contact barrier, she continues:

I don't think sex or affection is a need in his life right now. I don't think that he realizes that sometimes it is a need for me. When we reached that point in the counseling, he quit. I think he is afraid to talk about it. I would be willing to talk, but he is not. I am letting him go at his own pace.

In terms of her biographical coming out, Mrs. Marston has this to say:

I've started doing things more the last six months. Going to school requires my forcing myself to do a lot of things, because I know that if I don't I am going to be in trouble. I am forcing myself to do things like being a den mother. I came to realize that if anything happened to my husband that I could not support myself or my kids so I am going back to college so that I have something to fall back on in case something happens.

Then she comments on some repercussions from this: "The kids don't like it; they don't want me to go to school. They didn't mind my going to work. It is funny but going to school is really different. I said to them, 'You realize why I am going back to school?' And they replied, 'Because you are going to get a divorce.'"

Marital uncertainty also marks this period for Mrs. Marston.

It has gotten somewhat better and I don't think it will get worse. It is up to him. He either has to want it or not want it. If he doesn't, I will know because it will get worse. I can only do so much. He keeps saying, "If something happens between us, I will take care of you." I say, "What do you mean by that?" He says, "Drop it." . . . Now that he has become more independent, it is important to me that he find out where he is, what he wants to do with his life.

Mrs. Marston continues with her sentimental and identity
work.

> I encourage him to talk about the things that he does.
> When he goes to the rehab center I ask, "How much
> weight did you lift today?" I encourage him to do
> things with the boys. When one of the children asks
> me for help with math, I say, "Ask your dad." I buy
> him things that I know he likes, like finding the right
> lightweight backpack to put on his chair. . . . Some-
> times I put my arms around him and say, "It is okay."

She also continues to push her husband, but with modera-
tion.

> It is important to me that he get out and do things.
> I have to watch myself because I have expectations of
> him that may not be his. It is important to me to see
> his progress. It gives me hope when I see him trying
> and constantly working at it. I know he is not going
> to fall back; he is going to keep doing. I told him to
> keep going, let me do all the falling back.

Now Mrs. Marston attempts to assess the consequences of the
stable trajectory phase.

> In some ways the disability has torn us apart . . . we
> are not so much husband and wife anymore. It is more
> like we are live-in companions. The loving relation-
> ship is completely gone. It is very stressful. I just
> practically fall apart. The boys understand what is
> happening. One time we were driving home from
> somewhere and the older one said, "Mom, it is just not
> the same between you and Dad is it?" "No." "It is not
> very fair." I said, "No, it is not." But what can I do?
> I've tried to put my arms around him and kiss him,
> but if I touch him the wrong way he goes into spasms

and is frustrated. I have to be careful about what I do and what I say.

Still, in the following comments we see the beginnings of partial change for the better, some coming back and opening up.

> I don't feel as guilty anymore. I started coming back because I couldn't take acting like I was anymore. I think the counseling has helped in that I was able to talk about it. Talking helped me to realize a lot of things about T. No matter how much I wanted him to change, I realized he wasn't going to change unless he wanted it. No matter how much I tried to be the perfect person, it wasn't going to make any difference. It is up to him. Once I realized that, then I could start thinking about what I wanted to do, what has to be done, and what makes me happy and the kids happy. It has helped me to come back some, but I still am not where I was before. I was always very organized. I am not now. . . .
>
> He is starting to talk more about what he is doing, not about the relationship but other kinds of things. I am beginning to understand more of what he likes and dislikes. He asks me about my classes. He doesn't ask too much. He still doesn't want to know too much.

Case Summary. In this case we see a dedicated wife and mother trying to hold onto her marriage and to do what she believes is best for her husband and children, though at considerable cost to herself. Three years after the accident, she is attempting to break out of the downward cycle that she is in and to gain some control over her life. Trajectory progression through three phases—acute, comeback, and stable—is illustrated here, although the disabled mate has not yet fully come back emotionally from his accident. Of course, this case also highlights many theoretical points relevant to illness trajectory, its work, and its impact on the well spouse.

Case 2: Living Through Subphases of a Downward Trajectory

Trajectory experience can take many directions, depending upon the nature of the illness and/or disability, the marital relationship, religious beliefs, life stage, and so forth. Consider the situation of the Daughertys, a situation that is in direct contrast to the Marstons' in terms of its downward trajectory and also in family relationships and other structural conditions. This second case highlights the experience that work and life are not so much affected by trajectory phase as they are by type and subphase of trajectory.

The Daughertys are a middle-class, middle-aged couple. Mr. D. owns his own insurance business. Mrs. D.'s life has always centered around the home, her husband, and the raising of their six children. Only one child is still at home. Always close, the couple have drawn even closer together since his diagnosis of melanoma three years ago. They have been able to talk about the illness and its implications and therefore to help each other come to terms with what this inevitably means.

Here is the story from Mrs. D.'s perspective. (Mr. D. covered essentially the same points from a similar perspective.) Mrs. D. first noticed a slight change in a mole on her husband's back so she suggested he see a doctor, who did "burn it off." Then another mole appeared, and this, too, was burned off. The couple trusted their doctor's judgment. They thought no more about it until one day a lump appeared under Mr. D.'s arm. He was put into the hospital, the mole was removed, and a biopsy was finally done. "This was the first time I heard the word *melanoma*. I didn't associate it with cancer. When the doctor said it was 'all out,' we thought that was the end of it."

Not long afterward, another lump appeared. It was quite large and down to the bone. The couple were both a little shaken and prayed that all would be well. The lump was surgically removed. At this time, Mrs. D. still didn't realize the full impact of what was to come even though the physicians did tell her that they didn't know the source of the cancer, that it was now in the blood stream, and that there was no cure. "For days I walked around feeling like there was a 'brick' in my stomach."

Then a lump appeared on Mr. D.'s back. Since they were planning a vacation, the doctor told them to go ahead. While on vacation, a trajectory projection first crystallized: "I said to myself, perhaps next year at this time I won't have a husband. It was the first time I started entertaining this kind of thought." Mr. D. was aware of what she was thinking, so they talked about it. In spite of, or perhaps because of, the looming potential, the couple had a wonderful time on this vacation. Afterward, the lump was removed, but Mrs. D. had doubts about having delayed treatment and blamed herself for the delay. "I never dreamed it would be this serious."

When lumps later appeared under both of Mr. D.'s arms, their physician referred them to a major medical center. The physician who saw them there decided to take a wait-and-see attitude, for he judged the lumps were not yet large enough to warrant removal. The Daughertys asked about chemotherapy, but the physician pointed out that it was only 30 percent effective. Surprisingly, the lumps spontaneously disappeared. The physician continued to observe Mr. D. Then, in the middle of summer, another lump appeared. It was not until late in the fall that the physician believed surgery was called for.

When the couple next returned to the medical center, for some reason they were seen by another physician. They were given an appointment to return in two weeks. When they did, they were told that the lump was now too large to be removed surgically.

> He laid it right on the line; he didn't pull any punches. He said no way could he operate, it was too large an area, wouldn't heal properly. He was almost saying, maybe a few months, maybe a lot less.

Stunned, the Daughertys were told they would have to see an internist, who would decide upon the next mode of intervention.

> They had kind of implied . . . in our minds we had thought this disease is not so bad, maybe once a year or in nine months he would go in and have surgery. We just thought it would go on and on. I mean, you don't put a time frame on it like it will go on for two

years, then this will happen. I have an optimistic
nature, perhaps too much so. I guess we both kind of
felt that way. In fact, the doctor told us early in June
that he would rather carve than radiate. I can't say
they misjudged. It is all in God's hands. You can't
look back and say if . . . that tears you apart. You can
only go forward and trust in God.

When they returned the next week, they were told that the
treatment of choice was now chemotherapy. The couple did not
give up hoping or stop living, but they realized death was inevitable, though still in the distant future. "We always thought the
illness was something we could live with, that we had the option
of surgery. The door was closed, slammed."

What did this new trajectory projection mean for Mrs. D.,
Mr. D., and their relationship? It meant they had a lot of prepara-
tory work to do in planning for her future; they also had to readjust
and come to terms with the new treatment, its side effects, and their
now foreshortened future together. "Whenever you have change you
have to work it out and then fit it into your pattern of living and
thinking. He is facing the reality that he has to have things in
order."

We shall limit the rest of this narrative to what the foregoing
knowledge has meant for Mrs. D. and the kinds of work she has to
do (aside from learning the business, in all its many details, and
how to handle the couple's financial matters).

In terms of information work, Mrs. D. states: "At first we told
everyone that there would be occasional surgery and that is the way
it would be. Now I have to tell everyone. He has three sisters back
East, then there are the children."

And in speaking of identity and comfort work:

I know when he is just marking time, trying to get
through a period. He does things, but he just kind of
does them because they are expected. I've learned how
to handle it when he gets down. He gets grumpy. I let
him know I don't approve of the way he is behaving,
and he knows he needs my reminder. You can't let

them get away with things just because they are sick. It wouldn't be a happy situation for him because he would hate himself and I can't let that happen. But I also know that he only does this when he is very tense and under a great deal of pressure and it just kind of comes out that way. I encourage him to watch TV, something to relax him. . . .

I find that when I am bothered, I go out into the yard and walk around in the grass. It is very comforting. I walk around and sometimes kind of pray. I tell the children he is not afraid, he is very peaceful, that he feels that there is a purpose to all of this.

Projecting a future in which she is alone is a forward review that is part of the coming to terms process and the beginning of reconstituting Mrs. D.'s new single identity. "Once in a while it just kind of hits me. I think, I'll probably be alone some day. I'll be a widow. What is it going to be like? My routines won't be changed, but I will be doing it alone. I don't look forward to it, but it is easy to push the thoughts away; it is morbid."

Reminiscing involves a backward review and a storing of memories for future backward reviews, a type of closure act, a coming to terms with past life as well as potential death.

We've always had mornings together because he doesn't have to be to work until late. Mornings were always precious to us. Now we get up and go to church together, walk, and talk. It is a wonderful time. We were talking [about] how blessed we are to have had that time together. And I do spend time with him at the office.

Of juggling treatment options and planning for potential side effects, Mrs. D. says: "When you think about an option, you have to juggle the side effects against its value. I know that he will lose some hair, and he has very nice hair. But that is just a vanity thing. I did say, 'Perhaps it will change your personality?' We talked about that. . . . We planned our vacation so that it would not coincide with the treatments."

Spouses of the ill must also prepare for the next downward step, anticipating the future and marking the downward progress of trajectory in terms of treatment. According to Mrs. D., "Now chemotherapy is the option replacing surgery, the next step down. That is the way I categorize it in my mind. Radiation will be the last resort, when there is nothing else."

Normalizing and keeping up hope (Knapfl and Deatrick, 1986) are what sustain the Daughertys in continuing the illness work and keeping their lives going. "Our life is perfectly normal. He goes to work, plays tennis. He is very loving, and we have a good relationship all the way around. Always there is that hope."

This very collaborative couple were able to pace their coming to terms together, probably because of their ability to talk to each other about the trajectory and its potential course and because of their strong religious faith. Then, too, Mr. D. is still active, receiving and responding to treatment, and so death still seems off in the distance.

There is another aspect of well spouses' experiences with illness that is too important to overlook. It is what might be called the *tug-of-war phenomenon:* their experiences of being torn between two conflicting sets of feelings. These experiences occur especially when they care for partners who are slowly deteriorating and becoming progressively very debilitated. On one hand, the spouses feel depleted emotionally and physically from the work— the physical tasks to be done for the ill mate coupled with the everyday tasks and biographical work to be done for the self and others. Tired and drained by the long duration of the illness, the heaviness of the work load, and the need to hold up and be strong, their own solicitous and tender concern is replaced by urges to yell at their ill mate, to handle the ill mate roughly, to delay in responding to his or her requests, and so forth. There are days when the burdened spouses may even wish the ill would hurry up and die.

On the other hand, spouses of the ill feel guilty and angry with themselves because of their thoughts and/or actions. After all, they may have been married for forty or more years, been more or less happy in their marital relationship, and had an agreeable division of labor. Deep down there may still be strong emotional ties, and in many instances a strong sense of duty and obligation. For some, the caretaking tasks give a reason to live and to keep going day after day. Many have had to relinquish outside contacts, almost wholly, because of demands on their time and energy. Thus, while wishing to be out of the present situation, they do not necessarily want to be deprived of their mate. So the well partners are caught up in a no-exit situation: the only way out seems to be a physical or mental breakdown or temporary respite from caretaking duties through social programs or the assistance of relatives and friends. When the ill mate finally dies, the other may experience both relief and a tremendous sense of loss.

Summary

Theory. This chapter opens with the observation that the stress experienced by spouses and other caretakers of the ill is well documented in the literature. Why, then, are there not sufficient resources for caretakers to call on? We suggest several reasons in this chapter, including that caretakers may not be aware of available resources or believe they must pay for them. Another factor may be that a sense of family responsibility is so paramount to many caretakers that they are reluctant to call on other people except in an emergency. As well, stress in their lives may be so cumulative that even they are not aware of how great it is until too late.

Some of the impacts of a partner's illness and its management on the well spouse are illustrated using personal accounts, each in its own very expressive language. These excerpts reflect the consequences of the spouse's deep involvement: overwork, exhaustion, frustration, strained marital relationships that may be essentially reduced to work relationships, and so on. Two longer case illustrations are also presented. The first follows the progress of a couple through a paraplegic trajectory as it passes through the acute, early comeback, and later comeback phases, and then, finally, stabilizes. Through it all, the well spouse struggles to keep her marriage together and her children psychologically secure, but at much expense to her personal life. The second case follows a man with cancer through several subphases of a deteriorating trajectory and presents some of the couple's experiences, especially those of the wife. We show, for instance, her reactions to the first appearance of the disease and to each new sign of further deterioration. We also illustrate the formation of new biographical projections and the altered life plans that accompany them. The wife's anticipated stance toward becoming a widow is expressed clearly, as are the kinds of biographical reviews associated with this stance and other changed and changing self-conceptions.

Applications. Ill people and their spouses usually live in locales where the other people living around them are relatively or completely unaware of their difficulties. The motto of these couples seems to be: "Don't burden other people with your problems." Sometimes this motto even describes how they feel about revealing the depths of their problems to their own adult children. At the same time, these couples may be relatively unfamiliar with the range of home care services available to them, may reject these services for one reason or another, or may not find their way in the home care agency maze. Various case illustrations and excerpts from our interviews bring out the need of these couples for different kinds of services when they experience different kinds of trajectories and subphases. The major practical question—for both health care policy makers and providers—is how to create a match between services and trajectory phases and subphases. Indeed, the primary question may be how to get the services to these couples at all.

One clear implication is that closing the gap between services and need should begin in hospitals and clinics. Staffs should begin to think in terms of acute care being followed by comeback—as indeed some staffs already do—and anticipate that movement through phases. Health personnel who are out in the community and visiting the homes of the chronically ill ought to be thinking not only in terms of acute care, but in terms of chronic illness trajectories. They should also be concerned about the spouses and children of the chronically ill. Future health care policy can surely include the creation of mechanisms to bridge the gap between health facilities and the homebound ill. It can also make financing available so that burdened caretakers can get time off for respite, help with housekeeping services, and so on. Most of all, perhaps, changes can be made in the direction of matching services to trajectory types and subphases and making existing services much more visible.

13

The Unending Work
and Care Associated
with Chronic Illness

At the center of our theoretical formulations in this book are two concepts: *work and trajectory*. Their relevance can be grasped quickly by the following considerations. When illness appears, its management involves more or less work and care by some person or persons, this work and care entailing tasks and usually work relationships in order to get the tasks performed. However, illnesses have courses, and chronic illnesses have courses of life-long duration that may go through any number of phases (comeback, stable, unstable, deteriorating, dying). It follows that the specifics of the illness work can, and usually will, vary considerably according to the phase of illness. As we noted in Chapter Three, "illness course" as a concept (derived from medicine) does not at all satisfy the aims of a sociological interpretation of how illness is managed even by the primary physician, let alone when the management of an illness moves into the home. The concept of illness trajectory encompasses not only the course of physiological illness but all the associated work; it also includes the work relationships and worker experiences, which in turn affect the work of managing the illness. (Also implicitly it includes at least various interactional and organizational conditions that affect the work.) At home, the management is carried out within an ongoing context embracing the daily lives and biographical concerns of the entire family. This context is quite different from that found in hospitals and other health care facilities.

318

Unending Work and Care

In a general sense, this entire book is a spelling out answers to a set of fascinating theoretical, and pragmatical important, questions, including the following: What work i involved in this illness management at home? How does it relate to the work entailed in living a normal, everyday life? How does it relate to the biographical concerns (which obviously can be affected by and then affect the illness work—and also involve a species of work)? How does this interrelated work actually get *done?* When done effectively or ineffectively, then why and with what consequences—specifically, for the illness management? Over the long course of the illness (however stable), how are the everyday lives and biographies shaped by the entire illness trajectory, and with what consequences for the illness management and thus potentially for the physiological course of the illness?

Unless a chronic illness is genetic, it first appears within the ongoing context of the daily activities and biographical concerns mentioned above. (If it is genetic, the child grows up with an awareness of illness as a part of everyday life and biography.) In Chapter Two we noted the frequency of prediagnostic work inevitably occurring unless the diagnostic signs are simply noticed by an alert physician or picked up fortuitously when diagnostic tests (such as blood tests) are being done for other reasons. The diagnosis made, the physician typically has a prognosis (*trajectory projection* in our specialized terminology) in mind, though of course the patient may disagree and seek another one, given certain conditions for that. The physician's prognosis involves both the probable natural course of the illness if no interventions are made and what the course will probably be if specified interventions are made. The physician then lays out a treatment involving a regimen that calls for varying kinds and amounts of work. Thus, the total work of managing that more or less expected course of illness may include taking drugs on schedule, carrying out specified procedures (for example giving oneself insulin shots), following diets or adhering to dietary restrictions, visiting the physician's office or the outpatient clinic for scheduled checkups and tests or treatments, and so forth. The specific tasks and their combinations vary immensely according to illness, symptomology, phase of illness, and even the physician's medical ideology. At the same time, staying afloat of daily life also involves clusters of tasks—constitut-ing everyday-life work—such as housekeeping, cooking, child rearing, family financing, holding down an outside job, and so on.

As for the biographical concerns of the ill and their marital partners: the impact of the illness, the work associated with its management, and its sometimes radical alteration of the house-hold's division of labor taken together inevitably set into motion various biographical processes in the ill person and his or her partner. The more severe the identity impact, the more prolonged and "deep" will be those processes—and what we have termed the associated biographical work. These biographical processes and biographical work have been described in Chapters Four and Five. Briefly, the illness can, in various ways, lead to failure of body parts or systems. These body failures may result in failures of perfor-mance, which in turn can profoundly affect the self-conceptions of an ill person. Body appearance may also be affected, or so the ill may believe, and the perception of this change and of how people are reacting to it can, of course, have an impact on self-conceptions too. Usually the impact is negative. All such changes of self to body are not adequately captured by the usual phrase "changed body images," for there is a triadic relationship of body to self to environment that is disturbed by severe illness or the anticipation of even an annoying but extended illness. For this triadic relation-ship we have chosen the term *biographical body conceptions (BBC)* and noted how its disturbance involves and affects the ill person's sense of biographical time—a personal past, present, and future. The consequences of that are several biographical processes, including (1) contextualizing the illness into one's life, (2) coming to terms with one's body and activity limitations, (3) reconstructing one's identity, and (4) recasting one's biography. All of these processes involve strenuous cognitive and emotional work as the person struggles with the problems of contextualizing, coming to terms, and so forth.

Imagine now the ill man or woman who is simultaneously scheduling and carrying out regimens, holding down a job, doing his or her part of the housework and child rearing, and at the same time is going through one or more of the biographical processes. Imagine also that the well spouse is in a similar, though obviously not an identical, complex situation. Essentially, together and individually they are juggling the three major *lines of work* (illness, everyday, and biographical), each line composed of various types of work and their associated tasks. The work is carried out through a set of work processes: (1) discovering, drawing on, and maintaining various types of resources (manpower, time, money); (2) negotiating and maintaining a division of labor in which the work is parceled out; (3) mutually sustaining motivation for their common enterprise; and (4) articulating the many tasks. The relative success or failure of juggling the lines of work—and so illness management—depends largely on how these basic work processes are carried out. No matter how well activities are planned and contingencies anticipated, additional contingencies will arise from two sources. First, in a processually internal sense, they arise as consequences of the evolving work relationships themselves and from the biographical processes that are simultaneously going on. Second, they arise fortuitously from external sources, such as changes in economic climate or government relations, or in the conditions of work at one's job.

Another major source of contingencies, expected or not, is the diseased body itself as it moves along an illness course. Even merely symptomatic changes, not to mention systemic ones, may throw the ill person into a new phase. In a profound sense, the physiological course will shape, even if it does not totally determine, the trajectory That is, the illness status affects the work that principal actors perceive they must do and also their work relationships; the status simultaneously affects their everyday work and biographical work, which in turn affect the illness management and its associated work The illness course cannot totally determine the trajectory because that is affected by those other dynamics, as well as by contingencies external to them. The important point, then, is that there exists a complex interplay between illness and its management with the other lines of work plus the inevitable contingencies that occur *over time* to affect that interplay. This is why we call this type of management management in process: it never stands still.

But how is the work actually carried out? There is something analytically missing if one settles only for the foregoing formulations, despite their great complexity. The answer suggested by close scrutiny of the data is that *interactional processes* are also essential. There are not simply work, tasks, work processes; there are people who interact while doing that work and those tasks and who are engaged in those work processes. The interactional process that appears to be crucial pertains to what Blumer (1969) has called the *alignment* of actors' actions. In our analysis we noted how a couple's joint action can be perceived by one or both participants as more or less disaligned, and then how they evolve and carry out interactional strategies to achieve some measures of *re*alignment (Chapter Seven). We noted the crucial relevance of preinteraction internal processes (including anticipatory daydreams in which scenarios are acted out), postinteraction reviews (playbacks in memory), and evaluations. The last sometimes become part of the conscious reassessing of further realignment steps and strategies. This then results both in further "pre-views" of interaction and in strategies that are sometimes used, in some form or other, when future interactional scenes take place.

In Chapter Seven we also sketched a *conditional matrix* that can be of help in organizing the analysis of conditions affecting work-related actions and interactions and their consequences. The matrix consists of a set of concentric circles. The outer circle represents the macro conditions, the political-socioeconomic conditions that prevail at any given time. In the next circle are the more direct set of conditions bearing on work performance. These include the illness, the biographies, and the everyday-life conditions. Work as such makes up the next circle of the matrix: specifically, the three lines of work and their subtypes. Next is the structural context, which encompasses conditions that emerge from attempts to maintain control over the three lines of work. This context includes the work processes and the concomitant tendency toward competition among the lines of work for available resources, unbalanced work loads, disruption in the work flow, and the mutual sustaining of the partners. In the next circle are the interaction, the interactional conditions that arise from each interactant's interactional stance, an interactional context that involves the degree of alignment perceived by each interactant, and the developmental aspects of interaction. Finally, in the innermost circle is work performance per se and the degree to which it takes place. Flowing from work performance are consequences that arise depending on whether or not and how that work takes place. In turn, these consequences bounce back through the different circles of the matrix to affect each of them in varying degrees. Thus, they become conditions entering into the next phase of the action that is related to work performance. In short, this matrix is a diagrammatic way of picturing the structural and interactional elements of this complex work situation.

In Chapter Seven we concluded our cumulative outlining of this cluster of theoretical formulations, as derived from and utilizing the interview data. However, Chapters Eight through Eleven do not simply illustrate these formulations and the linkages among them; they develop them in further detail and as they pertain to different types of trajectory phases. The names of these phases suggest purely medical occurrences, but they are *trajectory*—not illness—phases, involving not merely shifts in the illness course but in work and work relationships and, consequently, in marital and biographical relations too. The phases are (1) comeback), (2) stable, (3) unstable, (4) deteriorating, and (5) dying. (We did not discuss another phase, the acute, which is managed mainly in hospitals or other health facilities.) Each phase has its own properties, processes and subprocesses, combinations of work, work relationships, problems in juggling the major lines of work, and also, understandably, the differing impacts on marital relationships and personal identities. As explained in Chapter One, the case presentations were chosen in accordance with theoretical criteria, including trajectory phase, complexities of relationships among the three main lines of work, and types of work relationships between the marital partners. This makes for much variation among the cases, both within and among the various chapters. Then in Chapter Twelve, we suggested some consequences of all of these factors for the lives of the well partners in order to highlight their special difficulties.

All of these chapters, replete as they are with extended case histories, bring out both the general patterns of illness work and trajectory management and the great variability *as it relates* to the general patterns. Given the complexity of phenomena and the variation of circumstances and situations of the couples, as pointed out by our theoretical formulations, no analysis that is faithful to this complexity could yield merely a list of "findings." Nor could an analyst offer a neat set of relatively verified properties or hypotheses. What happens or will happen in any given marital situation cannot be understood without comprehending both the overall relationships among our theoretical formulations *and* the specific circumstances of the case. For that reason, our theory of illness impact and management has deliberately taken a discursive rather than a propositional form (Glaser and Strauss, 1967; Glaser, 1978). (As we said at the outset of this section, the entire book is a spelling out of answers to the central questions about illness and work, meaning that the propositions are discursively embedded in the text.) In writing up qualitative analyses, researchers rarely use a propositional form, although many settle for a relatively descriptive level of analysis. Our analysis is much more abstract, conceptual, conceptually "dense," and, we hope, relatively integrated than most. By the use of many quotations, case histories, and précised references to specific data, we have attempted to remind readers that the theory is grounded in data but also to give a better sense of what the interviewers have experienced. The theoretical formulations are empty unless readers can supply similar experiences from their own lives or the observed (or read about) lives of others. We ourselves have had the additional but not totally necessary advantage of actually hearing the interviewees' voices.

This summary of our theoretical formulations or scheme has been complex. Because it does not readily lend itself to the presentation of a diagram or a single, clear model (useful as that might be), we shall break it into component parts that should be simpler to grasp diagrammatically. Moreover, it is probable that each component can be used fairly independently by readers who are interested either in studying chronic illness or in working as practitioners with the ill.

Think of the several components: (1) the contextual, (2) the work and interactional, (3) the biographical, and (4) the trajectory phasing, all of which, of course, are interrelated. The contextual component consists of the conditional matrix, which is pictured diagrammatically in Chapter Seven. Recall that it consists of multilevel and multiinteractional sets of conditions (including body failure) for the illness work. The work and interactional component consists of the following: the juggling of illness work, everyday-life work, and biographical work; the carrying out of the work through the several work processes (resources, division of labor, mutual sustaining, articulating); and the micromechanics of aligning and realigning. The biographical component consists of the complex, sequential but biographical processes. These processes were outlined at the close of Chapter Five. Finally, the trajectory phasing cases, which were presented and discussed in individual chapters, include several types of phases: acute, stable, unstable, comeback, deteriorating, and dying. Any given ill person's total trajectory, of course, can be diagrammed as a kind of trajectory profile for its past and present phases. The total theoretical scheme or model embraces all these components and their complex relationships.

Trajectory: Final Definition and Some Research Implications

Definition. Early in this chapter, we summarized the definition of trajectory with which our research began—what this central concept encompasses in terms of elements and their relationships. However, it is important to understand that concepts as they are used in research are instrumental to the research: hence their definitions are *working* and therefore usually *evolving* definitions. A concept and its definition guide the researcher, enabling him or her to focus on a particular phenomenon, to raise questions about it (such as when does it appear, what are its properties, how does it relate to other phenomena), to collect relevant data, to analyze these data in terms of the very same questions just mentioned. When a substantial body of theory has evolved, these interrelated concepts and their associated definitions have become quite elaborated, their contents more specified.

Perhaps in some limited kinds of research enterprises—say, a short series of experiments or some survey research projects—the definitions that are utilized will remain relatively unchanged throughout the study. More characteristically, scientists employ concepts and their associated definitions instrumentally, changing their boundaries and their interrelationships as a given research project progresses. As Herbert Blumer (1969, p. 161) has succinctly written about this alteration in initial formulations of a concept: "When experiment [actually any research] is pushed into new domains along the line of the concept, one must expect to encounter new facts which, in turn require a revision of conceptions and so of the content of the concept. Scientific concepts have a career." Or as Abraham Kaplan (1964, pp. 77-78) has so eloquently written about what he calls the "process of 'successive definition' ":

> The closure that strict definitions consists in is not a precondition of scientific inquiry but its culmination. To start with we do not know just what we mean by our terms, much as we do not know just what to think about our subject matter. . . . The questions a scientist puts to nature and the answers she gives have the form of a Platonic dialogue, not an Aristotelian treatise; we do not know just what has been said till we have done—and then new questions crowd in on us.

In this book the alteration of content and the definition of trajectory should be evident. The summary definition would now need to include subsidiary phenomena pointed to by the secondary concepts and their relationships as developed chapter by chapter. These include the three major lines of work, the work processes, the alignment process, the conditional matrix, the BBC chain, the several kinds of trajectory phases and their subsidiary biographical processes, and so forth. A simple or precise definition would be difficult to offer at this point. However, perhaps the following definitional statement will help to summarize this concept's current content.

> The concept of trajectory encompasses not only the course of illness but all of the associated illness work carried out through the work processes. Inclusive in this work and the work processes are types and lines of work and modes of articulating them, as well as various biographical processes that are set in motion

by the illness course itself and the work of managing
it and are affected and in turn affect the carrying out
of work done via the work processes.

Research Implications. A number of research directions and
studies can be drawn by implication from this central concept. We
shall suggest a few.

1. Studies of specific illnesses, carried out in depth. Currently there are useful monographs on illnesses such as epilepsy
(Schneider and Conrad, 1983) and arthritis (Locker, 1983) and
numerous papers on others. However we have in mind studies that
concentrate more directly on the nature of the trajectories and
phases typically characteristic of each illness and the characteristic
patternings of the illness work for each illness.

2. Studies of single people who have neither spouses nor
immediate family to aid in the illness management and associated
work. Especially needed is research on elderly women, whether
unmarried or widows. Our point here, aside from the practical
aspects of studying this population, is that its members are more
likely to lack certain of the resources that are available to people
who have marital partners. Consequently, there are many theoretical questions to be addressed in terms of the operation of the
various work processes under the condition of potentially fewer
material and psychological resources.

3. Studies of entire families, one or more of whose members
are ill. This could include families in which two or three members
are suffering from the same or different illnesses and in which the
illness is genetic (diabetes) or not. Again, the emphasis would be on
complications in the resource picture, as well as complications in
work and biographical processes brought about by the plurality of
illness courses.

4. Studies of chronically ill children and their families,
whether the illnesses are fatal (cystic fibrosis) or not. The emphasis
would not be on coping or stress or grieving and other psychological concepts but on phenomena associated with the interrelation-
ship of age and trajectory phase.

5. Comparative studies of people who are ill from the same
diseases but who are from different age-groups. We suggest studying

these populations especially from the standpoint of the biographical processes precipitated by the illness courses and the ways these affect the illness management.

6. Studies of organ transplant patients in which the resource focus would be not only on the work and experiences of the ill and supportive spouses and relatives but also on the elaborate medical organization (surgical service, outpatient clinic, physician's office, agency services), the components of which, working together in an elaborate division of labor, manage to keep the ill alive and relatively well or superbly "functioning" in predominantly stable phases.

7. Studies focused specifically on the biographical processes and experiences of the ill and their spouses, elaborating much further the kinds of formulations and findings offered in this book, for people suffering from different specific illnesses. This line of research would contribute additional depth to understanding the mutual influences of illness on identity and vice versa. Comparative studies of different illnesses would be also useful if done from this perspective.

8. In-depth studies (going well beyond our own research project) of the different trajectory phases. We believe that the stable and unstable phases would be of particular theoretical usefulness if only because they are so little understood in terms of trajectory (including work).

9. Comparative studies of disabled people who do *not* suffer from a chronic illness (that is, who have stable, unchanging body failures) and those who do have one or more chronic illnesses (for example, the quadriplegics and paraplegics whom we studied). The unchanging symptoms bring about another consideration and should add to our theoretical understanding of those people who do have changing symptoms or who must work hard at keeping them unchanging.

Practical Implications. Practitioners who are interested in using the concept of trajectory will find it has many implications. Aside from the various suggestions made in the summaries of each preceding chapter, we suggest the following. Of course, other implications can easily be added to our list.

1. *Chronic conditions are long-term.* What is the type and

extent of illness or disability, and what is its potential course? What are the usual physiologic manifestations, including symptoms, complications, associated physical and mental limitations? Is there an immediate or potential life threat? Where is the affected person in his or her life stage and how are his or her needs—affectional, social, educational, career, financial, sexual, and so forth—affected by the illness or condition? What might the affected person, spouse, family have to come to terms with? What aspects of their everyday lives are affected?

2. *Phasing should be taken into account.* In what phase and subphase of the trajectory is this person? What are this person's specific needs within this phase? For example, if the phase is a comeback phase, is it early, middle, or late? If early, what specific medical, biographical, and everyday-life needs does this person have? What kinds of comeback questions is the patient, spouse, family asking? How long is this phase expected to last? What can be expected of the next phase and the next? How can the patient and family be best prepared, helped to move on?

3. *Trajectory projection and scheme are important to understand.* What does each participant, health professional, ill person, spouse, family member, know about the condition—its severity, degree of limitation, potential course, and so on? What does each see as the management scheme? To what degree are the participants' projections and schemes similar or different? What else is going on either biographically or in their everyday lives that might affect their management (for example, willingness to follow or enforce a prescribed regimen)? To what degree have they come to terms with the condition: are they facing it realistically, denying it, unable to accept it? What biographical and everyday situations are likely to affect the rate and degree of their coming to terms with the illness?

4. *Work is central to illness management.* Based upon the phasing and identification of medical, biographical, and everyday needs within a particular phase, what specific types of illness, biographical, and everyday work need to be performed? For example, what specific types of work need to be done to prevent crises and complications or to carry out the regimen? Does the ill person need assistance with finding new career paths, working out

a sexual relationship, finding ways to socialize and to give and receive affection? What types of work need to be done in the home: care for children, keep up the house, bring in money?

5. *Work processes allow work to get carried out.* In terms of *supervising,* the following questions should be asked: Who is the most appropriate person to assess the conditions, monitor the work, and rectify errors for each type of work? For example, if the patient is an elderly diabetic with poor eyesight and lives alone, who is supervising his regimen? Is a public health nurse or other qualified person going into the home to set up the medication for him or checking to see whether he is taking the correct medication and dosage on his own? Is the patient, nurse, neighbor, or some other person monitoring for signs of hypoglycemia or hyperglycemia? Other questions to be asked here are Is all the work that is supposed to be performed actually being done? Is regimen work being shunted aside because of overbearing biographical needs? Is the biographical or everyday work being done superficially or not at all because the illness is getting in the way—for instance, is a wife so busy caring for her husband that she doesn't obtain needed medical care for herself? Are certain aspects of the regimen being omitted? What kinds of difficulties are being encountered in the work performance? Is someone taking responsibility for overseeing the process? If not, why not, and who should?

In terms of *articulating,* these questions are relevant: What types of work have to be coordinated and in what sequence? Who is responsible for their coordination? Are there any coordination problems? For example, the spouse who is taking care of her disabled mate must perform not only all or a large portion of her mate's activities of daily living but perhaps carry out the medical or rehabilitative regimens, provide sentimental and other types of biographical work for herself, husband, and other family members, and also clean house, shop, pay bills, and so forth. Has she established routines for the work performance? Are the tasks being done in the proper sequence, especially the regimen and rehabilitative? Are there more efficient ways of doing things, perhaps with outside assistance or helpful devices?

As to the matter of *resourcing:* What resources are needed to carry out each type of work? Do the participants have the knowledge, information, transportation, time, money, equipment, and manpower to do it? To what degree are these resources present or absent? How might the needed resources be acquired? How might resources be conserved so that they will be available for the next illness phase, when requirements might be greater? For instance, when the cardiac patient who needs blood pressure checks and a low-sodium diet is discharged from the hospital, the couple should be assessed with very pointed and directed questions about their knowledge and physical abilities to perform these tasks. Do they have the equipment at home? Are they anxious about carrying out the tasks? There should also be some follow-up once they get home to answer their questions and determine if they have encountered any problems.

The matter of *allocating tasks* elicits these questions: Who is performing what tasks? Does this person have the physical and mental abilities, knowledge, time, and willingness to perform the tasks? For how long should or can this person do the work? How does trajectory phasing shift the allocation of tasks (increase or decrease performance ability)? What is the nature of each person's work load? Is one person carrying the burden of the work? How long can this go on? What can be done to lighten this person's work load? For example, for how long can two elderly people, one of whom has a progressively deteriorating illness, continue to live alone and care for themselves? At what point is outside assistance called for or should the ill or disabled partner be placed in a nursing home?

Then there is the matter of *motivating:* What specific rewards are needed to establish and maintain motivation to do the work (seeing improvement, cooperation of the other person, an occasional break)? Is initial motivation being sustained? If not, why not? What is necessary to reestablish it? Is it possible to find ways to integrate the regimen into the person's life-style so that it is not so difficult to maintain? Could the establishment of routines, use of devices, proper equipment make the work easier? Is there a part of the work that someone else could do? For example, would it be better for the arthritic patient to have her spouse help her get dressed in the morning so that she might save her energy for other more rewarding activities?

6. *Interaction is crucial to carrying out the illness work.* What is the nature of the interaction between the participants? What stance have they taken toward each other: collaboration, cooperation, or conflict? On what issues? How is this stance manifested: behavior that is trusting, appreciative, demanding, domineering? If there is conflict, what is the source? For example, is the wife of the cardiac patient being overprotective, or is he being foolish in his behavior? Is the woman with a spinal cord injury having difficulty in being dependent and demonstrating this difficulty by being demanding and manipulative? Is a man using his illness to control others? Does the patient understand why a particular test, treatment, regimen has been ordered? Are the marital partners having sexual difficulties? Are they together too much?

7. *Contingencies that affect the illness management need to be understood and planned for.* What sorts of routines has this person, couple, family established for managing the illness around their biographies and everyday lives? Are they realistically planning ahead for the future? Do they have plans for handling medical crises? Do they have plans for development of acute or chronic conditions in the spouse that might interfere with his or her ability to be a caretaker or necessitate that he or she be taken care of? Do they have enough money to handle a household crisis or pay for a visiting nurse, attendant, or nursing home?

8. *Consequences of illness and its management need careful consideration.* Is the regimen working to control symptoms, prevent crises and complications? If not, why not? Is the marital or family relationship better, the same, worse? Why? Has the afflicted person let go of his or her former self and found new directions for living? Is all the everyday work getting done? If not, why not? And what can be done about it? Has the well spouse had to go out and find work or had to leave a job because of the illness or disability? Does the caretaker show signs of overload, of having reached the limits of tolerance? How can this be remedied? What situations provoke setbacks in the coming to terms process? How can the person be helped to deal with these situations?

9. *Context also raises issues for effective care.* What types of technology are available to manage this condition? Are they being used? What are some of the barriers to utilization of services by this

person or family? Do they need help filling out forms, finding transportation, locating housing, securing financial aid? Does this case present ethical considerations? If so, what are they? What kind of neighborhood does this person or couple live in? What are their social supports? Could relatives, neighbors, friends be brought in to help? What kinds of changes in the home are necessary to accommodate this illness or disability?

In this section, a number of implications of our central concept—trajectory—were offered. The discussion was organized around important components of the concept: the long-term character of chronic illness; trajectory phasing; trajectory projections and scheme; work; work processes; interaction; contingencies; and the consequences of trajectory management. Each of these components raises a number of practical questions; questions that could guide practitioners' efforts to assist in trajectory management at home—and perhaps help the ill and their families in their own efforts at management.

This Study's Location and Character

In the final pages of this book it might be useful to locate the substantive aspects of our study within the context of recent sociological research on the experiences of the chronically ill. This locational strategy should give the reader a clearer understanding of the contributions of this study—as we see them, of course—and where they fit into the technical literature. Conveniently at hand is a recent review by Peter Conrad in which he discusses the research trends most directly relevant to our subject.

Conrad entitles his review "The Experience of [Chronic] Illness: Recent and New Directions" (1987). He begins by noting the increasing interest in studying chronic illness from an "experiential or subjective perspective," that is, the perspective of the person suffering from illness. (For sociologists' autobiographical accounts of their own illness experiences, see Lefton, 1984; Zola, 1982.) But *experience*, as Conrad discusses it, turns out on closer reflection to be an omnibus term, as does such wording as "a sociology of illness experience must consider people's everyday living with and in spite of illness." What such a perspective would focus on includes several phenomena: the meaning of illness, the social organization of the sufferers' life world, and the strategies used in adaptation; it would also focus on sufferers' theories and explanations for making sense of the events happening to them, what they do about the illness, how they manage regimens, how they manage their relationships with relatives and friends and work associates, and so on. As we said early in this book, the work of managing illness is certainly far from all of the illness experience, but surely it is one of the central features in that experience. Putting the issue in such a way suggests fairly precisely what we did and did *not* set out to do in this book.

Conrad further notes seven central "concepts or focal concerns" of recent research on the illness experience. One is uncertainty—and there are different aspects of this: uncertainty about the diagnosis, the symptoms, the course of illness, the treatment and regimen; about how life will be affected; and so on (Bury, 1982; Commaroff and McGuire, 1981; Davis, F., 1963; Davis, M., 1973; Dingwall, 1976; Lefton, 1984; Plough, 1981; Schneider and Conrad, 1983; Wiener, 1975a, 1975b). In terms of uncertainty, our research has addressed all of these aspects. This is because the trajectory concept covers them all. Of course, we have related them to the work activities of the ill and their partners. A second concept used by some researchers is the illness career (Davis, 1963; Speedling 1982; Suchman, 1965a, 1965b). Conrad critiques this use—as in its implications that there are regular stages—and suggests that "illness trajectory may be more appropriate . . . since it encompasses process and change but does not assume linearity or orderliness." We agree, although we think it is a powerful concept for more reasons than these.

A third focal concern of some researchers has been the stigmatizing effects of illness (Goffman, 1963; Scrambler, 1983), such as from having epileptic fits (Schneider and Conrad, 1980, 1983) or paralytic strokes (Davis, 1963) or arthritis (Locker, 1983) or leprosy (Gussow and Tracy, 1965). We did not in our interviews ask direct questions that would uncover experience with or feelings about stigma, but even the paraplegics and quadriplegics and those people who had strokes or suffered from Parkinson's disease did not touch much on the issue of stigma. Their concern was with activity and performance, not with appearance. No doubt, if the interviews had been more focused on relationships with managing behavior in public places or with strangers or on the job, then such stigmatizing experiences would have surfaced and perhaps been viewed as major problems. Within the circle of the family and intimate friends, however, this kind of insult to identity is probably of minor concern to the ill. After all, they are intensely preoccupied with adequately performing despite their sometimes impeding or constraining body failures.

A fourth focal concern noted by Conrad, and one central to our own study, is biographical work and the reconstitution of self. (See also, Bury, 1982; Charmaz, 1980, 1983, 1985; Lefton, 1984; Williams, 1984; Schneider and Conrad, 1983.) A fifth concern, and one of great importance for us, is the management of regimens (Conrad, 1985; Corbin and Strauss, 1985; Hayes-Bautista, 1976; Zola, 1982). A sixth concern is information, awareness, and the sharing of information. This was of peripheral theoretical interest for us, although the case histories are rich in data bearing on these important issues. Conrad's seventh item is family relations (Bluebond-Langer, 1978; Commaroff and McGuire, 1981; Corbin and Strauss, 1985; Davis, 1963; Gerhardt and Briesekorn-Zinke, 1986; Maines, 1983; Strauss and others 1984). Here he distinguishes three subareas: the effect of illness on family relations, care giving, and the ill person's view of the family. Locating our own study against this listing, the care giving was of major importance, with the other two areas being secondary to their effect on the care giving.

Conrad also suggests several "issues" that he believes are important if the emerging perspective of illness experience is to be more fully developed. Our data touches on two of these, but they were not examined by us. One issue pertains to how jobs and money/costs affect the illness experience. A second issue relates to potential gender differences in the illness experience. Aside from matters of work and the division of labor, our study did not focus on this issue. However, Conrad lists these issues and another— social support—under the general heading of economic and social resources. We were at pains to make such resources a major item in our theoretical analysis of how illness management is carried out by the ill and their partners.

Conrad further suggests several sampling issues that "can be summarized as: who, where, how, when and how many?" His critical discussion here is astute and useful. We have addressed some, but not all, of his issues when discussing theoretical sampling in Chapter One. Theoretical sampling was, as we have said, integral to our analysis.

Among the most interesting discussions for us in Conrad's review were what he calls pitfalls that researchers should be aware of. Aside from sampling biases and problems, he mentions several pitfalls. One is "too much undigested data"—that is, description and case material presentation with little conceptualization. Second is "too many unintegrated perspectives." A third "stems from relying on 'outsider' concepts for renderings of insider's experience"—that is, using frameworks developed for other purposes. (To use today's common parlance: The approaches are unduly deductive rather than inductive.) Another pitfall is that of "unsystematic case presentation." And a fifth is the inaccurate language we use to present our findings. For example, "People are not their illnesses . . . it is more accurate to see people as having illnesses rather than being [totally] their illness." It should be clear that we pass the test of Conrad's pitfalls (and we agree with his criticisms of them).

The hallmarks of our presentation, whatever its defects, are the following: the development of systematic theory; the balance sought between insider's (the interviewees') perspective and outsider's (the sociologists') interpretation; systematic case presentation; and careful, as well as theoretically systematic, treatment of people's management of illness within the context of other aspects of their lives.

References

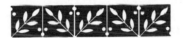

Ainley, S., Becker, G., and Coleman, L. (eds.). *The Dilemma of Difference: A Multidisciplinary View of Stigma.* New York: Plenum, 1986.

Anderson, J., Parsons, F., and Jones, D. (eds.). *Living with Renal Failure.* Lancaster, Pa.: MTP Press, 1978.

Archbold, P. "Impact of Parent Caring on Middle-Aged Offspring." *Journal of Gerontological Nursing,* 1980, 6 (2), 78–85.

Bayh, M., with M. Kotz. *Marvella.* New York: Harcourt Brace Jovanovich, 1979.

Becker, H. *Art Worlds.* Berkeley: University of California Press, 1984.

Becker, H., and Geer, B. "The Analysis of Qualitative Field Data." In R. Adams and J. Preiss (eds.), *Human Organization Research.* Homewood, Ill.: Dorsey, 1960.

Becker, H., Geer, B., Hughes, E., and Strauss, A. *Boys in White.* Chicago: University of Chicago Press, 1964.

Becker, G., and Kaufman, S. "Decision-Making in Rehabilitation." Paper presented at the annual meeting of the Gerontological Society of America, San Francisco, November 22, 1983.

Becker, H., and Strauss, A. "Careers, Personality, and Adult Social-ization." *American Journal of Sociology*, 1956, *62*, 253–263.

Bendifallah, S., and Scacchi, W. "Understanding Software Mainte-nance Work." *EEE Transactions on Software Engineering*, 1987, *13*, 311–323.

Benoliel, J. "Becoming Diabetic." Unpublished doctoral disserta-tion, School of Nursing, University of California, San Francisco, 1969.

Birrer, C. *Multiple Sclerosis: A Personal View.* Springfield, Ill.: Thomas, 1979.

Bluebond-Langer, M. *The Private Lives of Dying Children.* Princeton, N.J.: Princeton University Press, 1978.

Blumer, H. *Symbolic Interaction.* Englewood Cliffs, N.J.: Prentice-Hall, 1969.

Bray, G. P. "Positive Patterns in the Families of the Severely Dis-abled." *Rehabilitation Counseling Bulletin*, 1977, *20*, 236–239.

Brody, E. M. "Parent Care as a Normative Family Stress." *The Gerontologist*, 1985, *15* (1), 19–29.

Brooks, N., and Matson, R. "Social-Psychological Adjustment to Multiple Sclerosis." *Social Science and Medicine*, 1982, *16*, 2129–2135.

Brooks, N., and Matson, R. "Managing Multiple Sclerosis." In J. Roth and P. Conrad (eds.), *Research in the Sociology of Health Care.* Vol. 6. Greenwood, Conn.: JAI, 1987.

Bury, M. "Chronic Illness as Biographic Disruption." *Sociology of Health and Illness*, 1982, *4* (2), 167–182.

Cantor, M. "Families: A Basic Source of Long-Term Care for the Elderly." *Aging*, 1985, *349*, 8–13.

Caulkins, K. "Shouldering a Burden." *Omega*, 1972, *2*, 23–36.

Charmaz, K. "The Construction of Self-Pity in the Chronically Ill." In N. Denzin (ed.), *Studies in Symbolic Interaction*, 1980, *3*, 123–145.

Charmaz, K. "Loss of Self: A Fundamental Form of Suffering in the Chronically Ill." *Sociology of Health and Illness*, 1983, 168–195.

Charmaz, K. "Intrusive Illness: Meanings and Consequences in the Lives of the Chronically Ill." Paper presented at the annual meeting of the Pacific Sociological Association, Portland, Oregon, April 11–14, 1984. (Available from K. Charmaz, Gerontology Program, Sonoma State University, Rohnert Park, Calif. 94928.)

Charmaz, K. "Experiencing Chronic Illness as an Interruption." Unpublished manuscript, February 1985. (Available from K. Charmaz, Gerontology Program, Sonoma State University, Rohnert Park, Calif. 94928.)

Chester, M. A., and Barbarin, O. A. "Difficulties of Providing Help in Crisis: Relationship Between Parents of Children with Cancer and Their Friends." *Journal of Social Issues*, 1984, *40* (4), 113-134.

Cluff, L. E. "Chronic Disease, Function and the Quality of Care." *Journal of Chronic Disease*, 1981, *34*, 299-304.

Colman, H. *Hanging On*. New York: Atheneum, 1977.

Commaroff, J., and McGuire, P. "Ambiguity and the Search for Meaning: Childhood Leukaemia in the Modern Clinical Context." *Social Science and Medicine*, 1981, *15B*, 115-123.

Conrad, P. "The Meaning of Medications: Another Look at Compliance." *Social Science and Medicine*, 1985, *20* (1), 29-37.

Conrad, P. "The Experience of Illness: Recent and New Directions." In J. Roth and P. Conrad (eds.), *Research in the Sociology of Health Care*, Vol. 6. Greenwich, Conn.: JAI Press, 1987.

Corbin, J. "Women's Perception and Management of Pregnancy Complicated by Chronic Illness." *Health Care for Women International*, 1987, *8*, 317-337.

Corbin, J., and Strauss, A. "Collaboration: Couples Working Together to Manage Chronic Illness." *Image*, 1984, *16*, 109-115.

Corbin, J., and Strauss, A. "Issues Concerning Regimen Management in the Home." *Aging and Society*, 1985, *5*, 249-265.

Cowie, B. "The Cardiac Patient's Perception of His Heart Attack." *Social Science and Medicine*, 1976, *10*, 87-96.

Dalton, M. *Men Who Manage*. New York: Wiley, 1954.

Davis, F. *Passage Through Crisis: Polio Victims and Their Families*. Indianapolis, Ind.: Bobbs-Merrill, 1963.

Davis, F. *Illness Interaction and the Self*. Belmont, Calif.: Wadsworth, 1972.

Davis, M. *Living with Multiple Sclerosis*. Springfield, Ill.: Thomas, 1973.

de Mille, A. *Reprieve.* New York: Doubleday, 1981.

Dewey, J. *Human Nature and Conduct.* New York: Holt, Rinehart & Winston, 1921.

Dewey, J. *Art as Experience.* New York: Minton, Balch and Co., 1934.

Dewey, J. *Logic: The Theory of Inquiry.* New York: Holt, Rinehart & Winston, 1938.

Dingwall, R. *Aspects of Illness.* London: Martin Robertson, 1976.

Eckberg, J. Y., Griffith, N., and Foxall, M. J. "Spousal Adjustment to Chronic Illness." *Rehabilitation Nursing,* 1986, *25* (1), 19–29.

Ereackson, J., with J. Musser. *Joni.* Minneapolis: World Wide, 1976.

Erikson, E. "Identity and the Life Cycle." In G. Klein (ed.), *Psychological Issues.* New York: International Universities Press, 1959.

Estes, C. "Health Problems in Policy Issues of Old Age." In L. Aiken and D. Mechanic (eds.), *Applications of Social Science to Clinical Medicine and Health Policy.* New Brunswick, N.J.: Rutgers University Press, 1986.

Fagerhaugh, S. "Getting Around with Emphysema." *American Journal of Nursing,* 1973, *73,* 94–97.

Fagerhaugh, S., and Strauss, A. *Politics of Pain Management: Staff-Patient Interaction.* Reading, Mass.: Addison-Wesley, 1977.

Fagerhaugh, S., and Strauss, A. "Negotiation and Pain Management on Geriatric Wards." In D. Maines and N. Denzin (eds.), *Work and Problematic Situations.* New York: Crowell, 1978.

Fagerhaugh, S., Strauss, A., Suczek, B., and Wiener, C. *Hazards in Hospital Care: Ensuring Patient Safety.* San Francisco: Jossey-Bass, 1987.

Feldman, D. J. "Chronic Disabling Illness: A Holistic View." *Journal of Chronic Disease,* 1974, *27,* 287–291.

Fengler, A., and Goodrich, N., "Wives of Elderly Disabled Men: The Hidden Patients." *Gerontologist,* 1979, *19,* 175–183.

Fischer, W. *Time and Chronic Illness: A Study on the Constitution of Temporality.* Unpublished paper, University of Bielefeld, West Germany, 1983.

Fisher, B., and Galler, R. "Friendship and Fairness: How Disability Affects Friendship Between Women." In A. Asch and M. Fine (eds.), *Voices from the Margin: Lives of Disabled Girls and Women*. Philadelphia: Temple University Press, 1987.

Fitting, M., and others. "Caregivers for Dementia Patients: A Comparison of Husbands and Wives." *Gerontologist*, 1986, *26*, 248-252.

Forsyth, G. L., Delaney, K. D., and Gresham, M. L. "Vying for a Winning Position: Management Style of the Chronically Ill." *Research in Nursing and Health*, 1984, *7*, 181-188.

Freidson, E. *Medical Dominance*. Chicago: Aldine, 1970.

Freidson, E. "The Division of Labor as Social Interaction." *Social Problems*, 1976, *23*, 304-313.

Fujimura, J. "Constructing 'Do-able' Problems in Cancer Research: Articulating Alignment." *Social Studies of Science*, 1987, *17*, 257-293.

Gadow, S. "Body and Self: A Dialectic." In V. Kestenbaum (ed.), *The Humanity of the Ill: Phenomenological Perspectives*. Knoxville: University of Tennessee Press, 1982.

Gerhardt, U., and Briesekorn-Zinke, M. "The Normalization of Hemodialysis at Home." In J. Roth and S. Ruzek (eds.), *Research in the Sociology of Health Care*. Greenwich, Conn.: JAI Press, 1986.

Gerson, E. "On the Quality of Life." *American Sociological Review*, 1976, *4*, 266-279.

Gerson, E. "Scientific Work and Social World." *Knowledge*, 1983, *1*, 357-377

Gerson, E., and Star, S. L. "Analyzing Due Process in the Workplace." *ACM Transactions on Office Information Systems*, 1986, *4*, 257-270.

Gerson, E., and Strauss, A. "Time for Living." *Social Policy*, 1975, *6*, 12-18.

Glaser, B. *The Patsy and the Subcontractor*. New Brunswick, N.J.: Transaction, 1976.

Glaser, B. *Theoretical Sensitivity: Further Advances in the Methodology of Grounded Theory*. San Francisco: Sociology Press, 1978.

Glaser, B., and Strauss, A. "Awareness Contexts and Social Interaction." *American Sociological Review*, 1964, *29*, 669-679.

Glaser, B., and Strauss, A. *Awareness of Dying.* Chicago: Aldine, 1965.

Glaser, B., and Strauss, A. *Discovery of Grounded Theory: Strategies for Qualitative Research.* Chicago: Aldine, 1967.

Glaser, B., and Strauss, A. *Time for Dying.* Chicago: Aldine, 1968.

Goffman, E. *The Presentation of Self in Everyday Life.* New York: Doubleday, 1959.

Goffman, E. *Stigma: Notes on the Management of Spoiled Identity.* Englewood Cliffs, N.J.: Prentice-Hall, 1963.

Goffman, E. *Frame Analysis.* New York: Harper & Row, 1974.

Goldstein, V. "Caretaker Role Fatigue." *Nursing Outlook,* 1981, *29* (1), 24–30.

Griffith, C. "Sexuality and the Cardiac Patient." *Heart and Lung,* 1973, *2,* 70–73.

Gussow, Z., and Tracy, G. "Strategies in the Management of Stigma: Concealing and Revealing by Leprosy Patients in the U.S." Unpublished manuscript, Department of Psychiatry, Louisiana State University Medical Center, 1965.

Hayes-Bautista, D. "Modifying the Treatment: Patient Compliance, Patient Control and Medicine." *Social Science and Medicine,* 1976, *10,* 233–238.

Holaday, B. J. "Parenting the Chronically Ill Child." In P. Brandt and others (eds.), *Current Practice in Pediatric Nursing.* St. Louis: Mosby, 1978.

Hughes, E. C. *The Sociological Eye.* Chicago: Aldine, 1971.

Isaac, B. *A Breast for Life.* New York: Exposition Press, 1974.

"Javitz' 'Talk to Doctors.' " *San Francisco Chronicle,* May 12, 1984, pp. 1, 3.

Joas, H. "The Intersubjective Constitution of the Body Image." *Human Studies,* 1983, *6,* 197–204.

Kaplan, A. *The Conduct of Inquiry.* San Francisco: Chandler, 1964.

Kaufman, S., and Becker, G. "Stroke: Health Care on the Periphery." *Social Science and Medicine,* 1986, *22* (9), 983–989.

Kilmont, J., and Valens, E. G. *The Other Side of the Mountain.* New York: Warner Books, 1975.

Klein, R., Dean, A., and Bogdonoff, M. D. "The Impact of Illness Upon the Spouse." *Journal of Chronic Illness,* 1967, *20,* 241–248.

Knapfl, A., and Deatrick, J. "How Families Manage Chronic

Conditions: An Analysis of the Concept of Normalization." *Research in Nursing and Health,* 1986, *9,* 215–222.

Kotarba, J. "The Chronic Pain Experience." In J. D. Douglas and J. M. Johnson (eds.), *Existential Sociology.* New York: Cambridge University Press, 1979.

Kotarba, J. A. "Perceptions of Death, Belief Systems and the Process of Coping with Chronic Pain." *Social Science and Medicine,* 1983, 17 (10), 681–689.

Kübler-Ross, E. *On Death and Dying.* New York: Macmillan, 1969.

Labrie, V. "Lupus: Managing a Complex Chronic Disability." Unpublished doctoral dissertation, Department of Social and Behavioral Sciences, University of California, San Francisco, 1986.

Lefton, M. "Chronic Disease and Applied Sociology: Essays in Personalized Sociology." *Social Inquiry,* 1984, *54,* 476.

Levin, I.., and Idler, E. (eds.). *The Hidden Health Care System: Mediating Structures and Medicine.* Cambridge, Mass.: Ballinger, 1981.

Locker, D. *Disability and Disadvantage: The Consequences of Chronic Illness.* London: Tavistock, 1983.

Louie, T. "The Pragmatic Context: A Chinese American Example of Defining and Managing Illness." Unpublished doctoral dissertation, School of Nursing, University of California, San Francisco, 1975.

Lubkin, I. *Chronic Illness: Interventions for Health Professionals.* Boston: Jones and Bartlett, 1986.

McCready, M. "Young Disabled Adults and their Personal Care Attendants." Unpublished doctoral dissertation, Department of Social and Behavioral Sciences, University of California, San Francisco, 1984.

Madruga, L. *One Step at a Time.* New York: McGraw-Hill, 1979.

Maines, D. "Time and Biography in Diabetic Experience." *Mid-American Review of Sociology,* 1983, *8,* 103–117.

Mead, G. H. *The Philosophy of the Present.* Chicago: Open Court, 1932.

Mead, G. H. *Mind, Self and Society.* Chicago: University of Chicago Press, 1934.

Merleau-Ponty, M. *Phenomenology of Perception.* London: Routledge & Kegan Paul, 1962.

Miller, J. (ed.). *Coping with Illness.* Philadelphia: Davis, 1983.

Moos, R., and Tsu, V. "The Crisis of Physical Illness: An Overview." In R. Moos (ed.), *Coping with Physical Illness.* New York: Plenum, 1977.

Nasaw, J. *Easy Walking.* Philadelphia: Lippincott, 1975.

Olesen, V., and Schatzman, L. "Trust in the Body: Preliminary Notes from a Study of Self-Care." Paper presented at the British Sociological Association meeting, Manchester, England, April 1983. (Available from the authors, Department of Social and Behavioral Sciences, University of San Francisco, San Francisco, Calif. 94143.)

Plough, A. "Medical Technology and the Crisis of Experience: The Cost of Clinical Legitimation." *Social Science and Medicine,* 1981, *15A,* 89–101.

Riemann, G. *Biographieverlaufe Psychiatrischer Patienten Aus Soziologisher Sicht* [Biographical careers of psychiatric patients from a sociological view]. Munich: Fink, 1987.

Rosenberg, M. L. *Patients: The Experience of Illness.* Philadelphia: Saunders, 1980.

Rustad, L. "Family Adjustment to Chronic Illness and Disability in Mid-Life." In M. Eisenberg and others (eds.), *Chronic Illness Through the Life Span: Effects on Self and Family.* New York: Springer, 1984.

Ryan, C., and Ryan, K. *A Private Battle.* New York: Simon & Schuster, 1979.

Schatzman, L., and Olesen, V. "The Physical Self in the Context of Mundane Ailments." Paper presented at the Pacific Sociological Association meeting, San Diego, Calif., Spring 1983. (Available from the authors, Department of Social and Behavioral Sciences, University of California, San Francisco, San Francisco, Calif. 94143.)

Schatzman, L., and Strauss, A. *Field Research.* Englewood Cliffs, N.J.: Prentice-Hall, 1973.

Schilder, P. *Psychoanalysis, Man and Society.* New York: Norton, 1951.

Schmitt, R. "Breast Identities: A Topical Life History Investigation of Stone's Version of Appearance and the Self." Paper presented at the American Sociological Association meeting, San Antonio, Texas, 1984. (Available from the author, Department of Sociology, Southern Illinois University, Carbondale, Ill. 62901.)

Schneider, J. "Disability as Moral Experience: Epilepsy and Self in Routine Relationships." Unpublished paper, Department of Sociology, Drake University, Des Moines, Iowa, August 1985.

Schneider, J., and Conrad, P. "In the Closet with Illness: Epilepsy, Stigma Potential and Information Control." *Social Problems,* 1980, *28,* 32–44.

Schneider, J., and Conrad, P. *Having Epilepsy: The Experience and Control of Illness.* Philadelphia: Temple University Press, 1983.

Schuetze, F. "Prozessstruckturen des Lebensablaufs" ["Process structures of the end of life"]. In J. Mattes and others, *Biographie in Handlungswissenschaftlicher Perspectiv* [Biography from the perspective of action science]. University of Nürnberg, 1981.

Scheutze, F. "Biographieforschung und Narratives Interview" ["Biography research and narrative interview"]. *Neue Praxis,* 1983, *3,* 283–293.

Scrambler, G. "Being Epileptic: The Sociology of a Stigmatized Condition." Unpublished doctoral dissertation, University of London, 1983.

Selye, H. *The Stress of Life.* New York: McGraw-Hill, 1956.

Speedling, E. *Heart Attack: The Family Response at Home and in the Hospital.* London: Tavistock, 1982.

Stur, S. L. "Simplification in Scientific Work: An Example from Neuroscience Research." *Social Studies of Science,* 1983, *13,* 205–228.

Star, S. L. "Scientific Work and Uncertainty." *Social Studies of Science,* 1985, *15,* 391–427.

Steele, T., Finkelstein, S., and Finkelstein, F. "Hemodialysis Patients and Spouses, Marital Discord, Sexual Problems, and Depression." *Journal of Nervous and Mental Diseases,* 1976, *162,* 225–237.

Stone, G. "Appearance and the Self." In A. Rose (ed.), *Human Behavior and Social Processes.* Boston: Houghton Mifflin, 1962. (See also the revised version, "Appearance and the Self: A Slightly Revised Version." In G. Stone and H. Farberman (eds.),

Social Psychology Through Symbolic Interaction. Waltham, Mass.: Xerox, 1981.)

Stoner, M. H., and Kranfer, S. G. "Recalled Life Expectancy Information, Phase of Illness and Hope in Cancer Patients." *Research in Nursing and Health*, 1985, *8*, 269-274.

Strauss, A. *Mirrors and Masks: The Search for Identity.* New York: Free Press, 1959. (Reprint. San Francisco: Sociology Press, 1969.)

Strauss, A. *Negotiations: Varieties, Contexts, Processes, and Social Order.* San Francisco: Jossey-Bass, 1978.

Strauss, A. "Work and the Division of Labor." *Sociological Quarterly*, 1985, *26*, 1-19.

Strauss, A. *Qualitative Analysis for Social Scientists.* New York: Cambridge University Press, 1987.

Strauss, A. "The Articulation of Work: An Organizational Process." *Sociological Quarterly,* in press.

Strauss, A. Fagerhaugh, S., Suczek, B., and Wiener, C. *The Social Organization of Medical Work.* Chicago: University of Chicago Press, 1985.

Strauss, A., and Glaser, B. *Anguish.* San Francisco: Sociology Press, 1970.

Strauss, A., and Glaser, B. *Chronic Illness and the Quality of Life.* St. Louis: Mosby, 1975.

Strauss, A., and others. *Chronic Illness and the Quality of Life.* (2nd. ed.) St. Louis: Mosby, 1984.

Stuifbergen, A. K. "The Impact of Chronic Illness on Families." *Family Community Health*, 1987, *9* (4), 43-51.

Suchman, E. "Social Patterns of Illness and Medical Care." *Journal of Health and Human Behavior*, 1965a, *6*, 2-16.

Suchman, E. "Stages of Illness and Medical Care." *Journal of Health and Human Behavior*, 1965b, *6*, 114-128.

Voysey, M. *A Constant Burden: The Reconstitution of Family Life.* London: Macmillan, 1975.

Waddell, C. "The Process of Neutralization and the Uncertainties of Cystic Fibrosis." *Sociology of Health and Illness*, 1982, *4*, 210-220.

Wertenbaker, L. *Death of a Man.* New York: Random House, 1957.

Westbrook, M., and Viney, L. "Psychological Reactions to the

Onset of Chronic Illness." *Social Science and Medicine,* 1982, *16,* 899–905.

Whitehead, A. *Process and Reality.* New York: Macmillan, 1923.

Wiener, C. "The Burden of Rheumatoid Arthritis." *Social Science and Medicine,* 1975a, *9,* 97–104.

Wiener, C. "Pain Assessment, Pain Legitimation and the Conflict of Staff-Patient Perspectives." *Nursing Outlook,* 1975b, *23* (3), 508–516.

Williams, G. "The Genesis of Chronic Illness. Narrative Re-Construction." *Sociology of Health and Illness,* 1984, *6* (2), 174–200.

Willis, J., and Willis, M. *But There Are Always Miracles.* New York: Viking, 1974.

Zarit, S., and Anthony, C. "Subjective Burden of Husbands and Wives as Caretakers: A Longitudinal Study." *Gerontologist,* 1986, *26,* 260–266.

Zarit, S., Reever, K., and Bach-Peterson, J. "Relatives of the Impaired Elderly: Correlates of Feelings of Burden." *Gerontologist,* 1980, *20,* 649–655.

Zola, I. *Missing Pieces: A Chronicle of Living with a Disability.* Philadelphia: Temple University Press, 1982.

Index

A

Accommodation: to chronic illness, 5-7; concept of, 6, 50; in performance, 58

Action, performance as, 55-56

Acute trajectory phase: concept of, 46; spouses in, 299-301; unstable phase distinct from, 237

Alignment: concept of, 2-3, 131; and interaction, in work performance, 131-135; levels of, 159-160; phases of, 132-133; work of, 322; in work performance case, 152, 153-154, 157, 162-163

Allergies, in unstable phase, 243-249

Allocation, issues of, 331

Alzheimer's disease: and conditional motivation, 16; and spouse's problems, 295

Aphasia, and failed performance, 58

Appearance: concept of, 56; responses to, 59; and stigma, 334-335

Applications: of biography, 87-88; of body failure, 66-67; of comeback phase, 204-205; of diagnostic quest, 31-32; of downward phase, 286-288; of interaction, 164-165; for spouses, 316-317; of stable phase, 235; of trajectory, 48; of unstable phase, 251-252; of work, 125-126

Archbold, P., 289

Aristotle, 326

Arthritis: lines of work for, 91-92; and performance, 58, 64, in stable phase, 46, 210-219; in well spouse, 304; and work load imbalance, 113

Articulation: of body work with outside work in stable phase, 231-233; concept of, 11, 120; of division of labor in stable phase, 222-223, 226, 229-230; issues of, 330; of resources, 121; of work, 120-122; in work performance case, 155

Asthma, in unstable phase, 243-249